T0324969

database technology for life sciences and medicine

editors

Claudia Plant
Technische Universität München, Germany

Christian Böhm
Ludwig-Maximilians Universität München, Germany

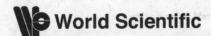
World Scientific

NEW JERSEY · LONDON · SINGAPORE · BEIJING · SHANGHAI · HONG KONG · TAIPEI · CHENNAI

Published by

World Scientific Publishing Co. Pte. Ltd.

5 Toh Tuck Link, Singapore 596224

USA office: 27 Warren Street, Suite 401-402, Hackensack, NJ 07601

UK office: 57 Shelton Street, Covent Garden, London WC2H 9HE

British Library Cataloguing-in-Publication Data
A catalogue record for this book is available from the British Library.

DATABASE TECHNOLOGY FOR LIFE SCIENCES AND MEDICINE
Science, Engineering, and Biology Informatics — Vol. 6

Copyright © 2010 by World Scientific Publishing Co. Pte. Ltd.

All rights reserved. This book, or parts thereof, may not be reproduced in any form or by any means, electronic or mechanical, including photocopying, recording or any information storage and retrieval system now known or to be invented, without written permission from the Publisher.

For photocopying of material in this volume, please pay a copying fee through the Copyright Clearance Center, Inc., 222 Rosewood Drive, Danvers, MA 01923, USA. In this case permission to photocopy is not required from the publisher.

ISBN-13 978-981-4307-70-3
ISBN-10 981-4307-70-X

Printed in Singapore by World Scientific Printers.

database technology for
life sciences and medicine

SCIENCE, ENGINEERING, AND BIOLOGY INFORMATICS

Series Editor: Jason T. L. Wang
(New Jersey Institute of Technology, USA)

Published:

Preface

Most complex challenges of today cannot be addressed by single disciplines but require interdisciplinary collaborations. Providing high-quality and affordable health care to all people or understanding and curing multi-factor diseases are such tasks which require close integration of medical scientists, biologists, and experts in data management and analysis from informatics.

Technological progress allows us to cheaply produce more and more data. To fully exploit the information potentially contained, effective and application-specific database solutions for data organization, storage, management and exchange are required. On top of these database techniques guaranteeing privacy, accessibility and data quality, data mining techniques allow us to explore complex patterns in the data, which often represent novel, valuable knowledge.

To bring forward interdisciplinary approaches involving database management and data mining on the one side and systems biology, medical imaging and high-throughput screening technology on the other, we have organized the *First International Workshop on Database Technology for Data Management in Life Sciences and Medicine (DBLM)* associated with the 20th International Conference on Database and Expert Systems Applications (DEXA), which took place on September 1st, 2009 in Linz, Austria.

Inspired by the great success of this venue we decided to invite the authors of the top workshop contributions to submit full papers as chapters of this book. In addition, we invited researchers from databases, data mining, biology and medicine to submit original research papers. An international committee selected from a total of 42 submissions 14 for publication.

We are grateful to the following reviewers who contributed with constructive comments to compile this excellent book:

- Elske Ammenwerth[1]
- Christian Baumgartner[1]
- Frank Fiedler[2]
- Katrin Haegler[2]
- Bettina Konte[2]
- Nikola S. Müller[3]
- Annahita Oswald[2]
- Michael Plavinski[2]
- Valentin Riedl[4]
- Michael Seger[1]
- Junming Shao[2]
- Michael Springmann[5]
- Bianca Wackersreuther[2]
- Peter Wackersreuther[2]
- Afra Wohlschläger[4]
- Andrew Zherdin[4]

[1] University for Health Sciences, Medical Informatics and Technology, Hall in Tirol, Austria
[2] University of Munich, Germany
[3] Max Planck Institute of Biochemistry, Martinsried, Germany
[4] Klinikum Rechts der Isar der Technischen Universität München, Munich, Germany
[5] University of Basel, Switzerland

We would like to thank Roland Wagner from University of Linz for giving us the opportunity to set up a workshop on this exiting topic at DEXA. We additionally thank Gabriela Wagner for supporting the review process and helping with the workshop organization.

Particular thanks go to Junming Shao who helped a lot with formatting and arranging the book chapters.

Further thanks to our affiliations and funding institutions: The Department for Neuroradiology at Klinikum Rechts der Isar, Munich headed by Claus Zimmer, the Alexander von Humboldt Foundation, the Institute for Informatics at University of Munich and the Department of Scientific Computing at Florida State University.

June 2010
Tallahassee, FL and Munich, Germany
Claudia Plant and Christian Böhm

Contents

Chapter 1

Biomedical Databases and Data Mining

Claudia Plant[1], Christian Böhm[1,2]

[1]*Florida State University, Tallahassee, FL, USA*
[2]*University of Munich, Germany*

Medicine, biology, and life sciences are very data intensive disciplines. All kinds of data are produced in tremendous amounts, e.g. text, semi-structured data, images, time-series, data streams, and often very high dimensional feature vectors. Modern devices for data acquisition allow to record more and more information. High resolution mass spectrometry, for example, allows us to measure and quantify hundreds of metabolites or peptides from one biosample. At the level of raw mass spectra even hundreds of thousands of features are measured per sample. A further application scenario is patient monitoring: Modern wearable sensors record various parameters of vital functions and are suitable for long-term patient monitoring.

The data explosion in biomedicine challenges the database community to provide solutions for effective data storage, processing, and exchange. A major additional challenge is to support the so called *knowledge discovery process*, i.e. to extract as much as possible useful knowledge from the data. Data from proteomic spectra for example has shown the potential of superior results for early stage cancer detection than traditional biomarkers [Petricoin *et al.* (2002b,a)]. However, only very few among several thousands of features are relevant for diagnosis. One challenge in the emerging field of proteomics is to identify biomarkers for various diseases, characterizing e.g. different types and stages of cancer. It is still a long way towards to the clinical use of diagnostic tests but one important goal is to identify

1

significant features (biomarkers) from very high dimensional biological data sets. In the monitoring scenario, it is essential to efficiently identify unusual patterns in streaming time series of sensor measurements. These suspicious observations can be shown to an expert for further analysis.

Going beyond the original intention of the data acquisition, biomedical data may contain valuable, previously unknown information which even can be out of the scope of the original study. The inspiration behind the research area called *data mining* is to reveal such information. High-dimensional data, for example in proteomics and metabolomics, may exhibit various groups of instances, representing unknown sub-stages of a complex disease. In time series of sensor measurements there may be undiscovered correlations between patterns which are characteristic for an abnormal physiological process.

1.1 Databases and Knowledge Discovery in Biomedicine

It is a long way from the masses of raw data to information useful to biomedical research and patient management. As foundation for all further steps, the data needs to be suitably organized to guarantee accessibility and long term conservation. Since the earliest days of electronic computing, the need for software systems structuring and organizing data has promoted vital research activities in the area of databases. In biomedical applications, huge amounts of data need to be organized preserving privacy and allowing for efficient search and retrieval. The data are commonly of various sources, type, quality and format. For biology, the community of bioinformatics has identified the design, development and long-term management of biological databases as a core research area [Birney and Clamp (2004)]. Biological databases typically contain raw and aggregated data from scientific experiments and literature from the areas of genomics, proteomics, metabolomics, and phylogenetics. Medical databases, as well as clinical and health information systems typically contain phenotypic data from patients and are managed by local hospitals or on a national basis. Medical databases are often focusing on a certain disease and tend to be less standardized than biological databases. Information exchange across health care providers or even across countries is still often difficult. Recently, much research effort is spent towards standardization and exchangeability of medical data, as reflected by numerous projects focussing on the electronic patient record.

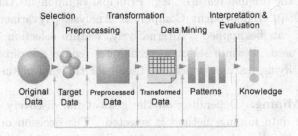

Fig. 1.1: The KDD process.

To support biomedical research on complex diseases, typically data from several biological and/or medical databases need to be integrated.

To meet the requirements of huge amounts of data, the research areas of *knowledge discovery in databases (KDD)* and *data mining* have emerged in the recent years, with multiple books, e.g. [Ester and Sander (2000); Witten and Frank (2005); Han and Kamber (2001)] and numerous papers, e.g. [Fayyad *et al.* (1996); Ng and Han (1994); Ester *et al.* (1996); Papadimitriou *et al.* (2003)], surveys and theses, e.g. [Murtagh (1983); Pan (2006)] to mention a few. Often the terms data mining and knowledge discovery are used interchangeably, however, in the strict sense data mining is one step in the KDD process, which is defined as follows in [Fayyad *et al.* (1996)]: ***Knowledge discovery in databases** is the non-trivial process of identifying novel, potentially useful, and ultimately understandable patterns in data.*

Figure 1.1 gives an overview on the KDD process which comprises five major steps:

(1) **Data Selection.** As a first step the data needs to be carefully selected. Selection criteria include e.g. data availability, quality, type, format, semantics. The selection of high quality data semantically corresponding to the goal of the discovery process is essential for the following steps.

(2) **Preprocessing.** The target data often requires preprocessing. Suitable strategies on scaling and normalization of the features and strategies to handle missing attribute values have to be selected and applied.

(3) **Transformation.** To reduce the dimensionality of the data, dimensionality reduction techniques, which derive transformed representa-

tions of the original features, e.g. Principal Component Analysis [Jol-liffe (1986)], Independent Component Analysis [Hyvärinen and Oja (2000)], can be applied. Alternatively, feature selection techniques can be used. Feature selection techniques reduce the dimensionality by identifying features which are useful for the goal of the discovery process.

(4) **Data Mining.** Depending on the goal of the discovery process, a suitable data mining method is selected. The decision on the data mining algorithm is not easy, since for most tasks there is a huge variety of possibilities. The selected algorithm is applied on the preprocessed and transformed data. For most data mining algorithms it is also a non-trivial task to find appropriate parameter settings.

(5) **Interpretation and Evaluation.** The results of the data mining algorithm are analyzed and interpreted. If the results are not satisfactory, there may be the need to go back one or more steps. In fact, the KDD process is an iterative process.

As a crucial step of the KDD process, data mining requires the selection of a suitable data mining algorithm w.r.t. the goal of the discovery process. Following a common characterization [Han and Kamber (2001)], the diverse data mining methods can be categorized as follows:

- **Clustering:** Find a partitioning of the objects of the data sets into groups (clusters) while maximizing the similarity of the objects in a common cluster and minimizing the similarity of the objects in different clusters.
- **Outlier Detection:** Find objects in the data set which are exceptional, i. e. which do not correspond to the general characteristics or model of the data.
- **Classification:** Learn a function, model or other method from a subset of the data objects to assign a data object to one of several predefined classes.
- **Association Analysis:** Find subsets of the attributes or subsets of attribute ranges which occur frequently together in the data set (called frequent item sets). Derive so called association rules from the frequent item sets. The association rules describe common properties of the data.
- **Evolution Analysis:** Discover and describe regularities or trends for objects with properties that change over time.
- **Characterization and Discrimination:** Summarize general proper-

ties of the data set or of a set of features (characterization). Compare different subsets of the data to other subsets (discrimination).

Another common characterization is to distinguish between *supervised* and *unsupervised* data mining methods. Supervised data mining requires that an attribute is selected by the user which has to be learned by the system for future prediction. The attribute to be learned is often called the class attribute. Specifying suitable values for the class attribute requires domain knowledge and is often done by human experts. The most prominent example for supervised data mining is the task of classification. A classifier is trained on a data set of labeled instances with known values of the class attribute, the so-called training data set. From the training data set, the classifier extracts information to learn a method to predict the value of class attribute of a novel unlabeled instance.

For unsupervised data mining, no class information is required. The most familiar example is clustering. Clustering algorithms aim at finding unknown classes of the data set without any a priori knowledge. This book provides contributions to supervised and unsupervised data mining.

An important issue, especially in the context of biomedical applications, is the performance of data mining methods. In the definition of data mining given in [Fayyad *et al.* (1996)] the performance aspect is explicitly highlighted:

Data Mining is a step in the KDD process consisting of applying data analysis algorithms, that, under acceptable efficiency limitations, produce a particular enumeration of patterns over the data.

1.2 Outline of this Book

This book features research contributions from internationally leading experts addressing various aspects along the way from data to knowledge in biomedicine. Chapters 2 to 8 are dedicated to biomedical databases, data warehouses, and information systems. Central aspects discussed include modeling of such systems, privacy, data exchange data integration, and data quality.

Chapter 2 by Darshan S. Dillon et al. presents a methodology for modeling multi-agent systems. Multi-agent systems are distributed software systems consisting of autonomous intelligent components called agents which allow supporting complex high-level tasks including data collection and information retrieval. The DYNASTAT methodology purely relies on the standardized modeling language UML 2.2. The authors demonstrate the potential of DYNASTAT in three scenarios: information retrieval on diseases, data collection and data mining, and a system for the general health care practitioner.

In Chapter 3 Fusheng Wang et al. propose SciPort, an extensible data management platform for biomedical research. The web-based platform allows researchers to collect, manage, browse and exchange scientific data. Based on native XML, SciPort supports comprehensive user-friendly queries implemented with XQuery. By using ontologies, SciPort provides semantic enabled data management. To share data, SciPort provides a central server-based light-weight approach to integrate data sources across distributed research institutions. SciPort has been successfully used for translational biomedical research consortia and large scale research collaboration.

Grigorios Loukides et al. focus in Chapter 4 on the challenges of anonymizing and integrating clinical and genomic data which is essential for knowledge discovery. The authors outline DIANOVA (Data Integration ANOnymization and View Auditing), a framework for privacy preserving data integration and exchange. DIANOVA is intended to support anonymized integrated views of the database which are useful for genome wide association studies.

In Chapter 5 Mahesh Visvanathan and Gerald H. Lushington provide insights into the challenges emerging from combining mathematical modeling and biological knowledge. For the long-term goal of drug target discovery, the authors integrated biological knowledge from online databases and mathematical knowledge about pathways into a common database. This database allows to systematically study the basic nature of pathways, taking the TNFα-pathway as an example.

Chapter 6 by Sandra Geisler et al. presents a case study in ontology-based data integration. For data management in clinical trials, OnTrIS is presented, an ontology-based data integration system. Based on a core ontology, the user can derive an adapted ontology which triggers the creation of an integrated database. The system has been successfully tested on a pilot trial within the project 'MyHeart' on prevention and monitoring cardiovascular diseases.

In Chapter 7 Francesca Cordero et al. introduce the BIOBITS data warehouse for comparative genomic studies. In particular, a computational genomic comparison of the Ca. Glomeribacter Gigasporarum Bacterium and the Arbuscular Mycorrhinza Fungi genome is supported by BIOBITS. The genomic and proteomic components of the biological problem are represented by a double star schema. The data warehouse also contains two data mining modules: a case-based reasoning and a clustering component. Case-based reasoning is essential for retrieving information at various levels of abstraction and clustering provides the possibility to annotate genetic sequences.

Matteo Bertoni et al. present in Chapter 8 a real life case study on data quality in medicine: A large scale medical database containing several ten million records of clinical and administrative data from hospitals in the Bologna area (Italy) is subjected to a extensive analysis of data quality. Clinical data are privacy-sensitive, heterogenous, produced by different information systems and mainly intended for patient care. Major quality problems have been found, e.g. wrong genders, missing data, inconsistencies, and useless database columns which are mostly due to low motivation and training of the personnel and missing database constraints. Data quality deserves more attention when designing hospital databases.

Chapters 9 and 10 present solutions for efficient similarity search in large biomedical image databases. Efficient similarity search is building block for knowledge discovery and data mining. Chapter 9 by Marc Wichterich et al. proposes an approach for efficient computation of the Earth Movers Distance (EMD) which is an established measure for for effective image retrieval but very time consuming to compute.. The EMD between two images is defined as the minimal amount of changes required to transform the feature representation of one image to the other and the evaluation required solving a linear optimization problem. To speed up computation, the authors propose a dimensionality reduction technique for EMD incorporating domain-specific aspects. The evaluation demonstrates that the approach successfully supports evaluating the EMD on two biomedical image data sets with very different characteristics.

In Chapter 10 Andreas Wichert and Pedro Santos present a system supporting similarity search on clinical records. The system comprises the Subspace Tree, an indexing structure to support content-based image retrieval. In contrast to comparison methods, the Subspace Tree does not partition the data space but the distances among subspaces. Experiments with X-ray images on the prototype system demonstrate that the indexing technique successfully copes with the very high dimensionality of the image data.

Chapters 11 to 15 present contributions implementing various stages of the KDD process in a large variety of exciting biomedical applications. As an approach belonging to the data transformation step, Michael Netzer and Christian Baumgartner present in Chapter 11 a framework for ensemble feature selection in biomedical applications. Stacked feature ranking, a recently developed ensemble feature selection technique is applied for distinguishing alcoholic from non-alcoholic fatty liver disease from breath gas analysis. Both diseases are generally difficult to distinguish but require different treatment. Breath gas samples have been analyzed by mass-spectrometry. The feature selection approach yielded some breath gas maker candidates well corresponding to domain knowledge as well as several novel findings.

The following two chapters are dedicated to unsupervised data mining for investigating the very complex mechanisms in certain diseases: breast cancer and somatoform pain disorder. Chapter 12 by F. Javier Lopez et al. is dedicated to fuzzy association rule mining from breast cancer genomic data. For breast cancer some well studied major prognostic factors exist, including e.g. the size and the histological grade of the tumor. The authors integrate the prognostic factors with whole genome microarray data to study the associations between these two types of data. An analysis on 2,751 patients revealed several interesting rules partly confirming and partly extending previous knowledge.

Bianca Wackersreuther et al. present in Chapter 13 a graph-mining approach to detect co-activated networks in the human brain. Different anatomical regions of the human brain form distinct functional networks fulfilling certain tasks. Functional magnetic resonance images from a study on somatoform pain disorder have been studied. After modeling the brain of each subject as a graph, the proposed algorithm searches for so called motifs, which correspond to frequently occurring sub-graphs. The evaluation demonstrates that certain motifs are much more prevalent in patients than in healthy controls which supports the hypothesis that somatoform pain disorder manifests itself in altered brain function.

Chapters 14 and 15 focus on supervised mining medical data in two scenarios for highest importance to the health care system especially considering the demographic shift. Chapter 14 by Marie Persson et al. studies the interesting question whether it is possible to predict the need of surgery of a patient send to hospital from the referral documents issued by the general practitioner. Sufficiently accurate predictions would allow estimating the surgery demand for different departments of the hospital and thus more efficient resource planning for the hospital and less waiting time for the patients. On a sample data set from Blekinge hospital in Sweden promising results have been obtained with different classifiers.

Philipp Kranen et al. present in Chapter 15 an adaptive multi-step approach for scalable emergency detection from remote health monitoring data. To minimize communication costs and energy consumption of the mobile devices, a technique combining several index-based Bayes-tree classifiers is presented: Potentially critical events are identified by an efficient pre-classifier. Only for critical events, detailed sensor data are sent to a more powerful classifier at the next layer. The experimental evaluation demonstrates that this approach is suitable for multi-step anytime classification of huge amounts of streaming data.

Chapter 2

DYNASTAT: A Methodology for Dynamic and Static Modeling of Multi-agent Systems

Darshan S. Dillon, Maja Hadzic, Tharam S. Dillon

Curtin University of Technology, Perth, Australia

2.1 Introduction

Multi-agent systems are distributed software systems where each agent is represented by a process that may be either single or multi-threaded. These agents are able to cooperate and may use regular data sources such as databases and files. The collection of agents is generally designed so that they collaborate in order to fulfill a particular purpose in a particular domain. We have focused on the application of multi-agents systems in the medical domain. The use of agent-based systems enables us to propose and design intelligent and dynamic medical information systems [Hadzic and Chang (2005b)].

Any multi-agent software system must have a collection of agents that have a number of characteristics. Usually, the term *intelligent* agent reflects the fact that the agent is able to perform intelligent actions within a society which consists of both computer agents and human agents. As such, agents have an environment in which they operate and objectives they are programmed to achieve, and thus, there is usually some way to measure their effectiveness and run-time success. They are able to reason in a procedural way and also use knowledge to make decisions in order to act. There are different triggers for agent decisions which can be internal or external. Agents are able to plan different courses of action to achieve their goals and make choices from these plans. Importantly, agents are social. The social interaction may include cooperation, coordination, communication or negotiation, all of which are means whereby agents interact in groups to fulfill system goals. Finally, there are a number of ways to implement agent-based systems on the various devices over which a multi-agent system may be distributed.

Existing methodologies to cover the modelling of multi-agent systems yield a number of points:

(1) Most existing methodologies to model multi-agent systems do not define an overarching model from which they choose agent characteristics to include in their scope.

(2) These methodologies cover a broad spectrum in relation to what percentages of agent characteristics are represented. Some methodologies cover a small subset in depth, while others are more complete.

(3) Some of these methodologies are abstract, and others define a concrete modelling language as a part of their process. Those that define a language, frequently have authors who create their own symbols and semantics, rather than using a standard language like UML.

The aim of this chapter is to address these issues. We will present an overarching conceptual overview of the things to be modelled in a multi-agent system, specified in DYNASTAT. We select a subset of agent characteristics from the overall conceptual framework that DYNASTAT will model. We define the phases for the conceptual modelling effort. Having defined DYNASTAT as an abstract methodology, we then use UML to work through an example of DYNASTAT in practice. Readers may choose to select a different language, but we have used UML.

In Section 2, some examples of the existing medical multi-agent systems and an overview of current progress in the modeling of multi-agent systems are provided. In Section 3, we discuss the main features of the DYNASTAT methodology. In Section 4, basic UML concepts and a number of UML diagrams that will be further used within DYNASTAT framework are discussed. In Section 5, a number of illustrative examples of the use of UML to model medical multi-agent systems are explained. Some of the advantages of medical multi-agent systems are summarized in Section 6. Finally, the chapter is concluded in Section 7.

2.2 Literature Review

2.2.1 *Multi-agent Systems in the Medical Domain*

Multi-agent systems are increasingly being used in the medical domain. Some of these systems are designed to use information available through specific medical and health institutions, while other systems use information from the Internet.

Examples of institution-specific multi-agent systems examined included Agent Cities [Moreno and Isern (2002)], AADCare [Huang *et al.* (1995)] and MAMIS [Fonseca *et al.* (2005)]. The Agent Cities [Moreno and Isern (2002)] agents enable the user to access his/her medical record, to search for medical centres on the basis of a given set of requirements, or to request and make appointments. AADCare [Huang *et al.* (1995)] is a decision support system used by physicians. It matches the patient's record against the predefined domain knowledge. This domain knowledge can contain knowledge regarding a specific disease, clinical management plans, patient records etc. MAMIS [Fonseca *et al.* (2005)], Multi-agent Medical Information System, provides ubiquitous information access to physicians and health professionals.

BioAgent [Merelli *et al.* (2002)], Holonic Medical Diagnostic System [Ulieru (2003)] and Web Crawling Agents [Srinivasan *et al.* (2002)] are examples of internet-based multi-agent systems. BioAgent [Merelli *et al.* (2002)] is a mobile agent specifically designed to retrieve information about genome analysis. It travels to multiple locations, collects information from each location and integrates information before despatching an answer to the user. Holonic Medical Diagnostic System [Ulieru (2003)] matches the comprehensive computer readable patient record (computer readable patient pattern, CRPP) against the information available through the Internet in order to provide enough evidence for correct diagnosis of the patient. Different web crawling agents [Srinivasan *et al.* (2002)] use information available on mutated genes to fetch information about associated diseases.

The need for the design of a multi-agent system for the purpose of dynamic information retrieval regarding common knowledge of human diseases has been explained in [Hadzic and Chang (2005b,a)]. The BioAgent system could be used for this purpose but it needs to be significantly modified as we are interested in information about human diseases and not genome analysis. Holonic Medical Diagnostic System does not retrieve information about human disease but it uses information specified in the patient record to provide enough evidence for correct diagnosis of this patient. Web crawling agents focus only on the genetic causes of human diseases. A large number of complex diseases are also caused by a number of environmental factors such as stress, family conditions, climate etc. Additionally, numerous human diseases are multi-dimensional not only in terms of their causes but also in terms of symptoms, causes and types. The availability of a systematic overview of the different aspects of human disease will make a significant contribution to the advancement of human disease research and practice.

2.2.2 *Methodologies for Modeling Multi-agent Systems*

We have examined a number of methodologies used to perform conceptual modeling of multi-agent systems. These include:

The methodology defined by [Malyankar and Findler (1998)] models three distinct areas of multi-agent systems including components (agent, system, environment, data and task model), processes (cooperative, competitive and neutral processes) and finally, constraints (identity, capability, class capacity and time constraints). The modeling constructs include the use of state-variables. The agent characteristics modeled for this methodology include autonomy, goals, connectivity, problem coverage and knowledge about other agents. There were no graphical diagrams in the chapter and so it appears this methodology is abstract and is not tied to a particular modeling language.

The BDI methodology [Rao *et al.* (1996)] models a system using three different types of models: object, dynamic and functional. Object models represent data structure, relationships and operations of objects in the system. States, transitions, events, actions, activities and interactions that describe system behavior are modeled using dynamic models, while flow of data during system activity, inside and between system components, are modeled by functional models.

In BDI methodology, agents are defined from an external perspective by defining an agent model (hierarchical relationships between agent classes) and an interaction model (responsibilities, services, control relationships between agent classes). From an internal perspective, agents are defined by belief model (the environment and internal state of an agent), goal model (set of agent's goals) and plan model (plan set). The modeling using this methodology includes an extension of object oriented techniques. The modeling language defined within the methodology has UML-like constructs for some diagrams, and OO type symbols for others. Most of these symbols appear to be author-defined.

The RoMAS [Yan *et al.* (2003)] methodology models agent roles and appears to have a single diagram type: use cases. In this respect the use cases are captured, roles are identified and agents are generated from roles. The notation for the diagram is a type of E-R notation and appears to have author-defined symbols.

We noted that most of the existing methodologies had a specific modeling language included in the abstract process defined to perform conceptual modeling. However, in most cases, this modeling language was not a standard one such as UML, which could be extended in a controlled way using stereotypes. Each language was usually author-defined, with the symbols used having no standard meaning from one paper to another.

2.2.3 *UML Modeling of Multi-agent Systems*

A number of researchers have attempted to use UML in modeling multi-agent systems [da Silva *et al.* (2005); Kavi *et al.* (2003); da Silva *et al.* (2004); de Maria *et al.* (2005); Odell *et al.* (2001)]. This research effort has contributed significantly to the development of a standardized methodology for modeling multi-agent systems. However, a number of issues have emerged from these research efforts that need to be addressed. These issues include poorly detailed presentations, modified semantics of UML diagrams without using stereotypes and limited use of stereotypes. Lack of detailed presentation is evident in [de Maria *et al.* (2005)] where VisualAgent presents some initial ideas, but does not use many existing UML diagrams or stereotypes. The semantics of UML diagrams has been modified by many researchers. For instance, Kavi [Kavi *et al.* (2003)] uses smiley faces, thought clouds, and the like, which have not been defined by the UML semantics. Da Silva [da Silva *et al.* (2004)] changes the semantics of rectangles without the use of a stereotype. Odell [Odell *et al.* (2001)] defines a rectangle to be an Agent/Role combination in sequence diagrams which means that a single Agent can be represented by multiple rectangles, each rectangle representing a single role. Again, this was done without the use of a stereotype. We also noted a limited use of stereotypes. For example, Odell [Odell *et al.* (2001)] did not use stereotypes to define an agent.

This chapter makes a number of contributions to the existing modeling approaches.

We show how different types of UML diagrams can be used to model different aspects of multi-agent systems. For instance, a Sequence Diagram is used to model the social nature of agents, Composite Structure Diagrams to model agent internals and an Activity Diagram to model the processes implemented by agents.

We do not change the semantics of existing symbols defined in the UML standard. No symbols are introduced into UML diagrams in this chapter that are not defined in the standard. The messages in the Sequence Diagram are an exception to this.

We use stereotypes to extend and modify the meaning of existing symbols in UML diagrams. Most often, this is done in order to have a symbol that usually represents a class or object, represent an agent instead.

2.3   DYNASTAT Methodology

The authors propose a methodology that is termed DYNASTAT. This stands for: Dynamic and static methodology for modeling multi-agent systems.

The methodology is a process that is independent of any particular conceptual modeling language and includes:

- An overview of what a multi-agent system is, and what individual agents are, in conceptual terms.
- A selection of specific agent characteristics that are to be modeled.
- A discussion of what is required in modeling terms, for each of these agent characteristics.
- Modeling phases.

2.3.1   *Conceptual Overview of Multi-agent Systems*

In conceptual terms, multi-agent systems have a number of characteristics [Parka and Sugumaran (2005); Tweedalea *et al.* (2007); Ren and Anumba (2004)].

Any multi-agent system usually has an environment in which agents operate. The agent may perform one task at a time, or it may multiplex many tasks. Each agent usually has the ability to observe the environment. Agents are usually able to observe part of the environment, but not all of it. The environment is *centralized* when it has a single controlling agent and *non-centralized* when many agents control the system. If changes in the environment are caused only by the agent itself, it is termed *static*, but if other things also contribute to the changes, the environment is called *dynamic*. If the action of an agent is unrelated to the past and future acts of the agent, we are speaking of an *episodic* environment. In a *sequential* environment, there is a relationship between current and past and/or future actions of the agent. In *deterministic* environments, the finish state of the environment can be uniquely predicted from the start state and the agent actions. Conversely, in *stochastic* environments, the finish state cannot be uniquely predicted based on the information above. The environment has either a finite number of states (*discrete*) or a very high number of states (*continuous*).

Every agent has a purpose, and so there is usually a need to measure agent effectiveness. *Performance measure* is used to measure how successful an agent is in carrying out its tasks. A rational agent is one that makes decisions to maximize its future performance. A performance measure must define the criteria of success. *Omniscience* is a characteristic that indicates an agent can predict the outcome of all its decisions and actions, under every circumstance.

Each agent has certain *beliefs* and plays different *roles*. It also has *goals*, particular outcomes the agent is programmed to achieve. The agent follows precisely defined *procedures* and also performs calculations based on formulas. The agent can *reason* and use knowledge to decide on a particular course of action in a particular environment. This usually means choosing a particular plan or path to a goal under certain conditions. An agent can *plan* a particular path to a goal. An agent makes use of *sensors* to observe the environment and effectors to act on the environment.

Every agent performs various actions. Usually, some event *triggers* an agent's actions. The trigger can be a request, a specific occurrence in the environment or an internal process. An agent usually uses *plans*, a collection of acts, ordered in a workflow with decision points. At each *decision point*, the agent will be able to *select* a particular plan. The agent will also *schedule* and *prioritize* its actions.

In addition to what an agent is, and what it does, each agent is capable of change. An agent is able to *learn* from the results of action and modify internal intelligence in order to make better decisions. Additionally, an agent can *adapt* and reconfigure itself in response to changes in the environment.

Agents are sociable and are often involved in *coordinations*, *cooperations*, *communications* and *negotiations*. Agents work together, cooperate to achieve particular goals, exchange information and come to agreements.

In terms of the implementation of agent-based systems as software, the *mobility* (ability of agents to move from machine to machine), *fault tolerance* (reliability of an agent), *distributed* (execution of a single agent over many machines with different threads of execution) and *persistent* (agent runs continuously) nature of agents need to be modeled.

The authors have chosen a subset of the agent characteristics to model in this chapter. They include agent's beliefs, roles, procedures, reasoning and decision making. We also model the sociable nature of agents including coordination, cooperation, communication and negotiation.

2.3.2 Modeling Phases

Regardless of the modeling language chosen for modeling, a number of steps have to be taken.

The specific diagrams to be used have to be identified. A mapping between particular characteristics and particular diagrams has to be established. The specific symbols in each of the diagrams to be used need to be identified and the meaning of each must be understood by the modeler.

The problem domain has to be understood in general terms. A specific application that is the subject for modeling needs to be identified. A number of scenarios would have to be analyzed in order to decide on what will be modeled. These scenarios are then worked through in the context of specific diagrams in order to complete the models for each case.

This completes our discussion of the DYNASTAT methodology. It is a methodology that applies to modeling multi-agent systems irrespective of the particular modeling language used. In this chapter, UML 2.2 is used to realize this methodology for the purpose of example. The next section discusses this modeling language as a prelude to a working example.

2.4 Use of UML 2.2 in the Framework of DYNASTAT Methodology

2.4.1 Overview of UML 2.2

The UML standard defines 13 different diagram types (http://www.omg.org/spec/UML/2.2/Superstructure). Each of these diagrams can contain a distinct set of symbols, which can be combined in a standard set of ways to model the system being examined. Each of these symbols has a specific meaning defined in the UML standard.

There are many versions of UML that have been released over time. The current version in use is UML 2.2 and this version is in beta. This is the version that has been used for diagrams in this chapter.

One important fact about UML is that it can be extended in a controlled way through the use of stereotypes. This essentially means that an existing UML symbol can be qualified to change the standard meaning it has in the standard. The symbol is qualified by a <<stereotype>> name text block somewhere in the symbol, or by defining a completely different icon. Either way, the idea is to allow modelers to effectively add an additional symbol to the pre-defined set in the UML standard and include that symbol in UML diagrams used in modeling.

2.4.2 *Usage of UML for Modeling Multi-agent Systems*

In some UML diagrams, there is at least one symbol that represents a class or object. Stereotypes are defined for some of these symbols to have them represent agents instead. Some diagrams also model messages between classes and objects, and these messages now represent inter-agent communication.

The Sequence Diagram and Composite Structure Diagram are two diagrams used in this chapter that fall into this category.

Other UML diagrams have a symbol that represents something independent of a class. For instance, a Use Case Diagram has a symbol to represent system functionality and an Activity Diagram has a symbol to represent an Activity in a process. In this case, stereotype symbols are not required to represent agents.

UML also models events that cause state transitions between a finite number of states. Although this chapter does not explore UML diagrams that use state machines, future work could further extend the paradigm shift above by having state machines model the internal state of an agent, the state of the agent environment, or the system as a whole. As above, this would require stereotyping some of the symbols used in state diagrams.

2.4.3 *Selected UML Diagrams*

This section discusses the basic diagram types in this chapter and defines the symbols used in the UML 2.2 diagrams drawn to model the multi-agent system used as an example. The symbols here are a subset of what is included in the UML standard, but provide a context so that the semantics of the drawn diagrams are clear.

Four basic UML diagram types have been included: use case, composite structure, sequence and activity diagram. They are discussed below.

Use Case Diagram

[Rumbaugh *et al.* (2004)]

This is a diagram that models the functionality of the system used by external end-users of that system.

The symbols most commonly used in this diagram type are shown in Figure 1 and include: (i) Actor, which represents an external person or system using the system being modeled; (ii) Use Case, which represents a unit of functionality; (iii) Association Relationship, which indicates the usage of a unit of functionality by an external actor; and (iv) Generalization Relationship, which indicates the inclusion of a specialization of the functionality in the parent.

In order to model a multi-agent system, stereotyping of these symbols was not required since the functionality of the system and its actors are not particularly centric to either classes or agents.

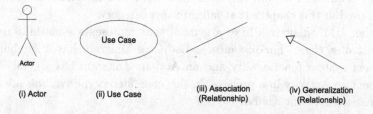

Fig. 2.1: Use Case Diagram (symbols).

Composite Structure Diagram

[Rumbaugh *et al.* (2004)]

This is a diagram defined in the UML standard to represent the internals of a class.

The symbols commonly used in this diagram type are shown in Figure 2 and these include: (i) Classifier, a rectangle to represent the class as a whole; (ii) Parts, rectangles inside the outer rectangle to represent different areas of processing of the class; and (iii) Ports, small squares at the borders of the outer rectangle and represent the connections between the class and the interfaces that are external to it.

In this case, the outer rectangle was stereotyped to represent an agent rather than a class. The inner rectangles were stereotyped to represent the parts of an agent, rather than a class. Finally, the ports were stereotyped to represent agent roles, rather than connectors to the external environment of the class.

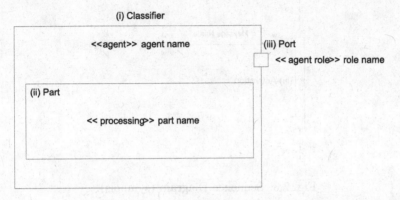

Fig. 2.2: Composite Structure Diagram (symbols).

Sequence Diagram

[Rumbaugh *et al.* (2004)]

This is a diagram defined in the UML standard that represents inter-object or inter-class interaction by way of messages.

Generally, the commonly used symbols are shown in Figure 3 and these include: (i) Heads, rectangles that represent the classes that are communicating and include a dotted line that goes down the page to represent time passing; (ii) Messages, arrows that go between the dotted lines and represent messages being passed between the classes that are communicating; and (iii) Activation - long rectangle that goes over the dotted line to represent the fact that the class has a run time instance that is operating.

In this case, the heads were stereotyped to represent agents, rather than classes. Ports were used at the edge of these rectangles to indicate roles played by the agents. This is a significant extension of the existing UML standard in semantic terms, and stereotypes were used to do it. Individual messages were not stereotyped, although they now represent inter-agent, rather than inter-class communication.

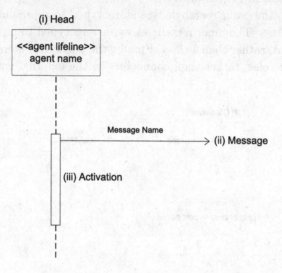

Fig. 2.3: Sequence Diagram (symbols).

Activity Diagram

[Rumbaugh *et al.* (2004)]

The UML Activity Diagram models any process in a system. A process may be implemented in a class, an agent, or any other type of construct.

Generally, the commonly used symbols are shown in Figure 4 and include: (i) Initial node which is represented as a black dot to indicate the start of the process; (ii) Activity node which is represented as a rectangle with rounded edges to indicate a unit of processing; (iii) Decision node which represents a decision or choice of an agent or class down different paths; (iv) Fork which is a heavy black bar with one arrow entering and many arrows exiting to represent one path of action diverging into many; (v) Join which is a heavy black bar with many arrows entering and one exiting to represent many paths of action converging into one; (vi) Termination node which is represented as a cross within a circle to signify the termination of a course of action, but not the completion of the entire process; and (vii) Final node which is represented as a black dot within a circle to indicate the end of the entire process.

In this case, it was not necessary to stereotype since the Activity Diagram that models a process independently of the process is packaged into a class, component or agent. Since this is the case, it is not necessary to change the semantics of the symbols using stereotypes.

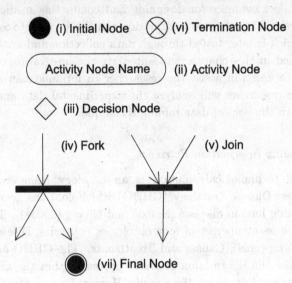

Fig. 2.4: Activity Diagram (symbols).

2.5   UML to Model Medical Multi-agent Systems

In building the system, the following two scenarios from the medical domain were used:

(1) medical researchers retrieving information from various information resources, and collecting evidence to design and conduct medical experiments, and

(2) general practitioners who have standard consultations with patients (primary care).

2.5.1   *Medical Researcher (UML Examples)*

The process of medical research is quite different from the day-to-day operation of the health care system. Most scientific medical research involves the use of certain rules to set up and conduct experiments and also the use of certain principles when analyzing the data collected to reach experimental conclusions. The system modeling for a medical researcher is focused on the intelligent retrieval of information from various information sources in order to collect evidence for designing and conducting medical experiments effectively. The retrieved information can also be used to formulate a hypothesis which is later tested through data collection and analysis. The system modeled in this chapter will automate the integration of existing sources of data and will assist the researcher to formulate an initial hypothesis. The researcher will analyze the experimental data and test the hypothesis with the help of data mining techniques.

2.5.1.1 *Modeling Information Retrieval*

The proposed technological solution is an ontology framework of the Generic Human Disease Ontology (GHDO) which contains generic information regarding human diseases [Hadzic and Chang (2005a)]. The ontology is designed as a superset of four ontologies capturing Disease Types, Phenotype (Symptoms), Causes and Treatments. The GHDO ontology is used to support the information retrieval process within the multi-agent structure. It is used to derive the Specific Human Disease Ontology template (SHDO template). The SHDO template specifies the information the user has requested in relation to a particular disease. For example, if a user is interested only in the causes of a specific disease, the SHDO template will contain only the causes sub ontology of the GHDO. When agents feed instances into this SHDO template after information retrieval, the SHDO template is converted into a Specific Human Disease Ontology (SHDO) which is presented to the user as the answer to his/her query.

Four different agent types within the GHDO-based multi-agent system are defined here:

(1) The <u>Interface Agent</u> constructs Specific Human Disease Ontology (SHDO) templates from GHDO. The SHDO template is sent to the Manager Agent once it has been generated.
(2) The <u>Manager Agent</u> assigns tasks to various Information Agents. The Manager Agent must have the appropriate expertise to do this; namely, it must have knowledge of the task structure. This is specified by the SHDO template.
(3) The <u>Information Agents</u> retrieve the requested information from a wide

range of biomedical databases. Depending on the requested information, an agent may be required to retrieve information about disease types, symptoms, causes and/or treatments. The Information Agents send the retrieved information to the Smart Agent.

(4) The <u>Smart Agent</u> collects and analyzes the information received from Information Agents, filters it for the relevant information and then uses the data to populate the SHDO template. The SHDO is sent to the Interface Agent to be presented to the user as the answer to his/her query.

Interaction between different agents is presented in the Sequence Diagram in Figure 5. The Sequence Diagram is used to model the inter-agent communication between all four agent types in the system. The diagram describes the process of a user querying the system about a particular disease. The generated SHDO template will be passed from Interface to Manager Agent, who will then message the Information agents to request data on the disease, symptoms, causes and treatments. This information will be gathered by Information Agents, who will then pass it to a Smart Agent that is responsible for integrating it into the SHDO template. Finally, that template will be returned to the Interface Agent, who will return it to the user. The agents themselves are modeled by head symbols that are stereotyped as <<agent lifeline>>. The Information and Smart Agents play more than one role and this is modeled by a port stereotyped as <<agent role>>.

In Figure 6, a Composite Structure Diagram is used to model the internals of the Smart Agent. It has a classifier stereotyped as <<agent>> to name the Smart Agent. It has four distinct areas of processing including: a controller to coordinate the actions of the agent, a part to analyze the data given to it by Information Agents, a part to filter that information for what is relevant and finally, a processing unit to assemble what is relevant into the SHDO template, before that populated template is returned to the user. These areas of processing are stereotyped using the <<processing>> stereotype. The two ports titled 'send' and 'collect' represent the roles played by the Smart Agent to send and receive data to other agents. They are stereotyped as <<agent role>>.

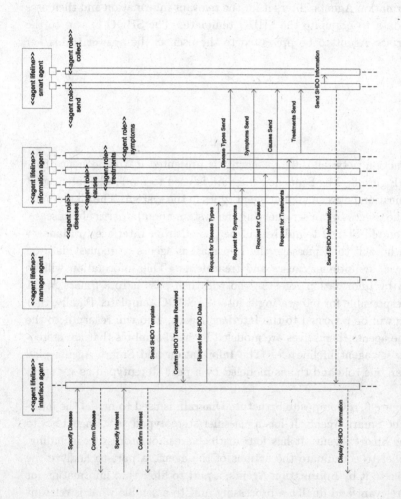

Fig. 2.5: Sequence Diagram representing interactions between different agent types in the GHDO-based multi agent system. The different agents are collaboratively working in this intelligent information retrieval system.

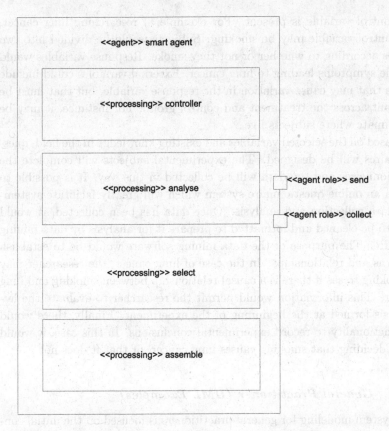

Fig. 2.6: Composite Structure Diagram to represent internal structure of Smart Agent.

2.5.2 *Modeling Data Collection and Mining Experiments*

In Figure 7, a Use Case Diagram illustrates the different functions involved in conducting a medical experiment. The medical researcher usually selects a category of experiment to be carried out. Various categories exist and they range from clinical trials to public surveys. Researchers also conduct a literature review which helps in formulating a hypothesis, which will be refined and verified by the experiment. A system such as that described in Figure 5 can assist the researcher in gathering relevant data. The researcher chooses a subject group and obtains their consent to participate in the experiment. There will be a functionality to assist the researcher to assign the subjects into different experimental groups according to whether or not the control variable is present. For example, if researching lung cancer, the control variable may be smoking. Subjects would be divided into two groups according to whether or not they smoke. Response variables would include symptoms leading to lung cancer. External variables could include things that may cause variation in the response variable, but that must be constant across the treatment and control group. For instance, it may be the climate where subjects live.

Based on the selected variables and existing knowledge in the field, questionnaires will be designed. The experimental subjects will complete the questionnaires and the data will be collected in this way. It is possible to design an online questionnaire system which will greatly facilitate systematic data collection and analysis. Once data has been collected, it would need to be cleaned and formatted to prepare it for analysis by data mining software. The purpose of the data mining software would be to establish patterns and relationships. In the case of lung cancer, the researcher may be looking to see if there is a causal relationship between smoking and lung cancer. This information would permit the researcher to evaluate the hypothesis formed at the beginning of the experiment. Finally, there would be functionality to record experimental conclusions. In this case, it would mean deciding that smoking causes lung cancer, or that it does not.

2.5.3 *General Practitioner (UML Examples)*

The system modeling for general practitioners is focused on the initial contact between doctors and patients and the establishment of preliminary diagnosis, prognosis and treatment of disease. It also includes following up to determine whether a recommended treatment has been effective and whether the patient has been cured of the disease. There is a health care system in most first world countries which includes a network of general practitioners and hospitals, both public and private. Usually, the initial point of contact for most patients who are ill is a general practitioner in a suburban clinic. After an initial consultation, the doctor usually makes some type of diagnosis and may ask the patient to give a sample of some type (for instance, blood or urine) which will be sent to a pathology lab for analysis. The results may refine or confirm the initial diagnosis. The doctor may also suggest some type of medical imaging technique for the same reason. One example of medical imaging would be a CT scan of the patient's brain to see if s/he has a brain tumor. If the patient has a certain type of disease, the general practitioner may recommend that s/he see a

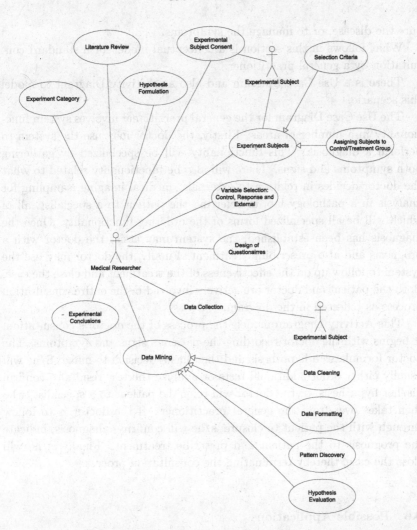

Fig. 2.7: Use Case Diagram representing the conducting of medical experiments including hypothesis formulation, data collection and data analysis.

specialist. The specialist may recommend surgery, and that would require the patient to be admitted to hospital.

Finally, the doctor may recommend some type of therapy from, for example, a clinical psychologist or physiotherapist. Whether the treatment modality is a drug, therapy or surgery, the goal of treatment is usually to cure the disease, or to manage the symptoms.

What follows in this section is a conceptual model for a standard consultation by a general practitioner.

There is a Use Case Diagram and also an Activity Diagram to model this scenario.

The Use Case Diagram for the general practitioner involves system functionality in a number of areas. Firstly, the doctor may use the system to perform a diagnosis. This functionality will be specialized by gathering both symptoms and signs. There will also be functionality related to what the doctor decides in relation to externals: medical imaging, sampling for analysis in a pathology lab, or referring the patient to a specialist, all of which will be all specialized forms of the ordering functionality. Once the diagnosis has been established, the system may assist the doctor with a prognosis and also prescribing treatment. Finally, the doctor may use the system to follow up on the effectiveness of the treatment and close the case. Both the patient and doctor are actively involved in the entire consultation process as reflected in the diagram.

This Activity Diagram models the process of the doctor's consultation. It begins with the doctor recording the patient's signs and symptoms. The doctor formulates a hypothesis and then has a decision to make. S/he will usually either order additional tests or analyze the test results to confirm his/her hypothesis, or the doctor will refer the patient to a specialist, who then takes over from the general practitioner. If the doctor is to follow through with the patient to closure, s/he will confirm a diagnosis, indicate the prognosis to the patient and prescribe treatment. Finally, s/he will close the case, thereby terminating the consultation process.

2.6   Possible Applications

In terms of medical research, multi-agent systems have the potential to provide evidence that will help the researchers obtain relevant information and progress with knowledge more rapidly. The information obtained through the intelligent GHDO-based multi-agent system can also assist in the formulation of hypothesis and provide foundational knowledge that will help obtain new knowledge in the field through the conduction of various medical experiments. An experimental process has been shown in which data is obtained through questionnaires and analyzed with the help of data mining algorithms. Data mining algorithms can analyze experimental data

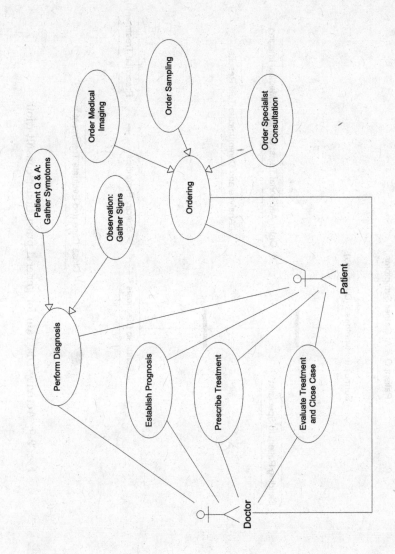

Fig. 2.8: Use Case Diagram for general practitioner consultation.

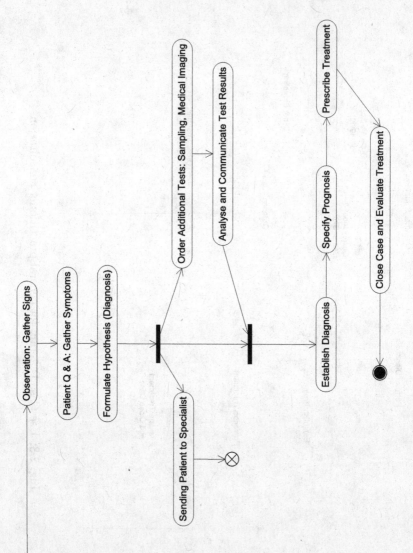

Fig. 2.9: Activity Diagram for general practitioner consultation.

and find patterns that a human researcher may easily miss. Additionally, the implementation of a multi-agent system also helps increase the control and simplifies the standard experimental process.

In terms of a standard consultation, the implementation of multi-agent systems has numerous advantages such as controlling the standard process of consultation, assisting the doctor to diagnose the patient illness, supporting decision-making processes in regard to requirements for pathology tests, medical imaging or specialist referrals and enabling data collection that will help doctors to improve the standard consultative process.

It is hardly conceivable that a software system can be designed to replace a human agent. Nevertheless, some interplay between the researcher/doctor and the system may refine the process being used and provide support for decision-making at various stages.

2.7 Conclusion

This chapter has established a methodology called DYNASTAT which provides a conceptual overview of multi-agent systems, a selection of agent characteristics modeled by the methodology and also a discussion of what needs to be modeled in particular for each agent characteristic.

After the presentation of this methodology, the authors chose UML 2.2 as a modeling language to realize DYNASTAT for a particular system in the multi-agent domain. We explained four UML 2.2 diagram types including: the use case, composite structure, and activity and sequence diagrams. A particular multi-agent system was then chosen from the medical domain in order to model these UML 2.2 diagrams.

Many of the areas of weakness in the current research have been addressed with a coherent example to permit the reader to follow a particular line of thought. It is to be noted that this chapter does not venture into the more complex paradigm of assigning roles to agent groups. The complexities of basic agent modeling have been explored before going further in order to build a solid foundation. Nevertheless, more complex paradigms in multi-agent systems such as modeling the environment, effectiveness of agents, change and adaptation of agents and implementation of agent systems may be considered in future work published by the authors.

Chapter 3

SciPort: An Extensible Data Management Platform for Biomedical Research

Fusheng Wang[1], Peiya Liu[2], John Pearson[2]

[1] *Emory University, Atlanta, GA, USA*
[2] *Siemens Corporate Research, Princeton, NJ, USA*

3.1 Introduction

3.1.1 *Overview*

Scientific data from biomedical research are proliferating in both heterogeneity and complexity. A biomedical data management system needs to address the following critical issues: i) modeling, authoring, storing and querying of complex scientific data; ii) data consistency among users; iii) a generic architecture adaptable for managing scientific data from different applications; and iv) integrating and sharing distributed data sources.

We develop SciPort, a Web-based extensible data management platform for biomedical research, where researchers can easily collect, represent, manage, browse, and exchange scientific data. SciPort provides a unified XML based generic approach to model and organize complex scientific data, where data schemas and hierarchies are customizable for different applications. By managing the data through a native XML database based approach, SciPort supports comprehensive user-friendly queries implemented with XQuery. By using ontologies, SciPort provides semantic enabled data management. To share data, SciPort provides a central server based light weight approach to integrate data sources across distributed research institutions.

3.1.2 Complex Requirements

The requirements for biomedical data management differ significantly between applications, from large scale data sharing, to laboratory data management; from biomedical research environment, to enterprise biomedical applications. With increased complexity of biomedical problems, biomedical research is increasingly a collaborative effort across multiple institutions and disciplines. Indeed, NIH provides large-scale collaborative project awards (U54) (http://grants.nih.gov/grants/guide/pafiles/PAR-04-128.html) for a team of independently funded investigators to synergize and integrate their efforts. For example, the Network for Translational Research: Optical Imaging (NTROI) (http://imaging.cancer.gov/programsandresources/specializedinitiatives/ntroi) is a large scale collaborative project award on the development for translational research through optical imaging. It requires not only managing the complex scientific research results, but also sharing the data across research collaborators.

As another example, in the Pathology and Laboratory Department of University of Pennsylvania, hundreds of students and researchers need to manage their experimental data, and the data have to be transparent to others. To reduce the cost, all the users are sharing a single data management system.

The user demands for biomedical data management systems have only increased with time (Anderson *et al.*, 2007). Unfortunately, it is still difficult for researchers to find biomedical data management solutions to support their research. The lack of viable solutions can be first attributed to the complexity and diversity of scientific data in biomedical domains. Biomedical data can be in heterogeneous formats such as structured data, DICOM images, non-DICOM images, raw equipment data, spreadsheets, PDF files, XML documents, and many others. Thus, the data are often a mix of structured data (often deeply hierarchical) and files. Meanwhile, the data structures of biomedical research data can be very complex, ranging from different primitive data types, to lists and tables, from flat structures to deep nested structures, and so on. The data values can also be constrained as single-value constrained data ("radiobutton"), multi-value constrained data ("checkboxes"), or values from controlled vocabularies. Although there are tools or applications developed for specific research disciplines, a common complaint is that "that tool only works for that lab" (Anderson *et al.*, 2007). The complexity of biomedical data demands an adaptable biomedical data management system that can provide generic data modeling and management of scientific experiments and be easily adjusted for different applications.

3.1.3 *Semantic Consistency*

Biomedical ontologies are being rapidly developed to specify domain concepts and their relations (Cimino and Zhu, 2006; Rubin *et al.*, 2007), such as RadLex (http:// radlex.org/), SNOMED (http://www.snomed.org/), NCI Thesaurus (https://cabigf.nci.nih.gov/tools/concepts/caCORE_overview), Gene Ontology (http://www.geneontology.org/), etc. Such controlled vocabularies or ontologies can be used to enhance structure based data management such as semantic enabled data authoring and queries. However, biomedical databases are mostly proliferated with structured data, and come with limited tools for leveraging controlled vocabularies or ontologies.

3.1.4 *Data Sharing*

An essential goal for biomedical research is to share experiment data to reuse experiments, pool expertise and validate approaches. Even having the data managed properly, researchers often find it difficult to share their data, due to the following reasons. i) The lack of data sharing infrastructure for convenient data sharing. Cyberinfrastructures such as Grid based systems (CaBIG (http://caBIG.nci.nih.gov/), Biomedical Informatics Research Network (BIRN) (http://www.nbirn.net/) focus on large scale data sources and are heavy weight for regular research sites; ii) Users' fear of losing control of their data. Researchers would rather have maximal control of their data on a server located on their own research sites, instead of "outsourcing" them somewhere else. Even when data are shared, the researchers may still want to have flexible sharing control – they keep the ownership of the data, and can revoke the sharing of the data at any time.

3.1.5 *Our Contributions*

These have motivated the development of *SciPort*, a unified Web-based platform for biomedical data management and sharing. SciPort provides i) a general and comprehensive scientific data model to represent, author, and organize complex scientific data, so researchers can quickly organize their data and experiments; ii) convenient tools to help data providers to author such data and automatically de-identify their data; iii) a system architecture that provides comprehensive management with tools to search, browse, report, and exchange data; iv) semantic enabled data management on authoring and querying using ontologies; v) high extensibility of the system for different applications and domains – "developed once, and used everywhere"; and vi) a lightweight, central server based data integration and sharing architecture to integrate and share distributed data sources.

3.2   Related Work

There is growing need of scientific data management systems [Anderson *et al.* (2007)], and much work on scientific management has been done in the past [Ioannidis *et al.* (1997); Kaestle *et al.* (1999); Keller and Jones (1996); Stolte *et al.* (2003); Chin and Lansing (2004)] (http://mirc.rsna.org, http://ncia.nci.nih.gov/) (Jakobovits *et al.*, 2002). Most of the work focuses on a specific application or discipline, e.g., [Keller and Jones (1996)] is used in environment and molecular sciences laboratory, and NBIA (http://ncia.nci.nih.gov/) is a cancer image archive. Thus, data models are tied and generalization is often limited. WIRM (Jakobovits *et al.*, 2002) is an open source toolkit for building biomedical Web applications based on relational based approach, and MyPACS (http://www.mypacs.net) is built on top of it to provide medical image management.

A context-based sharing system is proposed in [Chin and Lansing (2004)], which focuses on tools instead of data as in SciPort.

MIRC (http://mirc.rsna.org) is a popular pure-P2P based system for authoring and sharing teaching files, which is hard to extend for generic data management and suffers from security problems.

XML based data representation for biomedical data becomes increasingly popular. XNAT (Marcus *et al.*, 2007) is an XML based platform for managing neuroimaging and related data, and represents data in XML at the schema level. XNAT uses relational database engine as the backend storage, and provides data and query mapping between XML and RDBMS. In [Bales *et al.* (2005)], work has been done to provide unique XQuery based frontend for relational based data sources.

With the increasing collaboration of scientific research, collaborative cyberinfrastructures have been researched and developed in the past [Arzberger and Finholt (2002)]. Grid-based systems(such as caBIG – can-

cer Biomedical Informatics Grid (http://caBIG.nci.nih.gov/), Biomedical
Informatics Research Network (BIRN) (http://www.nbirn.net/)) provide
infrastructures to integrate existing computing and data resources. They
rely on a top down common data structure. This is difficult to get agreement upon and requires much effort and cost to setup and maintain such
systems. SciPort is lightweight and can be quickly customized for either
research labs or research networks.

3.3 Unified Scientific Data Modeling

An essential goal of managing biomedical research data is to capture all
the context information and results for an experiment or processing, such
as metadata about the data, the results (attributes, raw data, images),
parameters used in the experiment, and so on. To represent scientific data,
we model each experiment/processing as a document, and the relationships
of the documents are linked through document references. The data model
is discussed next.

3.3.1 *The Scientific Document Model*

One main characteristic of scientific data is its complex data structures,
which could be nested. Another main characteristic is their heterogenous
data formats, including both structural data and unstructured data. We
develop a generic scientific data model to represent all such information, as
shown in Figure 3.1.

The central entity of the data model is *SciPort Document*, which contains both *metadata* and *content*. Metadata include author generated metadata, such as title, description, and author information, and system generated metadata, such as creation date, modification date, hierarchy information, etc. Document content represents both structural data and
files/images. The latter are referenced through file links. The following
primitive objects are defined in the document content.

- **Primitive Data Types/Fields.** Primitive data types are used to
  represent structural data, including *integer*, *float*, *date*, and *text*. As
  SciPort is a Web based system, a few specialized data types are defined
  for the convenience of authoring and queries. These include *textarea*
  – multi-lines of text displayed in a block, *radiobutton* – single value
  constrained data type with options from a set of values, *checkbox* –

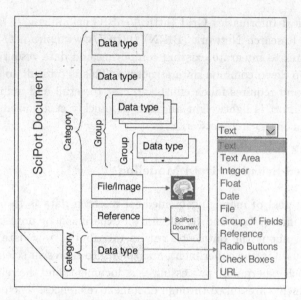

Fig. 3.1: SciPort scientific data model.

multiple value constrained data type with options from a set of values, and *URL* - a reference to a Web resource.

- **File.** Files can be linked to a document through the file object. Common file types are detected through file extensions. The system will also automatically detect if a file is of DICOM type. For an image or a DICOM file, the system will automatically generate a preview thumbnail.
- **Reference.** A reference type links to another SciPort document.
- **Group.** A group aggregates a collection of fields or nested groups. This could easily represent hierarchical structures. There can be multiple instances for a group, like rows of a table.
- **Category.** A category relates a list of fields, for example, "patient data" category, "experiment data" category. Categories are used only at the top level of the content, and not nested.

Figure 3.2 shows some content of a sample SciPort Document on medical image annotations. It includes categories "General Information", "Patient" for patient information, "Annotation", and "File". Inside Annotation category, there is a group field "TumorCollection", which has two instances. The TumorCollection group includes fields "name" and "UID", group "ImageObservationCharacteristicCollection", "DataCollection", "SpatialCoor-

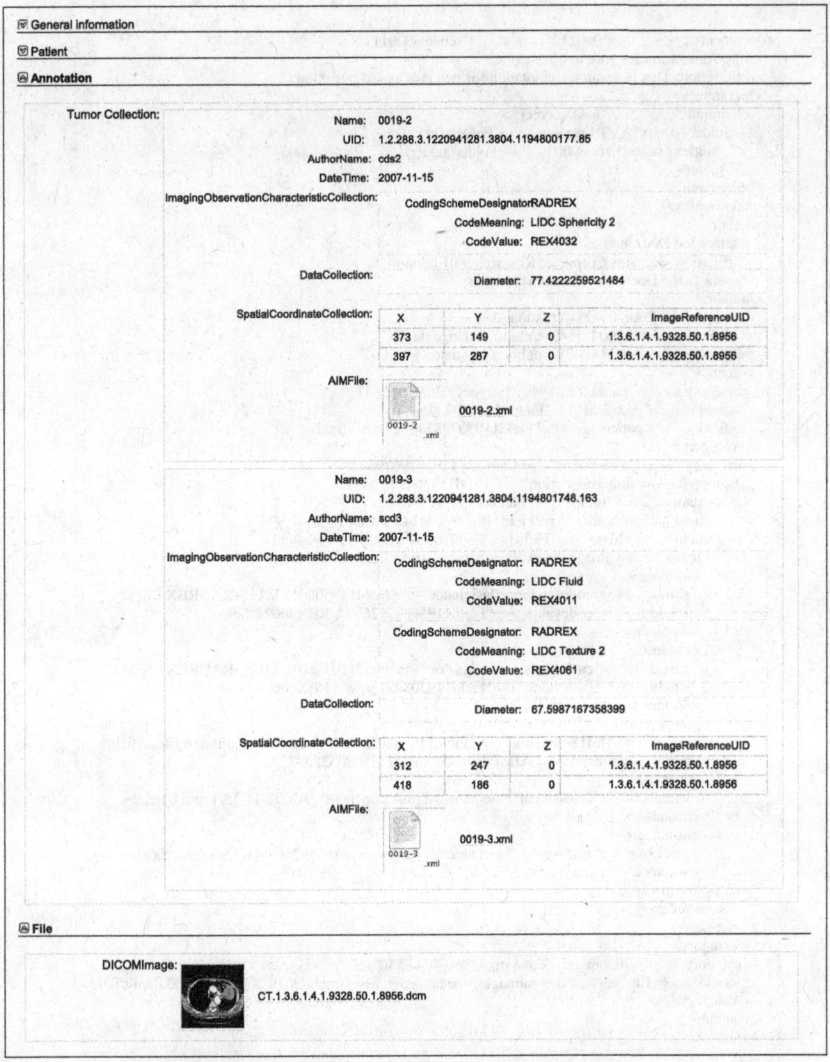

Fig. 3.2: A sample view of SciPort document.

dinateCollection", and a file type "AIMFile".

3.3.2 *XML Based Implementation of the Data Model*

The model can be best implemented as XML – we call it *SciPort Exchange Document*. The hierarchical nature of the data model fits perfectly with the

```
<document documentid="000112" schemaid="schema0001112">
  <title>Annotation for patient 0019</title>
  <description>This is a sample annotation for two tumors.</description>
  <hierarchies>
    <hierarchy sciportid="localserver1">
      <folder name="AVT Database" id="Folder0001">
        <folder name="patient 0019" id="Folder0023"/>
      </folder>
    </hierarchy>
  </hierarchies>
  <author>
    <name>Joe Doe</name>
    <affiliation>Siemens Corporate Research</affiliation>
    <contact>Joe.Doe@siemens.com</contact>
  </author>
  <creation_date>2008-05-25</creation_date>
  <modification_date>2008-05-28</modification_date>
  <publication_date>2008-05-28</publication_date>
  <content>
    <category name="patientinfo" id="Category1195079655778">
      <field name="patientid" id="Field1195079734541"/>
      <field name="patientage" id="Field1195079874032">68</field>
    </category>
    <category name="annotation" id="Category1195079679392">
      <group name="tumorcollection" id="Field1195079928800">
        <instance name="tumor" id="Field1195079928800">
          <field name="author" id="Field1195080028143">dsc</field>
          <field name="date" id="Field1195080070384">2007-11-15</field>
          <group name="imageobservationcharacteristiccollection" id="Field1195080130681">
            <instance>
              <field name="codingschemedesignator" id="Field1195080173813">RADREX</field>
              <field name="codevalue" id="Field1195080212689">REX4002</field>
            </instance>
            <instance>
              <field name="codingschemedesignator" id="Field1195080173814">RADREX</field>
              <field name="codevalue" id="Field1195080212688">REX4062</field>
            </instance>
          </group>
          <field name="AIMDescription" id="Field1195080538779">some description to files</field>
          <group type="file" name="AIMFiles" id="Field1195080538777">
            <instance>
              <field name="assessment">metadoc/avt_assessment/0019/2007-11-15/1.xml</field>
            </instance>
            <instance>
              <field name="assessment">metadoc/avt_assessment/0019/2007-11-15/2.xml</field>
            </instance>
          </group>
        </instance>
      </group>
    </category>
    <category name="dicom" id="Category1195079689556">
      <field type="file" name="dicomimage">metadoc/avt_assessment/0019/2007-11-15/56.dcm</field>
    </category>
  </content>
</document>
```

Fig. 3.3: A sample SciPort exchange document in XML.

tree based XML data model. Figure 3.3 shows a sample SciPort Exchange Document.

The structure of the XML document is shown in Figure 3.4. The XML document starts with a root element *document*. The attribute *documentid* of the root element is uniquely generated from the system, and the attribute

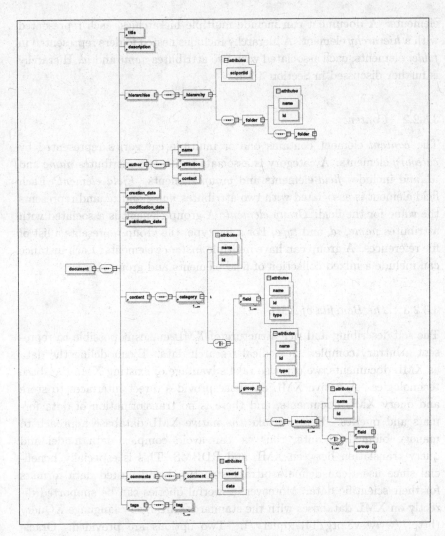

Fig. 3.4: SciPort data model diagram.

schemaid refers the ID of the corresponding schema.

3.3.2.1 *Metadata*

There is a list of metadata fields at the beginning of the XML document, including elements *title*, *description*, *author*, *creation_date*, *modification_date*, and *hierarchies*. The *author* element includes *name*, *affiliation* and *contact* elements. A document can include multiple hierarchies, each represented with a *hierarchy* element. A hierarchy includes nested folders represented in *folder* elements, each associated with two attributes *name* and *id*. Hierarchy is further discussed in Section 3.3.4.

3.3.2.2 *Content*

The *content* element contains one or multiple categories represented by *category* elements. A category is associated with two attributes *name* and *id*, and includes *field* elements and *group* elements. *Field element:* Each field element is associated with two attributes *name* and *id*, and represents the value for the field. *Group element:* A group element is associated with attributes *name*, *id*, and *type*. For a file type, the group represents a list of file references. A group can have multiple *instance* elements. Each instance can include a mixed collection of field elements and group elements.

3.3.2.3 *The Benefits of XML*

The self-describing and rich structure of XML makes it possible to represent arbitrary complex biomedical research data. By modeling the data as XML documents, we can also take advantage of existing XML database technologies. A native XML database provides direct interfaces to store and query XML documents, and there is no transformation of data formats and queries. Here we take the native XML database approach to manage biomedical data, thus we can avoid complex data model and query translation between XML and RDBMS. This is especially beneficial since users can define arbitrary structured and nested data formats for their scientific data. Moreover, powerful queries can be supported directly on XML databases with the standard XML query language XQuery (http://www.w3.org/TR/xquery/). Two options are provided: Oracle Berkeley DB XML (http://www.oracle.com/database/berkeley-db/xml/), an open source embedded XML database, and IBM DB2 with pureXML^{TM} support (http://www-306.ibm.com/software/data/db2/express/).

Document Atomicity: A SciPort document is atomic in terms of both access control and data exchange. Files linked in the document share the same access permission as the document. When the document is downloaded, the XML document including all the files linked in the document will be zipped as a single file for transportation. This excludes references to other documents which hold their own access control.

3.3.3   *XML-based Schema Definition*

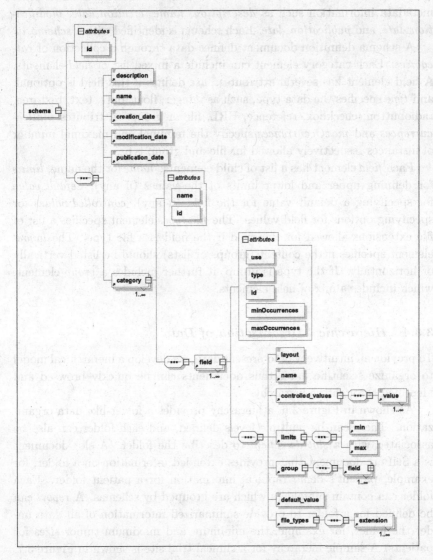

Fig. 3.5: SciPort schema model diagram.

Users can define their own schemas in an XML-based Schema Definition Language – *SciPort Schema Definition Document*. (XML Schema is not used since our approach is easier to implement and flexible to support

Web-based applications.) The structure of the Schema Definition Document is shown in Figure 3.5. A schema definition document includes some metadata information such as *description*, *name*, *creation_date*, *modification_date*, and *publication_date*. Each schema is identified with a *schema_id*.

A schema definition document defines data through a collection of *categories*. Each category element can include a mixed list of *field* elements. A field element has several attributes: *use* defines if this field is optional, and *type* specifies the data type, such as integer, float, date, text, textarea, radiobutton, checkbox, reference, URL, file or group. Attributes *minOccurrences* and *maxOccurrences* specify the minimal and maximal number of instances respectively allowed for file and group types.

Each *field* element has a list of child elements: *name* for the name, *limits* for defining upper and lower limits of the values (if any), *default_value* for specifying a default value for the field (if any), *controlled_values* for specifying options for field values. The *file_types* element specifies a list of file extensions allowed for this field if the field is a file type. The *layout* element specifies if the content (groups or lists) should be listed vertically or horizontally. If the type is group, it further includes a *group* element, which includes a mix of field elements.

3.3.4 *Hierarchical Organization of Data*

To provide an intuitive way to present data, we develop a hierarchical model to organize scientific data, thus documents can be quickly browsed and identified through the hierarchy.

As shown in Figure 3.6, a hierarchy provides a folder-like data organization. There can be multiple levels defined, and each folder can also be associated with a *slot document* to describe the folder. A slot document is a SciPort document that provides extended information on a folder, for example, patient's demographical information for a patient folder. Each folder can contain subfolders which are grouped by schemas. A *report* can be defined for a folder to provide summarized information of all data under the folder, for example, the minimum and maximum tumor sizes for patients. A sample hierarchy for a clinical trial site is shown in Figure 3.7.

The types and depth of a hierarchy is defined by *Level*, for example, "site", "patient", "measurement". A level can be pre-associated with schemas that confine documents or slot documents at the level.

Once the hierarchy and schemas are defined, users can conveniently author documents through SciPort authoring tools, where the interfaces

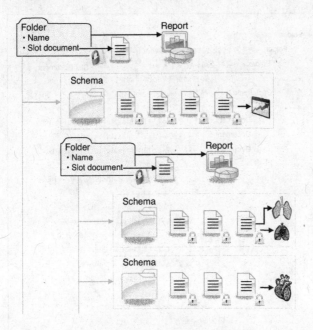

Fig. 3.6: SciPort hierarchy model.

are automatically generated based on the hierarchy and schemas.

3.4 Document Authoring and Searching

3.4.1 *Document Authoring*

SciPort provides comprehensive tools to support authoring, including document editor, file uploader, DICOM anonymizer (to automatically de-identify private data), and an import tool.

SciPort document authoring workflow is shown in Figure 3.8. There are two ways to author documents: import tool via Web Services, thus applications can send data into the system; Web based authoring tool, thus documents can be authored through a Web browser.

The workflow of authoring is as follows.

- A user either selects a hierarchy from the hierarchy browser, or selects a hierarchy from the document authoring tool.
- The user picks up a schema; once the schema is picked up, a Web form will be automatically generated based on the schema.

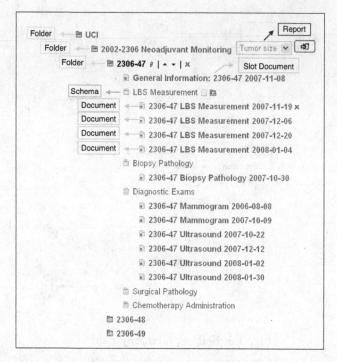

Fig. 3.7: A sample SciPort hierarchy.

- The user fills the Web form, and for file data type, the user links files from File Cabinet (Section 3.4.1.1), a temporary server folder for preloading files.
  A sample authoring page is shown in Figure 3.9c, and a sample file selection from File Cabinet is shown in Figure 3.9b.
- The user saves the document – the structured data are stored in the XML database server, and the linked files are copied from the File Cabinet to server data folders.

3.4.1.1 *File Cabinet*

File Cabinet is a personal folder on the Server, thus files can be preloaded and stored temporarily in it. The benefit is that it can separate structured data authoring from file uploading, which is often time consuming. Thus at authoring time, files are quickly transferred on the Server.

When a file is uploaded to the File Cabinet, if it is an image file (JPG,

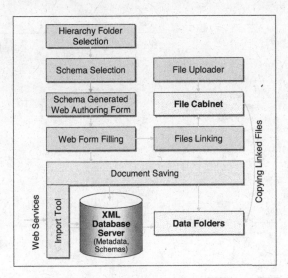

Fig. 3.8: Document authoring workflow.

TIF, PNG, GIF, or DICOM medical image), a thumbnail will be automatically generated, and DICOM files will also be automatically anonymized. If a zip file is uploaded, there is an option to unzip it or keep it as it is. Tags can also be added to files in the File Cabinet, so they can be quickly identified.

3.4.1.2 *Hierarchy and Schema Authoring*

SciPort provides high extensibility as users could conveniently customize the system to use in their applications without any programming. Hierarchy and schemas are among the components that could be authored and customized by users.

Hierarchy authoring includes level setup and folder creation. Level setup is performed at system configuration time, when a system administrator defines the levels to be used in the system. A level can be associated with schemas that will be inherited by all folders created later. Before any document is created in the hierarchy, users can adjust the depth of a level by moving it upwards or downwards in the hierarchy tree.

Once the hierarchy is ready, users can browse the hierarchy and create a folder directly inside the hierarchy. Once a folder is created, schemas defined at the corresponding level are displayed under the folder and can be used as the templates for authoring documents. A folder can be removed

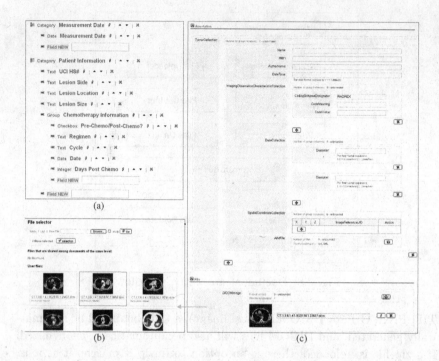

Fig. 3.9: Sample screenshots of authoring: (a) Schema editing. (b) File selection from a file cabinet. (c) Document authoring.

together with all its documents, or detached from the hierarchy. Documents can also be re-assigned to other folders.

SciPort also provides an Ajax based schema authoring tool for conveniently creating schemas with complex structures and data types. Users can create categories, define fields, groups and nested fields/groups under a group. Users can also define the constraints for each field, such as the minimum and maximum values, constrained values for radiobuttons or checkboxes, and default values. Figure 3.9(a) shows an example of schema authoring.

3.4.2 *DICOM Data Anonymization*

HIPAA compliance is a mandatory requirement for medical research, and one top task for this is to anonymize DICOM data, the most commonly used image format in clinical environments. DICOM headers include plenty of metadata of images. Metadata with private information of patients have to be anonymized before DICOM images can be used for research or sharing.

We develop an automated DICOM anonymization tool that will automatically detect if a file is a DICOM image and automatically anonymize it based on preconfigured anoymization settings. Once a file is uploaded to the server by a user, it will be stored in an internal temporary folder not accessible to users. The system will read the file header to check if it is a DICOM file, and anonymize it if it is. Zip files will be unzipped and checked as well for anonymization. Then the anonymized file is saved into the File Cabinet. When the user authors a document and links the file to the document, the file in the File Cabinet will be moved to the server document folder, which is available for access through the Web Server.

The workflow of the anonymization is shown in Figure 3.10. There are four use cases: configuring anonymization; uploading files to the file cabinet for anonymization; authoring documents with anonymized files from File Cabinet; and downloading anonymized files.

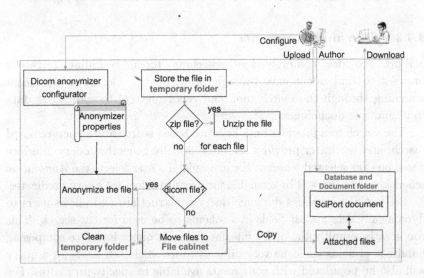

Fig. 3.10: The workflow of DICOM anonymization.

Figure 3.11 shows an example of DICOM anonymization configuration, where a user can configure what methods to use for anonymizing DICOM metadata fields.

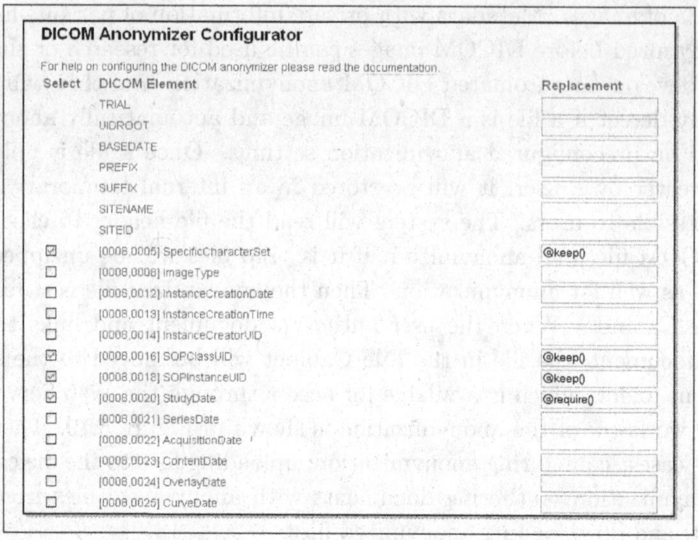

DICOM Anonymizer Configurator

For help on configuring the DICOM anonymizer please read the documentation.

Select	DICOM Element	Replacement
	TRIAL	
	UIDROOT	
	BASEDATE	
	PREFIX	
	SUFFIX	
	SITENAME	
	SITEID	
☑	[0008,0005] SpecificCharacterSet	@keep()
☐	[0008,0008] ImageType	
☐	[0008,0012] InstanceCreationDate	
☐	[0008,0013] InstanceCreationTime	
☐	[0008,0014] InstanceCreatorUID	
☑	[0008,0016] SOPClassUID	@keep()
☑	[0008,0018] SOPInstanceUID	@keep()
☑	[0008,0020] StudyDate	@require()
☐	[0008,0021] SeriesDate	
☐	[0008,0022] AcquisitionDate	
☐	[0008,0023] ContentDate	
☐	[0008,0024] OverlayDate	
☐	[0008,0025] CurveDate	

Fig. 3.11: A sample screenshot of DICOM anonymization configurator.

3.4.3   *Searching Documents*

SciPort provides comprehensive searching tools, including hierarchy browser to find documents through browsing the hierarchy, document searching through the search tool, and reporting tool to summarize data from multiple documents.

The search tool provides both keyword based search and structure based search, and the latter provides an automatically generated query interface based on user selected schema. For example, if a user selects the *Annotation* schema, a field list will be available for users to select for query predicates.

SciPort also provides dynamic query construction, and allows users to dynamically select what fields in a schema to be used for the search. This can greatly simplify the query interface, since a query interface composing hundreds of fields could be very difficult to use. Selected fields for a query will also be populated with constraints available to specify predicates. For example, if a *patientSex* field is selected for the *Annotation* schema, a list of constrained values ('M' and 'F') will be automatically generated as radiobuttons for the user to choose. Support of configurable queries makes it possible for users to personalize and reuse their own queries.

Besides structured fields, a hierarchy branch can also be used as a predicate. For example, a user can constrain the query on documents from one site only by selecting a site branch.

Search is automatically cached for reuse in one active session, or saved explicitly by users for future reuse.

Figure 3.12 is a sample search screenshot, and the functionalities of search are summarized as follows.

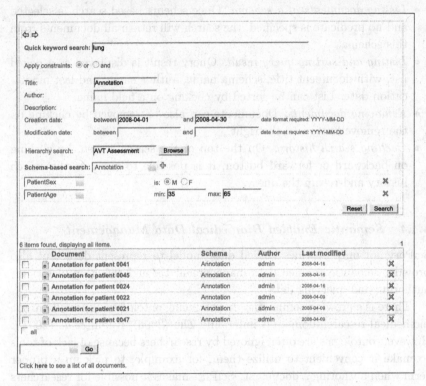

Fig. 3.12: Sample search screenshot.

- *Keyword search.* Global keyword search can be specified in the "Quick Keyword Search" field.
- *Global logic constraint.* There is a global "AND" or "OR" option to apply the combination logic to all the search predicates.
- *Common field search.* Common fields associated every document can be used to specify search conditions. The fields include *Title*, *Author*, and *Description*.
- *Hierarchy search.* Hierarchy folders can be selected thus only documents under certain folders are retrieved.

- *Schema-based search.* A specific schema can be selected to specify predicates on the fields from this schema. A user can interactively add new fields and specify predicates for each field, such as "equals", "range", "contains".
- *Listing all documents.* There is an option to show all documents.
- *Listing documents of a schema.* Once schema based search is selected and no predicate is specified, the search will return all documents from this schema.
- *Listing and sorting query result.* Query result is displayed as a paged list, with document title, schema name, author name, and last modification date. List can be sorted by clicking on a field name.
- *Removing documents.* Documents can also be removed by clicking on the remove button on the right.
- *Caching search history.* On the top of the search screen, by clicking on backward or forward button, it is possible to navigate the search history and re-run the query.

3.4.4   *Semantic Enabled Biomedical Data Management*

SciPort not only provides unified data model to represent data, but also provides semantic enabled data management through using ontologies for authoring and querying data.

There is a growing community on producing ontologies, especially in the biomedical research domain [Cimino and Zhu (2006); Rubin *et al.* (2007)]. However, ontologies are often ignored by researchers because of lack of tools to make it convenient to utilize them, for example, to pick up a proper term when authoring a document. SciPort makes it possible for researchers to precisely describe and query their data through semantic enabled data authoring and querying tools.

3.4.4.1   *Semantic Enabled Data Authoring*

The first objective of ontology integration with structured data is to enable data providers and authors to be able to access, navigate and pick up ontology terms easily at the time of authoring. Quickly identifying the right terms to use is one major hurdle preventing data authors on using ontologies, especially when ontologies are becoming huge (NCI Thesaurus defines nearly 40K concepts.)

To solve this problem, we first need an interface that can provide imme-

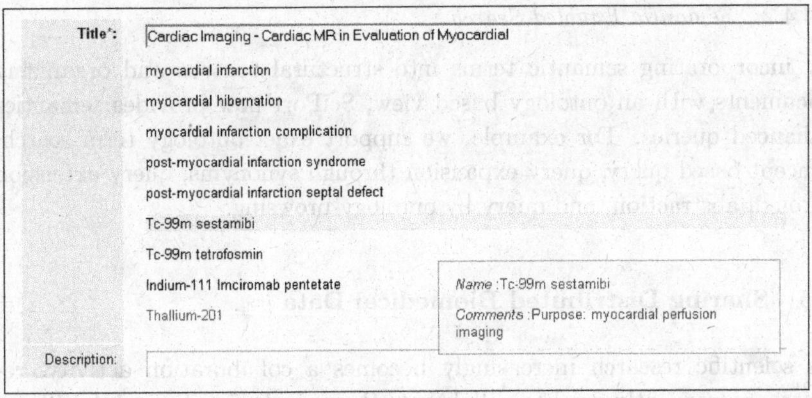

Fig. 3.13: A sample screenshot of ontology pickup.

diate response and also hints for users. For example, when a user types a keyword, he expects a list of related terms from an ontology being returned on the fly. This can be solved by leveraging the latest Ajax technology, which can support immediate data response without updating the whole Web page.

As shown in Figure 3.13, when an ontology is associated with a schema, the authoring interface will automatically provide ontology term pickup through Ajax. When a user types a keyword or a combination of keywords connected through "_", e.g., "breast_cancer", and then presses the *CTRL* key, the keywords will be automatically sent to the corresponding remote ontology server, and a list of related ontology terms will be returned. Once the user has a *mouseover* on one of the terms in the list, another overlay window will further show the description of this term. The user then identifies the right one and selects it as input.

Since each ontology has its own representation (OWL, Protege, OBO, or even XML) and APIs (HTTP requests, Web Services), we provide an ontology access layer (using LexGrid [Pathak *et al.* (2009)]) that provides a unified interface for accessing different ontologies. The process is as follows. When a user types in a keyword in the authoring Web page, it is sent through Ajax to the Server, which is translated into ontology API call through the Ontology Access Layer. The ontology server returns a list of related terms. When the user has a mouseover on one of the terms, another Ajax call is sent for the explanation of the term, and a similar process is performed.

3.4.4.2   *Semantic Enabled Search*

By incorporating semantic terms into structural content and organizing documents with an ontology based view, SciPort now provides semantics enhanced queries. For example, we support exact ontology term search, concept-based query, query expansion through synonyms, query extension through abstraction, and query by ontology browsing.

3.5   Sharing Distributed Biomedical Data

As scientific research increasingly becomes a collaboration activity, researchers frequently need to collaborate through sharing their data. There are several common requirements for data sharing: i) Convenience: data sharing should be a single step action; ii) Data ownership: researchers own and have full control of their data; iii) Flexible Sharing Control: while data can be shared, data sharing can also be revoked by researchers at any time; iv) Up-to-date of shared data. As data are updated or removed, corresponding shared data also need to be synchronized accordingly to stay current.

3.5.1   *Sharing Data through a Central Server*

To meet the above requirements and support closer collaboration and integration, we develop a distributed architecture to share and integrate data through a Central Server (Figure 3.14). In this architecture, each research site will have their own Local Server which itself functions as an independent Server for data collection, management, search, and report. In addition, there will be an additional Central Server upon which Local Servers are able to selectively publish their data (structured documents) (Figure 3.15). Images/files, which are often the major source of data volume, are still stored on corresponding Local Servers but are linked from the published documents on the Central Server. Once a user on the Central Server tries to download a document from the Central Server, actual data files are downloaded from the corresponding Local Server that holds the data.

Thus, the Central Server provides a global view of shared data across all distributed sites, and can also be used as a hub for sharing schemas among multiple sites. Since data are shared through the metadata (SciPort Documents), the integration is lightweight. Users on the Central Server will only have read access to the data.

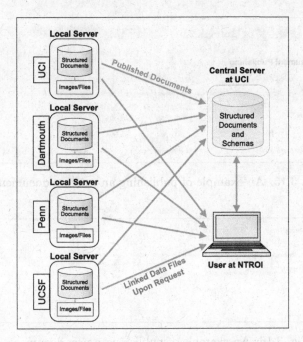

Fig. 3.14: The central server based architecture for data sharing.

Figure 3.14 illustrates an example SciPort sharing architecture formed by four Local Servers at four universities: UCI, UCSF, Dartmouth and Penn. Each Local Server is used for data collection and management of clinical trial data at its local institution. Since these clinical trials are under the same research consortium, they would share their data together by publishing their data (documents) to the Central Server located at UCI. Members at NTROI research consortium are granted read access on such shared data through the Central Server. Once the user identifies a data set from the Central Server and wants to download it, the user will be redirected to the corresponding Local Server that hosts the data to download the data to the client.

3.5.2 *Data Synchronization*

One requirement for the data sharing is to keep shared data up-to-date. The following operations are related to document synchronization.

- Create. When a document is created, the author has the option to publish this document (Figure 3.16). Once the document is published,

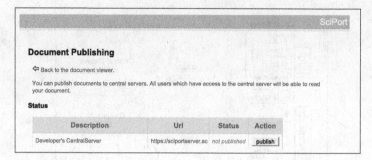

Fig. 3.15: An example of publishing an existing document.

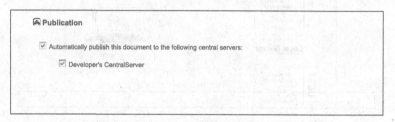

Fig. 3.16: An example of publishing a new document.

a "published" status is added to the document. A user can also set up an automatic publishing flag so all new documents will be automatically published.

- Update. When an update is performed on a published document, the document will automatically be republished to the Central Server.
- Delete. When a published document is deleted, it will also be automatically removed from the Central Server.
- Unpublish. A user can also stop sharing a document by unpublishing the document.

The Benefits. This data sharing architecture provides many benefits: i) data sharing is as convenient as a single click; ii) users have full control of their data, and can revoke the sharing at any time; iii) shared data on the Central Server always remain updated, and iv) the Central Server based sharing architecture makes it possible to conveniently share schemas, as discussed next.

3.6   The Architecture of SciPort

3.6.1   *Open System Architecture*

SciPort is built with a Web based architecture, and each server runs as a Web application server. The system is built with J2EE, XML and Web Services, running on Apache Tomcat Servers and Oracle Berkeley DB XML Database Server (http://www.oracle.com/database/berkeley-db/xml/) or IBM DB2 – a free version is also available as DB2 Express-C (http://www-306.ibm.com/software/data/db2/express/).

The system is OS neutral and can run on any Web browsers. It is built with standard protocols, including XML, XQuery, and Web Services.

3.6.2   *Rich Internet Based Application*

SciPort is a Web-based application, thus it is possible for users to use it at any place and at any time. Taking advantage of Web 2.0 technologies such as Ajax, SciPort provides rich capabilities close to those of desktop applications.

3.6.3   *The Architecture Components*

SciPort's architecture includes one or multiple Local Servers with an optional Central Server for sharing. Local Servers and the Central Server communicates through Web Services. The components of the architecture are discussed as follows (Figure 3.17):

- Authentication. Each Server has its authentication management, thus a login is required before accessing information on the Server.
- Administrative and customization. These include *User Manager* to manage users, roles and groups, *Hierarchy Management* to define and edit the hierarchy, and *Schema Management* to create and edit schemas. There is also an *Anoymization Configurator* to configure what information to be anonymized and in which way.
- Authoring Tools. These include *File Uploader*, which uploads files into a temporary user space on the Server to store uploaded files to be used for authoring documents; *Anonymizer* to anonymize private information; *Authoring Tool* to create, update, delete a document; and *Import Tool* to import a document.
- XML Database. This is the repository of scientific documents and

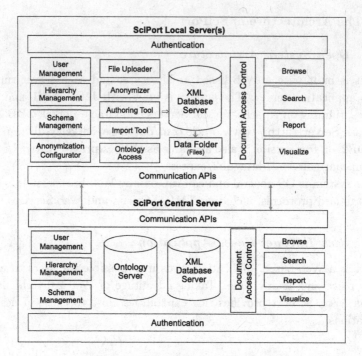

Fig. 3.17: SciPort architecture.

schemas, and provides storage, indexing and searching capabilities.

- File Folder. Files linked to documents are stored in the file folders and linked to the database.

- Document Access Control. When a document is authored, access permission to the document is assigned, and this manager will control the access for each document. Documents which are published to the Central Server will automatically be accessible from the Central Server where authentication is already checked.

- Search. The search tool provides keywords based search and structured based search, and returns a list of qualified documents. A document viewer displays a document, and also includes an *Export* function to download the document together with its linked files as a single zip file.

- Browse. This tool browses documents through the hierarchy.

- Report. A report will extract information and aggregate them into a table format, which can be exported into CSV or PDF formats.

- Communication APIs. The Server provides Web Services based APIs that can be used to access the server remotely. E.g., Import Tool can

be used with Web Services to integrate remote applications.
- Ontology Server. This provides interfaces to access terms from multiple ontology/vocabulary systems.

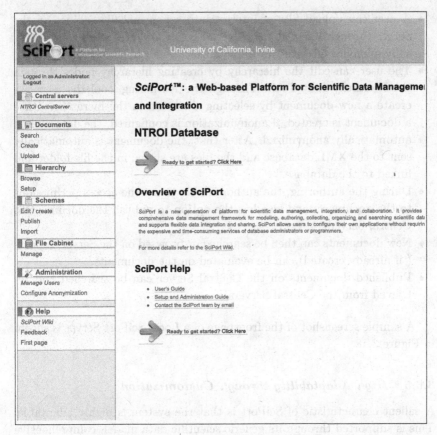

Fig. 3.18: A sample screenshot of a local SciPort server.

3.6.4 SciPort Workflow

Before SciPort is first used, administrative users on the Server will perform the following initial setup.

1) setup user accounts and assign privileges for each user.
2) Setup hierarchy level types.

3) Define schemas with the Schema Management Tool.

4) Configure anonymization rules with the Anonymization Configurator.

Once the setup is ready, the Server is ready to use by normal users.

- A user can upload files of interest into a personal file cabinet on the Server through File Cabinet. Uploaded DICOM files will be automatically anonymized with the Anonymizer.

- The user can edit the hierarchy by creating hierarchy nodes through the Hierarchy Edit Tool. Through the Authoring Tool the user can create a new document by selecting a schema in the hierarchy. Once a document is created, if anonymization is configured, the data will be automatically anonymized. After that, the document is automatically sent to the XML database and the files are stored in the file folder and linked to the database.

- During the authoring, the author is able to set the access permissions to the document, and also has the option to publish the document to Central Servers.

- New documents can then be searched or browsed on the Server; reports (if already created) can be evaluated on the documents.

- Published documents on the Central Server can be searched and retrieved from the Central Servers.

A sample screenshot of the frontpage of a Local SciPort Server is shown in Figure 3.18.

3.6.5 *High Adaptability through Customization*

A salient characteristic of SciPort is that the system is highly adaptable. This is supported through its generic scientific data model, comprehensive schema definition, hierarchy model, and the lightweight data sharing architecture. Convenient customization tools are provided thus SciPort allows users to configure their own applications without requiring expensive and time-consuming services or software development effort.

3.7 Conclusion

Biomedical research produces large amount of complex data and is moving towards multi-disciplinary, multi-institutional collaboration. These lead to strong demand for tools and systems to organize, manage, manipulate and share the data. This drives the development of SciPort – a Web-based generic biomedical data management and sharing system. By providing an XML based unified and effective means for data modeling, organization, management, authoring, searching and customization, SciPort provides a flexible and powerful system for managing biomedical research data. Its highly adaptable architecture makes it possible for researchers to use the system without any software development effort. By taking advantage of biomedical ontologies, SciPort enables semantic based data collection and queries. Through a Central Server based data sharing architecture, distributed data sources can be conveniently shared. SciPort has been successfully used for translational biomedical research consortia, large scale research collaboration at Siemens, and many other research organizations.

Chapter 4

An Integrative Framework for Anonymizing Clinical and Genomic Data

Grigorios Loukides, Aris Gkoulalas-Divanis, and Bradley Malin

Vanderbilt University, Nashville, TN, USA

4.1 Introduction

The integration of modern health information systems with high-throughput sequencing technologies has enabled the collection of detailed, person-specific, clinical and genomic data. Such data can be studied in the context of Genome-Wide Association Studies (GWAS) (i.e., studies that discover relationships between specific genomic variations and health-related phenomena) that have the potential to improve the diagnosis and treatment of an increasing number of complex diseases ranging from diabetes to schizophrenia [Donnelly (2008)].

In the past, such data was collected and analyzed by single investigators or institutions. Recently, however, it was recognized that the sharing of person-specific data can enable novel discoveries, improve the statistical power of existing GWAS and reduce both their time and cost [Gurwitz *et al.* (2006)]. In the United States, for instance, the National Institutes of Health (NIH) is drafting policy that will require scientists to share genomic data studied with NIH funding [1].

At the same time, preserving patients' anonymity becomes essential. Thus, a number of regulations and policies, such as the Privacy Rule of

---

[1] National Institutes of Health, Request for Information (RFI): Proposed Policy for Sharing of Data obtained in NIH supported or conducted Genome-Wide Association Studies, http://grants.nih.gov/grants/guide/notice-files/not-od-06-094.html

the Health Insurance Portability and Accountability Act (HIPAA) [2] and the NIH genomic data sharing policy [3], have been instituted. Nonetheless, these policies do not guarantee that patients' anonymity will be preserved.

To complement policies and regulations, several techniques that can provably preserve privacy by concealing patients' identity when data is collected [Zhang and Zhao (2005)] or disseminated [Aggarwal and Yu (2008)], have been developed. Broadly speaking, this is performed by: (i) removing *identifiers*, i.e. information that can explicitly identify patients, such as patients' names or Social Security Numbers, and (ii) ensuring that patients' *potentially identifying information*, such as demographics [Sweeney (2002b); Samarati (2001)] or diagnosis codes [Loukides *et al.* (2010)], cannot be exploited for patient re-identification. To illustrate how a patient can be re-identified based on his/her diagnosis codes, as well how this can be prevented, we provide Example 4.1.

Example 4.1. Consider a researcher who wants to share the record $\{John, \{157.0, 185, 493.00\}, TA...T\}$ in the context of a GWAS. This record corresponds to *John*, a patient diagnosed with *malignant neoplasm of head of pancreas, malignant neoplasm of prostate*, and *extrinsic asthma unspecified*, which correspond to the ICD-9CM (henceforth referred to as ICD) codes[4] $157.0, 185$ and 493.00 respectively. This record also contains John's DNA sequence $TA...T$. Releasing John's record after simply removing the name, allows an attacker, who knows that *John* is the only patient diagnosed with these particular ICD codes in the released data [Loukides *et al.* (2010)] [5], to associate *John* with his corresponding DNA sequence. This association reveals sensitive information about John and must be prevented.

To achieve this, the researcher could release $\{\{(157.0, 157.1, 157.2, 157.3, 157.9), (185), (493.00, 493.01, 493.02)\}, AT...C\}$, a transformed version of John's record. This record contains more general

---

[2]U.S. Department of Health and Human Services, Office for Civil Rights. Standards for protection of electronic health information; Final Rule. Federal Register, 2003 Feb 20; 45 CFR: Pt. 164.

[3]NIH, Policy for Sharing of Data Obtained in NIH Supported or Conducted Genome-Wide Association Studies (GWAS),http://grants.nih.gov/grants/guide/notice-files/NOT-OD-07-088.html

[4]The International Classification of Diseases, Ninth Revision, Clinical Modification (ICD-9-CM) is the official system of assigning codes to diagnoses associated with inpatient, outpatient, and physician office utilization in the United States.

[5]This knowledge can be derived from the Electronic Medical Record (EMR) system of a hospital from which John's record is derived, or from publicly available hospital discharge records.

clinical information in the form of transformed diagnosis codes. For example, (157.0, 157.1, 157.2, 157.3, 157.9) indicates that John is diagnosed with some forms of neoplasms, one of which corresponds to his actual diagnosis code 157.0. When the released data contains a "sufficiently" large number of patients' records that are indistinguishable from that of John, privacy protection is achieved. This is because it becomes more difficult for an attacker to link John's identity to his DNA using the released data [6].

4.1.1   *Challenges*

While most of the existing privacy-preserving techniques are useful when a single data owner (henceforth referred to as *owner*), such as a researcher or institution, attempts to publish patients' data, these techniques are inapplicable in a common scenario that arises when depositing patients' information in centralized repositories. In this scenario, information regarding a patient may be contributed by multiple owners, each of whom has knowledge of part of the patient's medical record, based on the interaction of the patient with the institution. Such information needs to be properly integrated, and made available for querying or analysis in a protected form. This setting presents three new challenges that need to be overcome.

First, data contributed by different owners needs to be integrated without revealing patients' identity. This involves the removal of identifiers and the transmission of data to a repository where the integration will be performed. An example of such a repository is the database of Genotype and Phenotype (dbGaP) at the U.S. National Library of Medicine [Mailman *et al.* (2007)] that facilitates the sharing of patient-specific records collected in the context of GWAS. While there is substantial research on how to remove identifiers [Uzuner *et al.* (2007)] and to securely transmit data [Katz and Lindell (2007)], data integration still remains a challenging task. This is because it requires merging large quantities of information that refers to the same patient, but is possessed by different owners. To make matters worse, this information often contains typographical errors, lacks standardization and is not organized based on a common schema (e.g., a patient's address may be stored under different column names, such as *address* or *home address*, in different datasets). Current approaches for data integration are inadequate to provide a practical solution to the setting we

---

[6]In this example, DNA sequences do not need to be modified, as it is assumed that they cannot be used for re-identification. We will further discuss this assumption in Section 4.2.2.1.

consider, as they are computationally expensive, do not scale well with the size of the data, and assume information that is free of errors, standardized and adheres to a common schema.

Second, the integrated data has to be transformed to guard against patient re-identification in accordance with data privacy and utility requirements. Privacy requirements determine which parts of clinical information are deemed as potentially identifying according to a certain policy. Existing policies involve limiting the probability of re-identifying a patient based on the released information [Sweeney (2002b); Samarati (2001)] (e.g., *John*'s transformed record), but assume a single policy for all data and data recipients (henceforth referred to as *recipients*). This is far from reality, however, because privacy requirements differ among studies, institutions and recipients. For example, such requirements can be determined based on the distribution of demographics of patients living in a certain area [Benitez and Malin (2010)], or on the level of trust to a certain recipient [Sun *et al.* (2009)]. Therefore, it is important to design methods that can guarantee privacy in the presence of various privacy requirements. Utility requirements, on the other hand, reflect whether the transformed data remains useful for the study or task it was collected and deposited for, and are typically agreed upon by owners before data integration. Most of the current research, however, implicitly assumes that minimizing the level of data transformation suffices to ensure that the released data is useful in specific applications. This is unsatisfactory in the context of GWAS, because it may distort the associations between clinical and genomic information, yielding inaccurate and potentially misleading findings [Loukides *et al.* (2009)].

Third, due to the detailed clinical and genomic information that is typically required for GWAS, data recipients may only be interested in querying parts of the deposited data. In this case, we can transform the clinical information retrieved by a query on-the-fly. This results in significantly better data utility in comparison to existing approaches that transform all the clinical information once and answer queries using a priori anonymized parts on the transformed dataset. However, achieving privacy in this scenario is challenging, because an attacker may stitch together parts that are anonymized on-the-fly (also called *views*) to re-identify patients, even when each of these views prevents re-identification when examined independently of the others.

4.1.2 *Contributions*

In this chapter, we introduce DIANOVA (Data Integration ANOnymization and View Auditing), a novel framework that facilitates the integration and querying of patient-specific data in a way that preserves patients' anonymity. To the best of our knowledge, DIANOVA is the first framework that is developed for, and can deal with, the complex real-world scenario mentioned above. In DIANOVA, multiple owners deposit their patient records along with their specific privacy requirements into the repository. The repository integrates these records, so that each record contains all the clinical and genomic information for a patient, as well as the privacy requirements, so that they reflect a global protection policy against re-identification. Furthermore, DIANOVA enables anonymized patients' records to be generated on-the-fly and in accordance with the specified utility requirements. As such, DIANOVA offers a number of important benefits:

(1) It aims at increasing data availability by allowing patient records from multiple owners to be securely transmitted and integrated.
(2) It allows patient records to be transformed in a way that preserves both privacy and utility to comply with the specified utility and privacy requirements.
(3) It minimizes unnecessary information loss by anonymizing patient records on the fly, while ensuring privacy preservation.

Besides presenting DIANOVA with a focus on architectural issues, this chapter makes the following specific contributions.

- We discuss methodologies that can be used to integrate patients' records. Moreover, we highlight a number of important properties that a record linkage algorithm should satisfy in order to be used in our framework, and show that none of the existing techniques satisfies all of these properties.
- We investigate how to release patient records in a way that they preserve privacy while remaining useful for GWAS. Towards this end, we survey existing anonymization algorithms with respect to their ability to produce data that satisfies detailed privacy and utility requirements, while minimizing data distortion. We conclude that most of the existing algorithms are inadequate to achieve practically useful anonymizations, as opposed to a recently proposed algorithm [Loukides *et al.* (2009)].

- We discuss properties that a practical approach for anonymizing views should have, and survey a number of existing methodologies by focusing on their usability for anonymizing views containing clinical and genomic information. We argue that, due to the semantics of patients' genomic information, it is possible to solve this problem with the use of an existing methodology [Byun *et al.* (2006)], originally proposed for anonymizing data after updates.

4.1.3 *Organization*

The rest of the chapter is organized as follows. We survey existing work on anonymizing data in Section 4.2. Section 4.3 provides an overview of the architecture of DIANOVA, while Section 4.4 discusses algorithms that can be used to implement the components of it. Finally, we discuss extensions of the proposed framework, which provide opportunities for data privacy methods development and deployment in Section 4.5, and conclude the chapter in Section 4.6.

4.2 Related Work

This section presents an overview of existing works for data integration and sharing, which are the two main operations of DIANOVA. Approaches for data integration are reviewed in Section 4.2.1, while a survey of works on privacy-preserving data sharing is provided in Section 4.2.2.

4.2.1 *Data Integration*

When patients' records contributed by multiple owners are deposited into the repository, there are often more than one records referring to the same patient. These records need to be identified to avoid introducing bias in GWAS by double counting the same patient, for example. However, this is challenging, because identifiers have been removed from the records, as discussed in the Introduction. To solve this problem, record linkage [Fellegi and Sunter (1969)] can be used.

Several record linkage approaches have been proposed [Winkler (1995)], such as those based on rule specification [Tejada *et al.* (2001)] and machine learning [Sarawagi and Bhamidipaty (2002); Winkler (2002); Cohen and Richman (2002)]. Most of these approaches suffer from poor scalability, because they cross-examine all possible pairs of records for detecting duplicates. To tackle this problem, approaches based on blocking [Newcombe and Kennedy (1962); Hernandez and Stolfo (1995)] have been developed. These approaches are able to deal with large amounts of data, because they operate in two steps. First, they cluster the patient records contained in the dataset of each owner using a commonly acceptable characteristic, and subsequently cross-examining the pairs of records that have a common value in this characteristic.

Record linkage approaches can be used to compare strings, such as gender or addresses. This is not straightforward, however, when these strings have typographical errors and syntax variations (e.g., when "13 Alpha Rd." also appears as "13, Alpha Road" in different records). To cope with typographical errors, approaches based on edit distance [Wei (2004)], n-grams [McCallum *et al.* (2000); Ravikumar and Cohen (2004)], and soundex [Sarawagi and Bhamidipaty (2002)] have been developed. Syntax variations are typically dealt with standardization methodologies [Winkler (1995); Borkar *et al.* (2001)], which operate by reducing the different spellings of a word (e.g., "Organization", "Org.") to a common spelling (e.g., "Organization"), typically through the use of lookup tables.

All of the aforementioned approaches assume that owners are willing to disclose their data. In some applications, however, owners may not be willing to disclose their data at all. In these applications, *privacy preserving record linkage* methodologies that perform data linkage in a way that the records contributed by each owner are not disclosed to others can be used [Verykios *et al.* (2009)]. These approaches are not directly related to the setting we consider, and thus we do not discuss them any further.

4.2.2 *Privacy-preserving Data Sharing*

Several privacy principles can be used to ensure that data is shared in a privacy-preserving manner [Aggarwal and Yu (2008)]. In our framework, we employ a well-established privacy principle called k-anonymity [Samarati (2001); Sweeney (2002b)]. This principle requires at least k records of a table to have the same values on a set of potentially identifying attributes (commonly referred to as *quasi-identifiers* or *QIDs*). A table that satisfies this principle is called k-anonymous. A k-anonymous table thwarts patient re-identification, because the probability of linking any of its records to a patient's identity through QIDs is at most $\frac{1}{k}$. Although k-anonymity concerns *QIDs*, not all attributes need to be of this type. In fact, the specification of which attributes are *QIDs* is left to the owner. For instance, a researcher may decide that a patient's DNA sequence should not be treated as a QID. To illustrate the concept of k-anonymity, we provide Example 4.2.

Example 4.2. Consider the two tables shown in Figures 4.1(a) and 4.1(b), respectively. The table of Figure 4.1(a) contains patients' ICD codes and genomic information (ID is an identifier used for illustration purposes only). Observe that this table does not satisfy 4-anonymity, when the combination of diagnosis codes $\{157.0, 157.1, 157.2\}$ is used as a *QID*, as there is only one record that harbors this combination of ICD codes in the table of Figure 4.1(a). The table of Figure 4.1(b) contains patients' records that have been transformed by replacing ICD codes with more general diagnosis information, as in Example 4.1. As can be seen, the table of Figure 4.1(b) satisfies 4-anonymity, because all of its records contain the combination of diagnosis codes $\{157.0, 157.1, 157.2\}$.

(ID)	ICD	DNA
(1)	157.0, 185, 493.00	TA...T
(2)	157.0, 157.1, 157.2,185	AC...A
(3)	157.1, 493.00, 493.02	CA...T
(4)	157.0, 185, 493.00, 493.02	GC...C
(5)	157.0, 157.3, 185, 493.01	AA...G

(a)

(ID)	ICD	DNA
(1)	(157.0, 157.1, 157.2, 157.3, 157.9), (185), (493.00, 493.01, 493.02)	TA...T
(2)	(157.0, 157.1, 157.2, 157.3, 157.9), (185)	AC...A
(3)	(157.0, 157.1, 157.2, 157.3, 157.9), (493.00, 493.01, 493.02)	CA...T
(4)	(157.0, 157.1, 157.2, 157.3, 157.9), (185), (493.00, 493.01, 493.02)	GC...C
(5)	(157.0, 157.1, 157.2, 157.3, 157.9), (185), (493.00, 493.01, 493.02)	AA...G

(b)

Fig. 4.1: (a) An example of a dataset containing patients' records. (b) A 4-anonymous version of the table of Figure 4.1(a).

Since concealing individuals' identities is essential to preserve privacy, k-anonymity has received much research interest. In what follows, we will briefly review some representative works on k-anonymity. Section 4.2.2.1 discusses anonymization approaches designed for different types of data, while Section 4.2.2.2 presents approaches for anonymizing the entire dataset or certain parts of it.

4.2.2.1 *Anonymization of Different Data Types*

The principle of k-anonymity is general and thus can be applied to different types of data. In this section, we discuss anonymization approaches with respect to the type of data they can be applied to.

Relational Data: Many works focus on applying k-anonymity to relational data. In this context, a relational table is a collection of records, each of which corresponds to an individual. A record has a fixed number of attributes that take values from a specified domain (e.g., all patients in a dataset are diagnosed with 5 ICD codes).

Transforming a relational table into its k-anonymous counterpart can be thought of a two-step process: (i) finding groups of at least k records that minimize the level of data transformation required to satisfy k-anonymity, and (ii) transforming these records to make the table k-anonymous. The first step can be achieved by employing various strategies, such as binary search [Samarati (2001)], data partitioning [LeFevre *et al.* (2005)], or clustering [Loukides and Shao (2007); Aggarwal *et al.* (2006)], to search for a "good" anonymization, as finding an optimal solution is NP-hard [Meyerson and Williams (2004)]. To perform the second step of k-anonymizing relational data, the techniques of suppression [Sweeney (2002a); Wang *et al.* (1988)] and generalization [Samarati (2001); Sweeney (2002b)] can be used. Suppression involves the removal of QID values or attributes, while generalization suggests replacing QID values with more general, but semantically consistent values.

The mappings between original and generalized values can be specified by hierarchies [Sweeney (2002a)] provided by owners. In the case of ICD codes, for example, a standard hierarchy is publicly available [7]. ICD codes are represented as leaf-level nodes and are ascendants of more general diagnosis information. For instance, 493.00 represents a diagnosis of *extrinsic asthma unspecified* and is a leaf-level node, while 493.0 represents *extrinsic asthma* and is the immediate ancestor of 493.00. The root of the hierarchy has a symbol which represents any ICD code.

Furthermore, there are a number of privacy principles that extend k-anonymity, such as l-diversity [Machanavajjhala *et al.* (2006)], t-closeness

---

[7]http://www.cdc.gov/nchs/icd/icd9cm.htm

[Li *et al.* (2007)] and tuple-diversity [Loukides and Shao (2007)]. All of these principles assume two types of attributes, QIDs and sensitive, and strengthen the protection provided by k-anonymity by additionally requiring values to follow a certain distribution with respect to the sensitive attributes. These principles are not applicable to the scenario we consider, because we do not adopt this classification. That is, diagnosis codes are partitioned into those that are potentially identifying or not.

Transactional Data: Another type of data that can be used to represent patients' records that harbor sets of diagnosis codes is transactional data [Loukides *et al.* (2010)]. That is, data comprised of records (also called *transactions*), each of which is associated with a set of items. Items are all drawn from the same domain and different transactions may have a different number of items, typically in the order of hundreds or thousands.

Some recent works consider applying principles that are similar to k-anonymity to transactional data [Terrovitis *et al.* (2008); Xu *et al.* (2008); Loukides *et al.* (2009)]. Items play the role of attributes in the traditional k-anonymity definition in the sense that they can be used to re-identify individuals. The underlying assumption of these works is that an attacker is constrained to use certain items (and not necessarily the entire transaction) to perform re-identification. This is a reasonable assumption, because, generally speaking, it may be quite difficult for an attacker to obtain knowledge about the items of a transaction containing hundreds of items.

Based on this assumption, [Terrovitis *et al.* (2008)] proposed k^m-anonymity, a principle to prevent attackers with the knowledge of at most m items from linking an identified individual to less than k published transactions. This principle is similar to k-anonymity in the sense that it guarantees that the probability of re-identifying an individual remains at most $\frac{1}{k}$. The principle of k^m-anonymity can be enforced using the Apriori-based Anonymization algorithm proposed in [Terrovitis *et al.* (2008)], which operates in a bottom-up fashion. This algorithm first enforces k^m-anonymity on items and then iterates on incrementally larger sets of items, stopping when k^m-anonymity is enforced on sets of m items.

Another privacy principle, called (h, k, p)-coherence, was proposed by [Xu *et al.* (2008)]. This principle is similar to k^m-anonymity in the treatment of potentially identifying items (i.e., it assumes that an attacker knows up to a specified number of items p), but it additionally ensures that the probability of associating an individual to some specified *private* items (e.g., diagnosis codes a patient is not willing to be associated with after his/her data is released) is limited to h. To satisfy (h, k, p)-coherence, the authors of [Xu *et al.* (2008)] proposed an algorithm that discovers all itemsets of minimal size that correspond to less than k individuals and protects them by iteratively suppressing the item contained in the greatest number of those itemsets. Since there are no fixed private items in the setting we consider, (h, k, p)-coherence degenerates to k^m-anonymity.

Furthermore, the work of [He and Naughton (2009)] assumes that an attacker can use all items of a transaction as QIDs and suggest applying k-anonymity. K-anonymity is enforced through a top-down, generalization-based algorithm. This algorithm starts by generalizing all items to their most generalized representation, and then replaces this generalized item with its immediate ascendants in the hierarchy if k^m-anonymity is satisfied. In subsequent iterations, generalized items are replaced with less general items one at a time, as long as k^m-anonymity is satisfied, or the generalized items are replaced by leaf-level items in the hierarchy.

Recently, [Loukides *et al.* (2009)] have proposed an approach for anonymizing transactional data using generalization of diagnosis codes under specific privacy and utility requirements. Although originally developed for a scenario involving an owner who anonymizes and then publishes his/her entire dataset, the approach of [Loukides *et al.* (2009)] can serve as a component in the DIANOVA framework.

The aforementioned approaches for anonymizing transactional data will be further discussed with respect to their ability to be used as components of our framework in Section 4.4.2.

Genomic Data: The release of person-specific genomic data raises serious privacy issues. Many patients fear that genomic information derived from their medical records will be used against them in employment decisions, limit access to insurance, or cause social stigma. As the relationships between genomic markers and disease are refined, the potential for discrimination will increase [Rothstein and Epps (2001)].

Protecting the privacy of genomic information has been attempted through removing [Stallings *et al.* (2006)] or encrypting [Gulcher *et al.* (2000)] patients' identifiers, before releasing data. However, patient re-identification may still occur based on aggregate genomic information [Homer *et al.* (2009)]. A number of recent works [Homer *et al.* (2009); Wang *et al.* (2009); Jacobs *et al.* (2009)] focus on determining whether certain genomic information about patients should be released, but are orthogonal to the problem of re-identification based on diagnosis codes we consider in this chapter.

4.2.2.2   *Anonymization of Different Data Sources*

Most of the work on data publishing assumes that the entire dataset is anonymized and disseminated once. In the case of depositing patient records to repositories, however, views of data may need to be published more than once. Many GWAS, for example, require accessing certain views that have been collected and deposited for a different GWAS, such as the "heart-healthy" population of a dataset [Donnelly (2008)]. Anonymizing views on-the-fly may achieve better data utility. Intuitively, this is because views have generally a smaller number of attributes than the dataset they are derived from, and the amount of data distortion required to make records anonymous increases significantly with the number of attributes that are anonymized [Aggarwal (2005); Xu *et al.* (2008)].

Several methods for releasing anonymized views in a way that prevents an attacker from combining views to perform re-identification, have been proposed. The work of [Yao *et al.* (2005)] investigated whether a set of views, derived by applying selection and projection operators only, violate k-anonymity when examined together. Furthermore, [Kifer and Gehrke (2006)] showed how to release a set of anonymized marginals, which are views in which duplicate values are preserved, in a way that preserves data utility and privacy.

Another line of research examines whether a new view can be safely released. [Wang *et al.* (2006)], for example, showed how to solve this problem for the case in which views are projections of the entire dataset based on the *lossy join* operator. This operator matches two values if one is an ancestor of another in a hierarchy. To solve the problem, [Xiao and Tao (2008)] introduced a privacy principle called m-invariance. Intuitively, m-invariance attempts to ensure that all released views have the same set of values in a sensitive attribute, and is enforced through inserting "counterfeit" values in the sensitive attribute. This allows the method of [Xiao and Tao (2008)] to guarantee privacy even when the underlying data from which views are derived is updated (i.e., new records are inserted and/or deleted). A method which works by ensuring that the set of records in which an individual's record may be contained is l-diverse was proposed by [Byun *et al.* (2006)].

In Section 4.4.3, we will examine whether the aforementioned methods can be used to anonymize views in our framework.

4.3   The DIANOVA Framework

In this section, we discuss the general architecture of DIANOVA. Sections 4.3.1 and 4.3.2, present the considered setting and the components of our framework, respectively.

4.3.1   *Setting*

In what follows, we discuss the parties that are assumed in DIANOVA and their corresponding roles, as well as the structure of data these parties contribute or access.

4.3.1.1   *Parties*

There are three types of parties in our framework: *(i)* owners, *(ii)* repository, and *(iii)* recipients. Owners deposit patients' records to the repository, which integrates patient records, and performs the view anonymization and query answering. Recipients are the parties who query the repository and obtain anonymized views. In DIANOVA, recipients may also be owners.

4.3.1.2   *Datasets*

We consider a dataset D, which is a collection of records each of which corresponds to a distinct patient. Each record is comprised of three parts: *(i)* a *relational* part, which contains demographics that are used for data integration and have been agreed upon by all owners, *(ii)* a *transactional* part, which contains diagnosis codes, and *(iii)* a *genomic* part, which contains a DNA sequence. We assume that each owner possesses a dataset D. An example of such a dataset is shown in Figure 4.2(a). After integrating all datasets of type D, we obtain a dataset D', which is stored in the repository. Since DIANOVA focuses on releasing diagnosis codes and genomic information, but not demographics, we consider that the integrated relational parts are not retained in D'. That is, D' contains diagnosis and genomic information only. As an example, consider Figure 4.3, which illustrates the result of integrating the datasets of Figures 4.2(a) and 4.2(b) respectively.

(ID)	Age	Address	ICD	DNA
(1)	41	15 Miller Rd	157.0, 493.00	TA...T
(2)	58	29 WE Ave	157.0, 157.1	(missing)
(3)	37	48 Country Road	493.00, 493.02	CA...T
(4)	64	255 Fairfax av.	493.00, 493.02	GC...C
(5)	29	19 Thomson Dr.	157.0, 157.3, 185	AA...G

(a) D_1

(ID)	Age	Address	ICD	DNA
(1)	41	15th Miller Rd.	185	(missing)
(2)	58	29 West End Ave.	157.2,185	AC...A
(3)	36	46 County Rd.	157.1	(missing)
(4)	46	255 Fairfax Ave.	157.0, 185	GC...C
(5)	29	19 Thomson dr.	157.0, 185, 493.01	(missing)

(b) D_2

Fig. 4.2: Examples of datasets that contain demographics, diagnosis and genomic information, and are contributed by different owners.

(ID)	ICD	DNA
(1)	157.0, 185, 493.00	TA...T
(2)	157.0, 157.1, 157.2,185	AC...A
(3)	157.1, 493.00, 493.02	CA...T
(4)	157.0, 185, 493.00, 493.02	GC...C
(5)	157.0, 157.3, 185, 493.01	AA...G

Fig. 4.3: Example of a dataset which is derived by integrating the datasets of Figure 4.2(a) and 4.2(b).

(ID)	ICD	DNA
(1)	157.0, 493.00	TA...T
(2)	157.0, 493.00	CG...C

(a) V

(ID)	ICD	DNA
(1)	(157.0, 157.1, 157.2, 157.3, 157.9), (493.00, 493.01, 493.02)	TA...T
(2)	(157.0, 157.1, 157.2, 157.3, 157.9), (493.00, 493.01, 493.02)	GC...C

(b) V'

Fig. 4.4: Examples of: (a) A view constructed from the dataset of Figure 4.3; (b) Its anonymized counterpart.

A view V is a projection of the records of D' on selected ICD codes and the DNA sequence. For example, the view illustrated in Figure 4.4(a) is constructed by retaining all records harboring the combination of ICD codes 157.0, 493.00 of the dataset of Figure 4.3. The counterpart of V after the transformation of ICD codes is denoted with V'. An example of V' for the view of Figure 4.4(a) is shown in Figure 4.4(b).

In addition, we assume a dataset P comprised of records that have only a transactional part. Each record of P, called *privacy constraint*, models a combination of diagnosis codes that are treated as potentially identifying. Privacy constraints are constructed by owners according to their expectations of adversarial background knowledge [Loukides *et al.* (2009)]. As we will explain Section 4.3.2, a number of datasets of type P are used to create a dataset P' that contains the adversarial background knowledge assumed by all the recipients. Datasets of type P, and the result of combining them into P', are shown in Figures 4.5 and 4.6 respectively.

ICD	Frequency
157.0, 157.1	1
157.2	1

(a) P_1

ICD	Frequency
157.2	1
493.00	3

(b) P_2

ICD	Frequency
493.00, 493.02	2

(c) P_3

Fig. 4.5: Examples of datasets that contain privacy constraints and are contributed by three different owners.

ICD	Frequency
157.0, 157.1	1
157.2	1
493.00, 493.02	2
493.00	3

Fig. 4.6: The dataset that results from integrating the datasets of Figures 4.5(a), 4.5(b), and 4.5(c).

Finally, the combinations of diagnosis codes that reflect GWAS-related diseases are represented as a dataset U'. We assume that these diseases are agreed upon by owners before data integration and that U' is stored in the repository. Each of the records in U' is called a *utility constraint* and has a transactional part only. Consider, for example, the dataset shown in Figure 4.7, which contains three utility constraints for *asthma*, *prostate cancer* and *pancreatic cancer*, respectively.

Table 4.1 presents a summary of the datasets presented in this section.

ICD	Disease
493.00, 493.01, 493.02	Asthma
185	Prostate cancer
157.0, 157.1, 157.2, 157.3, 157.9	Pancreatic cancer

Fig. 4.7: Example dataset U' that contains utility constraints agreed upon by owners.

Symbol	Dataset	Contributed by or Stored at
D	Dataset of patients' records	Owner
D'	Dataset of patients' records after integration	Repository
V	View of D'	Repository
V'	Anonymized counterpart of V	Repository
P	Dataset of privacy constraints	Owner
P'	Dataset of privacy constraints after integration	Repository
U'	Dataset of utility constraints	Repository

Table 4.1: Summary of datasets.

4.3.1.3 *Privacy and Utility Requirements*

Having presented the structure of datasets P' and U', we discuss their role in preserving privacy and utility, respectively. P' is used for testing whether anonymized records are sufficiently protected. This is performed by checking if the privacy constraints contained in P' either appear at least k times in the anonymized view that is released, or do not appear in it at all. In the former case, an attacker needs to distinguish among at least k individuals having a certain privacy constraint in the view to associate an individual's identity to his/her DNA sequence. In the latter case, re-identification is also difficult, because the released view contains no potentially identifying ICD codes.

The dataset U' is used for testing whether an anonymized view is useful in the validation of GWAS. This is achieved by checking if, for each utility constraint in U', the number of records harboring this utility constraint in V' is the same as the number of records harboring any of the ICD codes in the utility constraint in V. This guarantees that associations between utility constraints and DNA sequences are not distorted by data transformation, which is crucial to ensure the validity of GWAS. As an example, consider the utility constraint corresponding to *asthma* in Figure 4.7, the view of Figure 4.4(a), and the anonymized view of Figure 4.4(b).

Observe that the number of patients diagnosed with *asthma* (i.e., those harboring any of the ICD codes corresponding to *asthma*, which are shown in Figure 4.7) is two in both of these views. Thus, the anonymized view of Figure 4.4 can help validating GWAS for *asthma*.

4.3.2   Data Flow in DIANOVA

DIANOVA is comprised of three main components, each of which addresses one of the challenges mentioned in the Introduction. Specifically, data integration is performed by the *Data Integrator* (DI), anonymization of views by the *ANOnymizer* (ANO), and auditing of views by the *View Auditor* (VA), all of which are implemented in the repository. Clearly, the repository should be trusted by owners and recipients, and ensure data security, availability, and integrity [Verykios *et al.* (2008)]. An extended discussion of these issues is beyond the focus of this chapter.

We now walk through our framework and describe how it operates in a number of steps. Figure 4.8 provides a high-level perspective of the process.

(1) *Data Transmission*: This process involves the transmission of datasets D and P by an owner to the repository. To ensure that data is communicated in a secure way according to HIPAA legislation [8], owners use a symmetric key encryption scheme [9] to encrypt data, which is decrypted by the repository after transmission. We refer the reader to [Snyder and Weaver (2003)] for a technical discussion of encryption strategies in the context of biomedical data sharing.

(2) *Data Integration*: After transmitting and decrypting the datasets of type D, these datasets are merged into a single dataset D', which contains *one* record for each patient that appears in at least one of the contributed datasets. For each merging decision, DI identifies and combines the privacy constraints in P that involve the records currently being integrated. This process is repeated for all the contributed records, and results in creating a dataset P', which models the adversarial background knowledge assumed by all the owners together.

(3) *Query Handling*: Recipients query the repository asking for two types of information, namely diagnosis codes and DNA sequences. Such information is used to discover useful associations between clinical and

---

[8]Health Care Portability and Accountability Act, Public Law 104-191, http://aspe.hhs.gov/admnsimp/pl104191.html

[9]National Institute of Standards and Technology, Advanced Encryption Standard http://csrc.nist.gov/publications/fips/fips197/fips-197.pdf

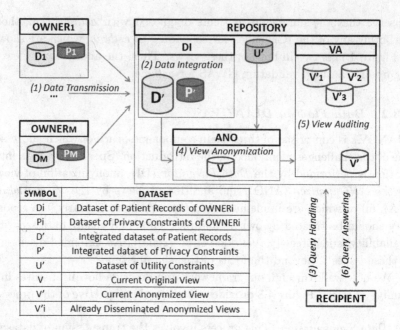

Fig. 4.8: General architecture of the DIANOVA framework. The database management system over which our framework is built, is not depicted.

genomic information in the context of GWAS. We assume that this information is modeled as an SQL query [10], which is handled by a database management system. The latter is also responsible for constructing a non-anonymous view V as an answer to the posed query. It is important to note that V is *not* provided to recipients, since this would breach privacy, but it is given as input to the ANO component instead.

(4) *View Anonymization*: ANO transforms a non-anonymous view V to its anonymized counterpart V'. Anonymization is performed by applying k-anonymity on the diagnosis codes (i.e., the transactional part of a record from D') in a way that is consistent with both the privacy and utility requirements, which are stored in datasets P' and U' respectively. While preserving privacy when examined independently of other views, an attacker can still use V' together with other anonymized views to re-identify individuals, as discussed in Section 4.2.2.2. Therefore, V'

---

[10]SQL is a language designed for querying data stored in database management systems

is provided as input to the VA component of our framework.

(5) *View Auditing*: Having obtained V', VA examines whether this view can be safely released. This is achieved by checking whether V' can be combined with other views corresponding to already answered queries (e.g, the views $V'_1, ..., V'_3$ of Figure 4.8). In this sense, VA simulates the operation of an attacker.

(6) *Query Answering*: In this step, a recipient's query is answered using either the anonymized view V' when it is safe to be released, or an answer indicating that the query cannot be answered. Alternative query answering strategies are discussed in Section 4.4.3.

4.4   Algorithms for Realizing DIANOVA

In this section, we examine whether existing algorithms can be used as components of each of the parts of our framework.

4.4.1   *Algorithms for the Data Integrator (DI)*

The DI component of DIANOVA is responsible for integrating patients' records coming from different recipients. As discussed in the Introduction, integrating these records is not trivial, particularly in the case of medical records, where several new challenges, specific to the nature of this data, arise. In this context, we present a set of properties that a record linkage algorithm should follow in order to be suitable for use in DIANOVA:

- *Good scalability for large datasets*: Datasets deposited in the repository are typically very large in size, containing millions of patients' records. Performing record linkage on so large datasets is a very challenging issue, since it requires to spend a trivial amount of time for each matching decision. As a result, an algorithm should be capable of performing the linkage efficiently.

- *Accountability for typographical errors and lack of standardization*: Patients' records contain typographical errors, and this severely obscures the process of their linkage. Furthermore, the lack of standardization among the fields of different records, further hardens the linkage of the data. This enunciates the need for transforming the data to a common, standardized format, prior to its linkage. Thus, a record linkage algorithm has to be capable of dealing with dirty and unstandardized data.

- *Accountability for different schemas*: Different hospitals may store their patients' records using different schemas. In this case, it is difficult for a record linkage algorithm to decide upon the fields that should be compared against each other, as they record the same patients' information.
- *High accuracy*: Since it is possible for patient records that refer to different patients to be erroneously merged together, a record linkage algorithm should be capable of minimizing this side-effect.

Unfortunately, none of the existing methodologies for record linkage is capable of satisfying all of the aforementioned properties, with the proposed approaches being mostly incapable of achieving good scalability [Winkler (1995)], as well as accountability for different schemas [Scannapieco *et al.* (2007)]. In particular, to cope with scalability issues, record linkage approaches need to benefit from using blocking techniques, as mentioned in Section 4.2.1. Furthermore, few approaches can operate on datasets with different schemas, as this line of research is currently in its infancy. For these reasons, we feel that more research has to be conducted to develop a record linkage algorithm that suits our framework.

4.4.2 Algorithms for the ANOnymizer (ANO)

Before proceeding to discuss an algorithm that can be used in the ANO component of DIANOVA, we outline a number of properties that we consider to be crucial for the design of such an algorithm. From our perspective, a practical algorithm should have the following properties:

- *Support various privacy requirements*: The privacy requirements are based on owners' expectations of which diagnosis codes are potentially linkable, and may be differ among owners. Thus, an anonymization algorithm should allow data that satisfies various privacy requirements to be produced.
- *Guarantee data utility in GWAS*: This implies that the associations between diagnosis codes and DNA sequences should be preserved to ensure that anonymized data can be useful in validating GWAS.
- *Minimize data distortion*: Patient records can be anonymized in many ways that achieve privacy. However, constructing an anonymization that minimally distorts data is computationally intractable [Meyerson and Williams (2004)]. Thus, an algorithm should be able to explore a large number of possible data transformations to find an anonymization

with "low" distortion.

We now examine whether existing algorithms can satisfy the aforementioned properties. As discussed in Section 4.2.2.1, the approaches of [Terrovitis *et al.* (2008); Xu *et al.* (2008)] are limited in protecting combinations comprised of a certain number of diagnosis codes only, while that of [He and Naughton (2009)] supports a single privacy requirement. This is an important shortcoming, because enforcing the privacy policies of these works results in excessively distorted data in practical scenarios.

At the same time, the implicit assumption behind the methods of [Terrovitis *et al.* (2008); Xu *et al.* (2008); He and Naughton (2009)] is that minimizing the level of data transformation suffices to ensure that the released data remains useful in practice. This is insufficient in the context of GWAS, because it has been shown to result in distorting the associations between clinical and genomic information, yielding inaccurate and potentially misleading findings [Loukides *et al.* (2009)].

In addition, the approaches of [Terrovitis *et al.* (2008); Xu *et al.* (2008)] explore a small number of possible data transformations. The work of [Terrovitis *et al.* (2008)] examines suppression only, while that of [Xu *et al.* (2008)] considers a generalization model in which entire subtrees of items are replaced by a generalized item in all transactions of the dataset. [He and Naughton (2009)] consider a generalization strategy in which original items can be replaced by generalized items in different transactions. Although this strategy is shown to be beneficial in terms of minimizing data distortion, it can degrade the accuracy of building data mining models [Xu *et al.* (2008)].

We now provide a high-level description of an algorithm called COnstraint-based Anonymization of Transactions (COAT) [Loukides *et al.* (2009)] that possesses all the aforementioned desirable properties. COAT works by iterating over the privacy constraints, attempting to satisfy each of them using generalization and suppression of ICD codes. This greedy strategy allows any privacy constraint (expressed as a combination of ICD codes) to be handled, and distorts data in accordance with utility requirements and no more than required to satisfy the privacy constraint. Furthermore, COAT has been shown [Loukides *et al.* (2009)] to yield better data utility than the alternative strategy of satisfying a large number of privacy constraints at once [Terrovitis *et al.* (2008)] using both benchmark and real-world patient records.

4.4.3 *Algorithms for the View Auditor (VA)*

We survey existing approaches on anonymizing views with respect to their ability to be used in the VA component. We identify the following properties that a practical approach should satisfy:

- *Guarantee k-anonymity on any combination of released anonymized views*: This prevents an attacker from combining the views he/she has obtained in order to breach k-anonymity.
- *Support views created on demand*: This ensures that a new anonymized view can be released to answer a query without violating privacy.
- *Preserve data truthfulness*: Records of an anonymized view should not contain false information.

While the works of [Yao *et al.* (2005)] and [Kifer and Gehrke (2006)] attempt to ensure that a set of views satisfy k-anonymity and preserve data truthfulness, they assume that all views are known to owners prior to anonymization. Therefore, these approaches would greatly restrict the ability of our framework to provide answers to queries that are not predicted a priori, should they be used to instantiate the VA component of our framework.

The approaches of [Wang *et al.* (2006)] and [Xiao and Tao (2008)] are able to satisfy the first two properties, but they do not preserve data truthfulness. This is because the lossy join operator inserts records that were not contained in the views prior to anonymization, while [Xiao and Tao (2008)] achieves privacy by inserting "counterfeit" sensitive values as discussed in Section 4.2.2.2. Violating data truthfulness is critical in the context of GWAS, because false information may lead to the invalidation of the findings of GWAS.

On the other hand, anonymizations produced using the approach of [Byun *et al.* (2006)] have all of the aforementioned properties. To explain this, we briefly discuss the approach of [Byun *et al.* (2006)]. We assume two anonymized views V_1' and V_2', the latter of which is the view corresponding to a query, and distinguish two cases in which further care for privacy is required [11]. In each of these cases, an attacker attempts to associate the identity of an individual with their corresponding DNA sequence using the diagnosis information contained in these two views.

---

[11]Additional cases in which privacy will always be preserved, as well as a scenario involving more than two views are discussed in [Byun *et al.* (2006)].

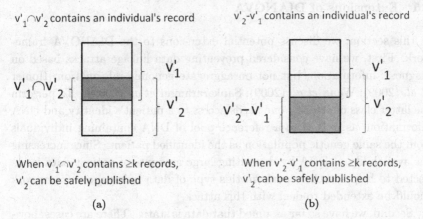

Fig. 4.9: The two cases in which the views need to be checked for potential violation of the privacy.

The first case involves an attacker who knows that both V_1' and V_2' contain an individual's record. In this case, we need to check whether there are at least k records contained in both V_1' and V_2'. While the approach of [Byun *et al.* (2006)] works by checking whether there are l distinct sensitive values in both V_1' and V_2', it suffices to check for k-anonymity in our case, because it is unlikely for two individuals to have the same DNA sequence [Lin *et al.* (2004)]. When this check succeeds, V_2' can be safely released, because there are at least k distinct DNA sequences in the intersection of V_1' and V_2', as discussed in Section 4.3.1. The second case assumes that an attacker knows that an individual's record is contained in V_2' but not in V_1'. In this case, we need to check whether V_2' contains at least k records that are not contained in V_1'. Similarly to the first case, a successful check implies that V_2' can be safely released. Figure 4.9 illustrates both of the cases.

Finally, we discuss the scenario in which the check in either of the cases fails. When this occurs, we can either deny the query or further transform the data contained in V_2' using generalization and suppression until achieving privacy [Byun *et al.* (2006)]. The former strategy is faster, but it does not help analysis as much as the latter strategy that still allows information about the queried records to be released.

4.5   Extensions of DIANOVA

In this section, we discuss potential extensions to the DIANOVA framework. First, we have considered preventing data linkage attacks based on diagnosis information, but not on aggregate genomic information [Homer *et al.* (2009); Wang *et al.* (2009); Sankararaman *et al.* (2009)]. To perform the latter class of attacks, one needs access to a patient's identity and DNA information, as well as to a reference pool of DNA containing individuals from the same genetic population as the identified patient. Since increasing the availability of DNA by depositing large amounts of patient data is expected to help attackers perform this type of data linkage, our framework should be extended to deal with this attack.

Second, we have so far assumed that data is static. There are cases, however, in which new data needs to be deposited into the repository and thus extending our framework to deal with data updates is necessary. Achieving this while preserving privacy, however, is a challenging problem, because the knowledge of updates can lead to patient re-identification. For example, attackers can breach k-anonymity by observing that a patient's diagnosis code has been further generalized after updates.

4.6   Conclusion

In this chapter, we presented DIANOVA (Data Integration ANOnymization and View Auditing), a framework for the integration and dissemination of patient records in a way that prevents patient re-identification. DIANOVA allows owners to securely transmit and integrate their patient records, and recipients to derive anonymized views of the integrated records that are useful in the context of GWAS. We have presented the main architectural components of DIANOVA, examined whether these components may be implemented based on existing algorithms, and discussed how DIANOVA can be extended.

Although this work provides the basis for designing a framework to integrating and querying patient data in a privacy-preserving way, more work is required to realize this framework in practice. First, while the algorithm of [Loukides *et al.* (2009)] has been shown to be able to anonymize patient records while preserving data utility in the context of GWAS fairly well, using this algorithm to instantiate the ANOnymizer component requires taking into account additional issues, such as its effectiveness for anonymizing representative query workloads. This is important, because query answering accuracy in practice may be "low" even when data distortion is minimized [Loukides and Shao (2008)]. Second, there are challenges related to implementation of the VA component. From a data utility perspective, the larger the number of disseminated anonymized views, or the detail of information contained in these views, the lower the level of data utility of these views [Byun *et al.* (2006)]. This issue may be addressed by adjusting the level of privacy based on the level of trust of recipients to ensure that untrusted recipients can only obtain a limited number of views or views containing "coarse" information only.

Acknowledgements

We would like to thank the anonymous reviewers for their valuable comments as well as Vassilios S. Verykios for helpful discussions. This research was funded by National Human Genome Research Institute Grant U01HG004603 and National Library of Medicine Grant 1R01LM009989.

Chapter 5

Data Integration Challenges Towards Combining Mathematical Modeling and Biological Knowledge: A Systems Biology Perspective

Mahesh Visvanathan, Gerald H. Lushington

University of Kansas, Lawrence, KS, USA

5.1 Introduction

Systems biology is a fusion of biology, computer science and other disciplines that enhances understanding of functional systemic relationships via integration of molecular profiling data (genomics, transcriptomics, proteomics and metabolomics) with genetic pathway information [Westerhoff and Palsson (2004)]. Modern data management tools are critical for analyzing and evaluating large molecular profiling datasets, but it is systems biology that truly provides the ability decipher complex biological implications of the data and enable systematic interpretation of dynamic biological processes. This marriage of state of the art separation and systematical analysis tools with systems biology provides a platform for pharmaceutical and biotechnology research to advance key health care pursuits such as drug development and personalized medicine.

Molecular profiling experiments (e.g., DNA microarray, LC-MS, etc.) have proven to be of exceptional value in identifying and characterizing biochemical pathways of importance to disease etiology and drug development. The phenomenal amounts of data acquisition produced by such methods has necessitated concurrent development of a variety of systematic approaches for biochemical data analysis. Systems biology is one such approach, whereby experiment, theory and modeling is synergistically applied toward understanding biological processes as a whole system. This requires an integrated software environment, comprised of tools for facile database access, formalized description of biological systems, visualization and modeling.

Many biological pathways have been painstakingly characterized based on molecular profiling studies, yet it is still difficult to assess the full range of biochemical implications of any pathway outside the obvious context of the genes specifically recorded within that pathway [Wittig and De Beuckelaer (2001)]. Several different approaches are being used to broaden this context. The most common approach is based on information gathered from pathway databases such as KEGG [Kanehisa *et al.* (2004); Kanehisa (1997)] Bio-Carta (http://www.biocarta.com/), WIT [Anderson *et al.* (2005)], BIND [Bader *et al.* (2003)], BioCyc [Karp *et al.* (2005)], DIP [Xenarios *et al.* (2002b)], PPI [Nakayama *et al.* (2002)], etc. The other approach entails building mathematical pathway models and simulating their response to different experimental conditions. Such models may be assembled within an integrated software environment that provides the mathematical constructs necessary to assimilate biological knowledge and provides a basis for validating the models relative to other experimental conditions.

5.2 Modeling Biological Systems

Mathematical modeling and dynamic simulation of biological pathways is one of the central themes in systems biology. While the concept is unquestionably robust, estimation of model parameters from experimental data remains the main bottleneck due to a shortage of sufficiently large and accurate experimental data sets, as reflects the high costs, tedium and logistics of such experiments. The kernel of any systems biology model is an intuitive conceptual representation of the system of interest normally called a biological cartoon, which contains the most significant and important nodes and vertices of a system under consideration. Biological cartoon maps provide an intuition of the overall dynamics and information processing in cellular systems, but are insufficiently descriptive to explain molecular dynamics quantitatively [Lodish *et al.* (2003); Schoeberl *et al.* (2002)]. To meaningfully assemble such an intuitive model and proceed to describe it quantitatively requires dynamic modeling.

In 2001 Phair reviewed a variety of different cellular dynamic modeling approaches [Phair and Misteli (2001)], noting the popularity of differential equations as a natural mathematical language for biochemical kinetics, membrane transport and binding events. While Petri nets [Murata (1989)] have been widely used to formulate and simulate biochemical processes (e.g., for modeling dynamic metabolic behavior [Hofestadt and Thelen (1998); Kuffner *et al.* (2000); Matsuno *et al.* (2003)], and analysis of gene expression patterns [Zien *et al.* (2000)]), the primary mode of pathway modeling remains ordinary differential equations: most of the mathematical models that have been developed are based on reaction kinetics and employ non-linear ordinary differential equations [Cho and O.Wolkenhauer (2003)].

Horenko deconstructed the modeling process by classifying biological processes into different categories [Horenko (2003)], a concept that has served as the basis for analysis and modeling of the intercellular communication response between membranes that transports and pumps the ions within a cell as studied using various approaches [Rivedal *et al.* (2003); Hayward (2002); Hao *et al.* (2003); MacKay *et al.* (2004); Darwish *et al.* (2001); Berry and Rumberg (2001); Sohma *et al.* (2000); Monk *et al.* (1994); McIntyre *et al.* (2002); LeBeau *et al.* (2000)], as well as the study of metabolism and signal transduction with in a cell cycle [Chen *et al.* (2004); McAdams and Shapiro (2003); Gagneur *et al.* (2003); Sorribas *et al.* (1995); Hoffmann *et al.* (2002); Ihekwaba *et al.* (2004); Barken *et al.* (2005)]. His formalism identifies discrete stochastic, and continuous deterministic modeling as two distinct approaches for biochemical pathway analysis. Dhar outlined an alternative modeling strategy (see Fig. 5.1), stating that systems biology is hypothesis driven, global, integrative, iterative and dynamic (http://www.bii.a-star.edu.sg/docs/education/lsm5194_03/notes/pawan_sysbio_lect11.pdf). Based on a fundamental hypothesis, existing global biological knowledge can be collected to construct an integrative conceptual model of the biological system. This conceptual model is then extended with more information to derive an analytical model. Simulation and analysis is performed on this extended model and the results are compared with data generated in subsequent experiments, permitting continual iterative model refinement and validation. The validated model can then be used for predictive or diagnostic purposes, or to explain non-intuitive phenomena.

Deville et al. classify biochemical pathways as metabolic, regulatory and signal transduction pathways [Deville *et al.* (2003)]. Several approaches exist for the mathematical modeling of metabolism [Edwards and Palsson (1997); Morgan and Rhodes (2002); Schilling *et al.* (1999)] and are reviewed elsewhere [Wiechert (2002)]. Metabolic flux analysis considers models that

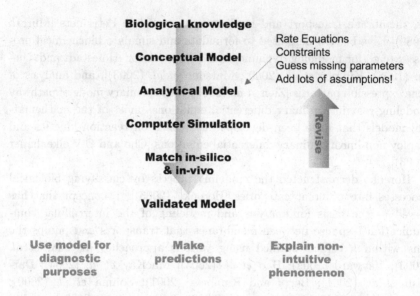

Fig. 5.1: Common strategy for analysis and modeling.

relate to the quantification of flux. It is based on the principle of mass conservation and requires specification of stoichiometry, i.e., metabolic and isotopic balancing, for which examples may be found elsewhere [Klamt and Stelling (2002); Klamt *et al.* (2002); Schuster *et al.* (1999); Mendes and Kell (1998)]. Metabolic flux analysis is an important tool in metabolic engineering as it allows detailed quantification of all intra-cellular fluxes [Wiechert (2001)], and has been modeled extensively via kinetic models [Bower and Bolouri (2001); Goryanin *et al.* (1999); Pfeiffer *et al.* (1999)].

5.3   Biological and Mathematical Data Sources

During the last 20 years there has been an increasing interest in applying databases to biological studies. Many exist that address protein, DNA, RNA and small molecules interactions, as befits the importance of such data. However, integrating the different of data representation paradigms, file formats, data architectures and license agreements into a common scheme is a daunting challenge. One can classify databases according to whether they connect back to primary experimental data in the literature (relatively rare but important), or are secondary sources of information based on review articles or curator knowledge (more common). Many databases have extensive information, but represent it in a form that precludes unambiguous correspondence to other databases. For example, some databases did not contain key data descriptors like sequence accession numbers, chemical compound numbers and PubMed (http://www.ncbi.nlm.nih.gov/entrez/query.fcgi?DB=pubmed) identifiers for publication references. This lack of context reduces the value of the information for large scale mining and broader understanding. Resources that adhere to sound database principles are critical for systematic understanding, thus it is important that resource developers strive toward a common standard representation.

Markowitz et al [Markowitz *et al.* (1997)] proposed a few criteria for evaluation and comparison of molecular biology databases. Most research has been concerned with genetic codes, amino acid sequences of proteins and 3-D protein structures that show usage of database in biological research [Paton (2001); Hammer *et al.* (1995); Bellahsene and Ripoche (2001)]. In this subsection we present a sample of the various available biological and mathematical data sources. The next subsection discusses different database export formats and the standardizations that are available for integration of biological and mathematical modeling data.

BIND: BIND stands for Biomolecular Interaction Network Database [Bader and Hogue (2000)], developed at Mount Sinai Hospital. As its name indicates, it describes interactions, molecular complexes and pathways. The database is freely available to both academics and commercial researchers.

DIP: The Database of Interacting Proteins [Xenarios *et al.* (2002b)] focuses on protein-protein interactions but recently began storing chemical reactions and chemical states of those proteins. It represents interactions via a binary scheme and uses a graph abstraction for its tools, but does not use a formal grammar for data specification. DIP data includes description of interacting proteins, experimental methods used to determine the interaction, dissociation constant, interacting amino acid residue ranges, and literature references. A visual navigation tool is provided.

CYGD: The Comprehensive Yeast Genome Database (CYGD) [Mewes *et al.* (2002)] presents a database that summarizes current knowledge of 6,200+ ORFs encoded by the yeast genome.

EcoCyc: EcoCyc [Karp *et al.* (2005)] is a private database (freely available to academics) that contains metabolic and signaling pathways from E. coli. EcoCyc is based on an object-oriented data model.

MINT: The Molecular Interaction Network Database is a manually curated relational database of literature-reported molecular interactions.

MINT has a simple schema for binary relations and reports protein post-translational modifications, cellular location, pathways, and complexes.

PPI: The Protein-Protein Interaction Database is a high-quality manually curated repository [Nakayama *et al.* (2002)] that includes data from single experiments that usually provide the most reliable PPI information.

KEGG: The Kyoto Encyclopedia of Genes and Genomes [Kanehisa *et al.* (2004)] is a curated repository of most known metabolic (and some regulatory) pathways rendered as diagrams. Each diagram (intended to represent all chemically feasible interactions in the pathway) is an abstraction onto which organism-specific enzymes and substrates can be mapped.

Recent efforts have been made to develop quantative mathematical models for biological pathways based on minimal biological information. Information from these models is available only through literature analysis, and the models cannot be interrogated for biological knowledge, hence both qualitative and quantitative information must be combined and stored in a database. A number of databases have arisen, to address this requirement, including those listed below.

Biomodels: Biomodels.net [Novère *et al.* (2006)] provides access to published, peer-reviewed, quantitative models of biochemical and cellular systems. Human curators annotate and cross-link components of the models to other relevant data resources, allowing users to identify the precise components of models, and helping them to retrieve appropriate models for visualization. In this way, all the models that are published in the public domain are made freely available to everyone.

DOQCS: The Database of Quantitative Cellular Signaling (http://doqcs.ncbs.res.in/) is a repository of signaling pathways models of use for managing and analyzing kinetic models of signaling networks [Sivakumaran *et al.* (2003)]. The DOQCS project aims to collect experimental data that can facilitate biologists / modeling collaborations to enhance biochemical understanding.

5.4 Various Data Exchange Formats in Systems Biology

Currently there are many pathway and protein interaction databases with broadly varying types of information, organisms covered, availability, and data formats. There are also various forms of mathematical models available for assimilating such data, including the following.

PSI MI: The Proteomics Standard Initiative Molecular Interaction

[Hermjakob *et al.* (2004)] attempts to define data representation standards for the proteomics community and facilitate comparison, exchange and verification. Some databases like DIP, TransPath support this type of standard.

BIOPAX: Biological pathway data exchange (http://www.biopax.org) format was designed to support metabolic pathway data and is implemented in OWL (http://www.w3.org/TR/owl-features/). The BioCyc [Karp *et al.* (2005)] database supports this standard.

MAGE-ML: The MicroArray Gene Expression Markup Language (http://www.geml.org/omg.htm) is part of a larger project that defines an object model (MAGE-OM) for gene expression data via OMG's Model Driven Approach (MDA).

SBML: The Systems Biology Markup Language (http://sbml.org/documents, http://www.cds.caltech.edu/ afinney/multi-component-species.pdf) was developed by Systems Biology Workbench Development group (SBW) to serve as a standard for exchanging mathematical molecular pathway models. SBML level 3 version 1already supports various systems that focus on modeling and simulation, such as JDesigner and Gepasi.

CELL ML: The Cell Markup Language [Catherine *et al.* (2004)] is an open standard based on XML that allows scientists to share models even if they are using different model-building software. CELL ML includes mathematics and metadata by leveraging existing languages such as MathML and RDFs.

KGML: The KEGG Markup Language is the export format of the dataset from KEGG database (http://www.genome.jp/kegg/docs/xml) format, reporting information contained in pathway graph objects.

SBML, PSI MI, and GeneXML are designed to be standards for pathway data exchange. In all three, the representation of interactions has at least one entity for representing subjects. For reaction specification, SBML has several dedicated subtypes, while PSI MI, BioPAX and KGML have only one. PSI MI specifies which molecule engages in interaction, a concept absent in SBML, BioPAX and others, but under consideration.

The principal structure of all formats is similar, reflecting the structure of a pathway graph, structured to represent interacting subjects. SBML represents the mathematical description of pathways. The PSI MI format allows cross-references and inclusion of pathway interactions. BioPAX focuses on molecule interactions in metabolic pathways, as expressed via OWL standards. Most other formats other than SBML and CELL ML support adding references to the databases to combine biological knowledge, while the latter two have the unique capacity of representing mathematical knowledge required for quantitative understanding of pathways. Both the biological and modeling knowledge (i.e., kinetics data) are important because they help to characterize pathway functionalities, but no standard format combines all relevant biological and mathematical modeling data into one syntax. A key challenge is thus to develop a common format to incorporate biological knowledge as per the PSI MI format with mathematical descriptions similar to that of SBML, and at this point we are unaware of any quantitative databases that fully address these requirements. XML is a natural choice for this standard, especially considering that BIND, DIP and PPI provide the protein interaction datasets in XML format (based on PSI MI standard) and thus is incorporated into our system.

5.5 Building an Integrative Framework to Combine Modeling and Biological Data Sources

As stated earlier, an integrative environment for biological pathway modeling should include a biological and modeling knowledgebase, and tools for describing biological pathways, structure and function. One platform under development aspiring to this goal is the Systems Biology Workbench (SBW) [Hucka *et al.* (2002)], which aims to link different systems biology research communities via tools for visualization and simulation of pathways, but lacks the comprehensive knowledgebase necessary for integrative model development [Visvanathan *et al.* (2004); Osprian *et al.* (2005); Visvanathan *et al.* (2007)] and validation [Bhalla and Iyengar (1999)].

5.5.1 *System Architecture*

As a first step, we analyzed the structure of existing metabolic and cell signaling pathway modeling tools such as Gepasi [Medes (1997)], Jarnac [Sauro (2000)], Stochsim (www.zoo.cam.ac.uk/compcell/StochSim.html) and Virtual Cell [Schaff *et al.* (2000)], as well as schematic tools like PATIKA [Demir *et al.* (2002)] for pathway cartoon model specification. This analysis led to selection of Vector Path-Blazer (http://www.iscb.org/ismb2003/posters/feodorATinformaxinc.com 468.html) as a platform for the Pathway Designing and Visualization Environment (PDVE), primarily because it enables the user to design and visualize pathway models and incorporate biological information. It also supports reaction and component drawing, and stepwise interactive pathway and protein-protein interaction network assembly, and permits pathway model export in XML format. The Pathway Simulation Environment (PSE) was developed using MATLAB 7.0 (http://www.mathworks.com/), a high level programming and interactive technical computing environment with diverse functionality. The core of the integrative environment is the Database for Modeling Signaling Pathways (DMSP) [Visvanathan *et al.* (2005a,c,b)] as implemented via MS-SQL Server 2000 (www.microsoft.com/sql), which communicates with the PSE and PDVE as part of a client-server architecture system (see Fig. 5.2). A user can design and visualize pathway models in the PDVE based on the information available to it from the knowledgebase. In the PSE, the user may then extract modeling knowledge and perform simulations and sensitivity analysis for pathway models of interest. Modeling results can be stored in the knowledgebase.

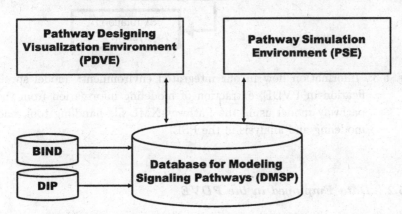

Fig. 5.2: Client-server architecture: Pathway Design Visualization Environment (PDVE) and Pathway Simulation Environment (PSE) coupled with a Database for Modeling Signaling Pathways (DMSP).

Vector PathBlazer (http://www.iscb.org/ismb2003/posters/ feodorATinformaxinc.com 468.html) is used in pathway model design by integrating modeling and biological data from the knowledgebase. The model is then communicated by the PDVE to the PSE in XML format. Modeling data required by the PSE is extracted from the XML file via a Pathway-XML modeling data handler developed in MATLAB. (see Results section for more detail). The PSE provides analysis tools for solving and analyzing mathematical pathway models. The results can be visualized in the PSE and stored in the knowledgebase. Relationships between pathway models designed in the PDVE, the process of extracting the modeling information using the Pathway-XML modeling data handling tool and subsequent PSE simulations and analysis is shown in Fig. 5.3.

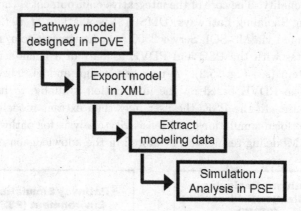

Fig. 5.3: Information flow in our integrated environment: model specification in PVDE, extraction of modeling information from the pathway model using the Pathway-XML file handling tool, and modeling and analysis in the PSE.

5.5.2 *Data Employed in the PDVE*

Achieving quantitative understanding pathways, a new fairly pursuit in molecular cell biology, entails addressing the challenge of integrating protein interaction data (as obtained for pathways from primary literature and databases) with mathematical models that quantify their associated interactions. The PDVE uses protein interaction data to qualitatively specify the network, but understanding the pathway dynamics and evaluating the role and relative significance of specific interations requires quantitative parameters such as kinetic rate laws for the specific interactions. Because kinetic characterization of interactions is sparse, literature curation was performed to identify parameters for specific pathways implemented in our system. A key goal in such studies is assessment of interaction modeling information within the context of information about the proteins involved and their known interactions. More specifically, signaling pathway modeling frequently requires fuse multiple pathway reactions to accurately quantify the associated kinetics. Fig. 5.4 depicts a reaction process within a pathway model designed in the PDVE. Mathematically it is considered a bipartite-directed multigraph structure, consisting of two types of nodes and directed arrows. A circle represents a protein and arrows represent association and disassociation of reactive proteins, as defined via the rate of reaction for product formation and complex dissociation. This process can be represented by a set of ordinary differential equations (ODEs) as will be discussed in the next section. Hence the PVDE considers the ontology of mathematical modeling of a signaling pathway [Kuroda *et al.* (2001)] in the pathway model design.

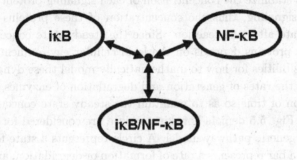

Fig. 5.4: A simple protein-protein interaction in a signal transduction pathway model designed in PDVE.

5.5.3 *Data Employed in Simulations*

Pathway or network models support experimental design, hypothesis generation and suggest suitable validation protocols. Data required for the simulations (i.e., kinetic constants, initial concentration and the kinetic parameters) is extracted into our PSE using Pathway-XML modeling data handler tool developed in MATLAB. MATLAB also provides various solvers for the numerical solution of differential equations (including ODEs with which biological pathways are most commonly modeled) as well as parametric sensitivity analysis (i.e., a systematic approach which can be applied to a dynamic biological interaction model to predict how the observed system will react to parameter changes) tools, which were thus implemented into our PSE. By varying a specific parameter, one can probe the kinetics in the modeled set of differential equations in a given range by calculating the dependence of the pathway component concentrations relative to the current parameter values. In the PSE we used *sens ind* (http://www.iwr.uni-heidelberg.de/sfb/PP/Preprint1996-19.ps.gz) (a subroutine written in MATLAB to extend the *odes15s* solver for simulation and analysis) to calculate ODE derivatives relative to kinetic parameters.

The framework of pathway models is typically based on standard enzymological constructs such as the Law of Mass Action (a formulation for balancing static equilibria or tracing outcomes of non-equilibria among competing processes) and the Michaelis-Menten model of enzyme kinetics [Sabau *et al.* (2002)]. For example, a signal transduction system usually behaves as a slowly time-varying nonlinear system during the reaction periods. Cells stabilize the concentration of each signaling protein before and after each signaling, thus the concentration of these proteins returns to a steady state after the reaction. Since the steady-state concentration of enzymes or proteins depends on the local cellular environment, there are several possibilities for how to mathematically model these dynamics. One is to model the rates of generation and degradation of enzymes or proteins as a function of time so as to maintain the steady state concentrations in the model. Fig. 5.5 depicts how kinetic data are considered for simulation based on a generic pathway model. A circle represents a state for the concentration, a bar represents a rate of formation or degradation, and directed arrows associate the circles and the bars. The relationship between the rate of catalysis and concentration changes for the substrate, enzyme, complex, and product is represented by the set of ODEs, and gives an appropriate dynamical description of the time-dependent concentration fluxes of these components.

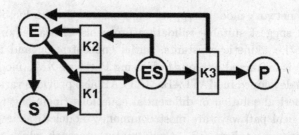

Fig. 5.5: Example of a simple enzyme kinetic reaction model.

As discussed in previous sections, some databases (http://doqcs.ncbs.res.in/) like DIP [Xenarios *et al.* (2002b)], MIPS [Mewes *et al.*

(2002)], BIND [Bader *et al.* (2001)] and PPI [Nakayama *et al.* (2002)] focus on biological (protein and gene) identification and interaction data, and do not provide mathematical modeling knowledge, while other databases like DOQCS [Sivakumaran *et al.* (2003)] maintain mathematical pathway models but lack comprehensive biological characterization. To support queries regarding the biological basis of signaling pathways, we combined biological and mathematical modeling information from the above resources into a database called DMSP [Visvanathan *et al.* (2005a,c,b)], comprising all requisite modeling data (kinetic constants, kinetic equations and initial concentrations) and biological information (descriptions of proteins and their interaction, and details concerning signaling pathways) required by our integrative environment wherein the data can be retrieved, analyzed and visualized in the PSE. DSMP is designed to represent different levels of data description, as shown in Fig. 5.6. The core basis of our knowledgebase is structured around components, reactions and pathways. In addition to basic component identification details (e.g. protein / gene, name / synonym, etc.), DSMP records reaction entities (in terms of components involved and their associated modeling data) and pathway entities (information about different representation models). The components that are involved in different reactions form different protein complexes, the identities of which are also maintained in the database. More detailed description about the DMSP schema will be presented in the Results.

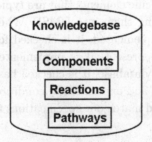

Fig. 5.6: Organizational structure of the knowledgebase contains components, reactions and pathways and their associated biological and modeling knowledge.

5.5.4 *Integration of Protein Interaction Data Sources*

The biological information in our knowledgebase is a curated compilation of data extracted (via XML or flat file formats [Constrium (2002)]) from different protein interaction databases. As depicted in Fig. 5.7, datasets were downloaded individually from their respective data sources, stored in dummy tables based on their XML schema specification, and converted to our standards by matching the individual attributes with our database schema specifications, and integrated into our system within a strict protocol that guards against data duplication.

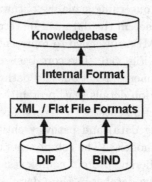

Fig. 5.7: Process of integrating biological from different protein interaction databases into the knowledgebase.

Fig. 5.8 show the specific elements that are typically identified from the DIP files when integrating them into DMSP. When there is a new interaction data set to be implemented, it is checked for unique identification. If the interaction is not present, it is implemented instantly; if it is already represented in the database, it is checked based on protein synonym names, protein sequence and experimental conditions. If the experimental conditions are unique and match our specifications then the entry is stored, otherwise it is ignored.

5.5.5 *Integration of Mathematical Modeling Data Sources*

DMSP considers the ontology of mathematical modeling of a signaling pathway [Kuroda *et al.* (2001)], and bases its modeling dataset curation on signaling pathway literature analysis. The main modeling elements that are required to model signaling pathways were identified as kinetic constants,

XML Source:

```
<node uid="DIP:3N" id="3" name="RA52_YEAST" class="protein">
...
<att name="organism">
  <val>Saccharomyces cerevisiae (budding yeast)</val>
</att>
</node>
```

The following table shows the XML tag that is parsed from the component part.

XML Tag	Description	Annotation
<node name=> </node>	Recommended name	Component Name **Note:** Components named "UNDEFINED", "UNKNOWN", "-", "Homo sapiens" or an empty value are skipped.
<node uid> </node>	Alternate name	Component Synonym Component Crosslink
<node class=> </node>	Molecule type. All molecules in the DIP database are proteins.	Component Class
<att name="organism">	Species	Component Organism
<att name="descr">	Description of the components	Component Synonyms
<feature name= >	Links to other databases	Component CrossLinks

Fig. 5.8: Representation of DIP XML datasets with component information.

kinetic equations and initial concentrations, thus relating the reaction components across different signaling pathways. Note that modeling knowledge must also consider complex associations among signaling pathways as identified from literature analysis. Currently DMSP considers mathematical models relating the EGF, Wnt, NFκB and TNFα signaling pathways, combined with their respective biological knowledge as integrated from the online protein interaction databases, as represented in Fig. 5.9.

5.5.6 *Database Schema Structure*

DMSP was built with key drug development requirements in mind, including a need for cartoon representation of pathways, qualitative details of specific proteins and their interactions, and quantitative assessment of the implications and sensitivity of the interactions [Kitano (2002)]. DSMP supports a variety of different pathway models via a schema representing different levels of modeling and biological data and various experimental conditions. The schema core reflects the PVDE workspace, with three

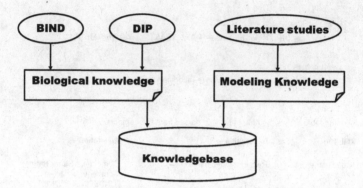

Fig. 5.9: The process of gathering biological and modeling knowledge from various sources integrating it into the knowledgebase.

distinct levels of entities: Components, Reactions and Pathways (see Fig. 5.10), thus DSMP tables are separated into component, reaction and pathway table entities. These entities inherit both the biological and modeling information, and each entry lists all relevant components and their respective involvement in reactions and pathways.

In the database the component table entities (Component Details Table, Component Attributes Table, Component Synonums Table) store a wide range of information that includes biological type (i.e., gene, DNA sequence, protein, sub molecule, etc.) of each component. A component can take part in a disease, which is stored in Component Details Table as a Component Disease column entity. The Component Formula column entity of the Component Details Table stores the chemical formula or protein complex information. A component can also have one or more synonyms and this information is stored in the Component Synonym Table. Component table entities also store information about component involvement in different reactions for different pathways. Each entry in these tables includes a unique component identifier. The reaction table entities store interaction specifics such as the components that are involved in a particular reaction for a pathway, the name of the reaction and reaction formula. The Reaction Attribute Table also considers different types of attributes relating to a particular reaction. For instance, one or more components can take part in a reaction with various kinetic constants. Every reaction is identified by unique reaction identifier.

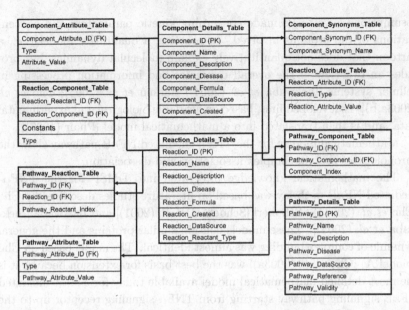

Fig. 5.10: DMSP database structure consisting of tables that store biological and modeling information for component, reaction, and
pathway entities.

5.5.7 *Pathway Model Implementation*

The TNFα-mediated NFκB-signaling pathway was used to test the requirements of the proposed integrative system. The biological data were extracted from DIP, BIND and PPI and integrated into DMSP with respect
to TNFα-mediated NFκB signaling pathway. The integrated modeling data
was extracted from literature studies [Cho and O.Wolkenhauer (2003); Cho
et al. (2003a)].

Exact description of the pathway is not an easy task. Various publica-
tions on this topic exist [Cho and O.Wolkenhauer (2003); Chen *et al.* (2004);
Cho *et al.* (2003a)] which attempt to integrate the interactions of all the
proteins in a pathway. Evidence for the substantial uncertainty about precise model structure is provided by many different biological cartoon models of TNFα-mediated NFκB-signaling pathway [Chen *et al.* (2004); Dixit
and Mak (2002); Karin and Lin (2002); Dempsey *et al.* (2003); Micheau and
Tschopp (2003); Pomerantz and Baltimore (2002); Baud and Karin (2001)].
The development of a precise mathematical model is also challenging. If
biological knowledge and the underlying experimental data are insufficient,

assumptions have to be made concerning kinetic parameters and concentrations of the proteins involved. In practice, a qualitative model (i.e., a cartoon that does not quantitatively explain molecular dynamics, but provides an overview of the overall dynamics and information processing in cellular systems [Ihekwaba *et al.* (2004); Barken *et al.* (2005); Cho *et al.* (2003a,b)]) is developed first, based on available biological and experimental data, and is then translated into a mathematical model [Phair (1997)].

Mathematical models for the TNFα-mediated NFκB-pathway show the chronology of protein complex association and dissociation.

The mathematical knowledge integrated into DMSP for the TNFα-mediated NFκB-pathway was based on literature studies described by Cho [Cho *et al.* (2003a)], Schoeberl [Schoeberl *et al.* (2001)] and Ihekwaba [Ihekwaba *et al.* (2004)]. These models contain similar proteins and the general dynamic of complex building was almost identical. The model based on Cho (model A) [Cho *et al.* (2003a)] was the best basis for extension because it is the most detailed mathematical model available today for TNFα-mediated NFκB signaling pathway starting from TNFα-signaling receptor up to the transcription factor AP1. The implemented TNFα pathway model contains 31 components (including proteins and protein complexes) that are involved in 19 different reactions (see Fig. 5.14). The biological description of proteins, protein complexes and genes that take part in TNFα signaling pathway was stored as component level entities in DMSP. The kinetic equations and kinetic constants pertaining to different reactions of the TNFα pathway model were inserted in the reaction level entities, and the complete structure of the TNFα pathway with the initial concentrations was stored in pathway level entities.

To illustrate the implementation, cIAP is a protein that takes part in TNFα pathway, thus information related to the cIAP protein was gathered from DIP, BIND and MIPS, and stored in DMSP. Details for all known reactions among TNFα signaling pathway components (including cIAP) were stored in the reaction tables. Kinetic equations and constants for these reactions were stored in the reaction tables. The complete structure of TNFα pathway (as characterized in [Cho *et al.* (2003a)] but including three additional components) with the initial concentrations was stored in the pathway tables. Collectively, the modeling knowledge is incorporated into the database schema at different levels, such that all datasets relating to the TNFα signaling pathway (and the role therein of cIAP and other proteins) can retrieved from the knowledgebase for use in PDVE where the TNFα pathway model is designed and visualized to provide the structure shown in Fig. 5.11. It should be noted that our system supports the concurrent presence of multiple distinct pathway model variants in the database. Different models of the same pathway help us in forming a better biological understanding by providing an expanded basis for validation and knowledge evolution as new data emerges.

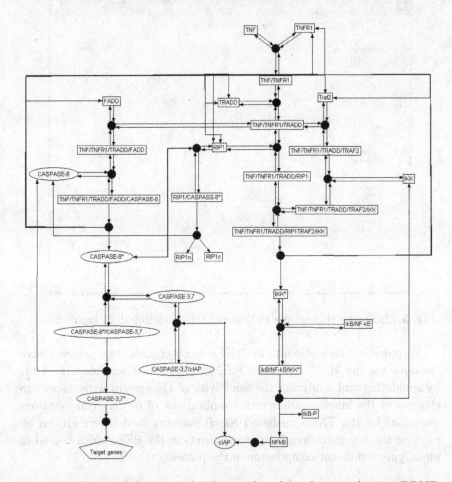

Fig. 5.11: TNFα-pathway model designed and implemented using PDVE based on biological and modeling information from DMSP.

Next, the TNFα-mediated NFαB-pathway model was exported from the PDVE to the PSE environment in XML format via a graphically interactive Pathway-XML modeling data handler tool in MATLAB (see Fig.

5.12). The tool loads the XML model, checks the modeling knowledge, then automatically extracts kinetic equations, rate constants and initial concentrations. This information is stored in individual MATLAB files as output according to the specifications required for performing analysis in the PSE.

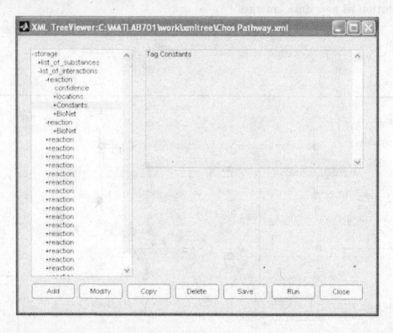

Fig. 5.12: Screen shot of the Pathway-XML modeling data handler tool.

Systematic examinations of the TNFα signal transduction pathway were the done via the MATLAB-based PSE graphical interface (see Fig. 5.13) by simulating and analyzing the sensitivity of the system with respect to changes in the kinetic parameters. Implications of protein concentration variations for the TNFα mediated NFκB pathway model were probed by plotting the concentration of the components in the PSE, which helped in identifying significant components in the pathway model.

5.5.8 *Exporting the Pathway Model*

After having analyzed the different XML formats for data exchange and export in previous section, the DMSPML export format was developed so as to effectively integrate biological knowledge from the online databases based on PSI MI standards. DMSPML also incorporates mathematical modeling

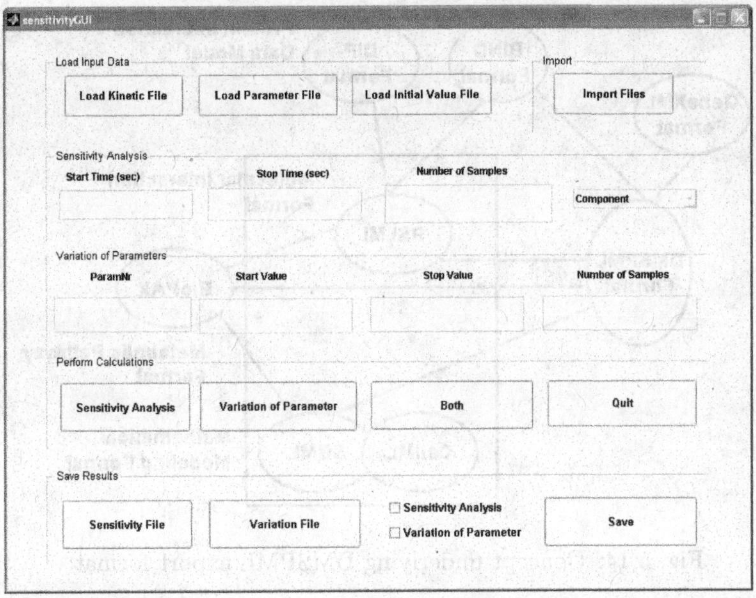

Fig. 5.13: Screen shot of the graphical user interface for running PSE simulations.

knowledge from literature studies and imposes a standard format (depicted in Fig. 5.14) that satisfies various community standards for exchanging biological and modeling knowledge.

The export mechanism provides a detailed perspective into the modeling ontology in terms of biological and mathematical information concerning pathways. Biological datasets extracted from online sources are based on OWL standards, hence this standard is incorporated into DMSP.

5.6 Analysis of the Developed Integrative Environment

DMSP is the core basis of our integrative systematic approach for analyzing pathways. Many projects focus on pathways, with a wide diversity and objectives, and the accumulation of more models with associated biological data is key for better understanding of pathways. Mathematical models provide more detailed insight into the components and reactions behavior within a pathway relative to experimental conditions that is absent from most protein interaction databases such as BIND

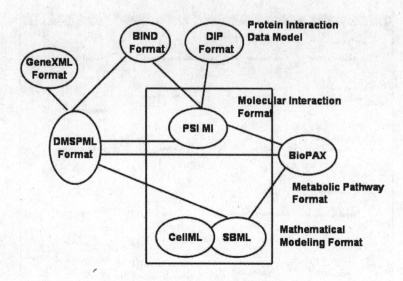

Fig. 5.14: Concept underlying DMSPML export format.

and DIP. Database projects like DOQCS [Sivakumaran *et al.* (2003)] and TRANSPATH [Schacherer *et al.* (2001)] have extensive information about chemical interactions in signaling pathways, but have thus far failed to facilitate integration of modeling information and simulation results with biological data. In contrast, GeneNet [Kolpakov *et al.* (1998)] and AFCS (Alliance for Cellular Signaling) (http://afcs.swmed.edu/afcs/letter to community.htm) have begun including quantitative pathway models and comprise excellent resources by providing enzyme level information.

While protein interaction databases try to provide qualitative datasets, but are not efficient in reporting mathematical modeling data required for signaling pathway simulations, DOQCS [Sivakumaran *et al.* (2003)] and SigPath (http://www.sigpath.org/) have recently begun maintaining mathematical models of cellular signaling pathways with few or no biological annotations. However quantitative modeling of signaling pathways is still a relatively new undertaking, and is subject to various challenges, including integration of biological information into a quantitative model based on current sources of information, such as the primary literature. DMSP was designed and developed to address these requirements, containing basic qualitative information gathered from protein interaction databases and the more specific quantitative mathematical knowledge from scientific literature. The protein interaction data that is gathered from BIND, DIP and PPI provides a detailed account of specific components and its interactions characteristics. The case of TNFα mediated NFκB signaling pathway model, that was implemented using this approach, is a demonstration of DMSP's success in addressing these requirements.

There are similar projects underway like SigPath (http://www.sigpath.org/) and Biomodels.net [Novère *et al.* (2006)] which support construction and annotation of pathway models. SigPath stores biochemical information with details for quantitative modeling on specific aspects of the cellular machinery. Biomodels.net [Novère *et al.* (2006)] provides access to published, peer-reviewed, quantitative models of biochemical and cellular systems. Human curators annotate and cross-link components of the models to other relevant data resources. This allows users to identify precisely the components of models, and helps them to retrieve and visualize models that are appropriate for their interests or observations. Collectively, these services aim to ensure that all the models that are published in the public domain are freely available for everyone. While Reactome [Joshi *et al.* (2005)] covers a more global view of providing more qualitative and quantitative information in terms of more biological information,.DMSP has a very specific aims of delivering more quantitative mathematical information that is required to model and to validate pathways. DMSP provides a novel service in that it addresses the issue of translocation, which is not implemented in existing protein interaction databases which provide only very basic qualitative information. To address this issue, DMSP specifically incorporates information derived from literature-reported pathways models in combination with biological knowledge, thus providing insight into the active roles played by specific proteins in various pathways.

5.7 Conclusion

Today there are still many challenges remaining in applying combined biological and mathematical knowledge toward understanding the dynamic nature of pathways. In this work, biological knowledge was accumulated from online databases and mathematical knowledge for pathways from the literature. Based on this, we have studied the basic nature of pathways using an integrative systematic approach. This systematic analysis still has limitations and further research must be pursued in order to derive results which can provide tangible guidance toward practical goals such as drug target discovery. A main focus of our ongoing research is to expand the database schema by incorporating more simulation results obtained for different pathways, which will aid in identifying key pathway components and reactions.

Further validation of the structure of a biological pathway can be achieved by complementary experimental and simulation studies, which are the next major focus of our ongoing work aimed at fostering a more physiological model. This can be attained by incorporating more data into the knowledgebase and re-analyzing the pathway models. We thus plan to expand the DMSP schema by interpreting information which helps to design protein complex representations in signaling pathways. A further objective is to include experimental data of specific experiments that are conducted for different signaling pathways.

Collectively these developments have interesting implications for future work in terms of opportunities for global information sharing. Plug-ins to open source tools like BIOUML [Bertalanffy (1973)] and Cytoscape [Mesarovic (1968)] are being developed through which DSMP pathways can be visualized. It would be also interesting to develop standards for query languages and database generators that can be used for enabling integrated databases and pathway discoveries. We further plan to investigate the work on ontologies and ontology integration that can be used to overcome the terminology problem when integrating data from different formats. An example of such an extension of terminology would be standardization based on Gene Ontology. Another possibility is to include user defined entities to provide more flexibility between these standards. It can be concluded that the approach that was developed and reported in the Visvanathan thesis is an important effort towards analyzing signaling pathways systematically by combining modeling and biological knowledge. Pathway models can be readily designed, visualized and simulated based on the knowledge stored in such a knowledgebase. Validation studies can also be performed by integrating experimental data into such a knowledgebase. This framework enables an iterative interplay between experimental analysis and modeling strategies: simulation results done on signaling pathways will enable us to interpret the biological system from a global systemic view, thus further enhancing the level of detail and sophistication with which we understand biological pathways, with practical implications toward important biomedical objectives such as drug target discovery and drug development.

Chapter 6

Ontology-based Data Integration: A Case Study in Clinical Trials

Sandra Geisler, Christoph Quix, Anke Schmeink, David Kensche

RWTH Aachen University, Germany

6.1 Introduction

Clinical trials are a common means in medical research to investigate new medications, medical devices, and other medical products. The data collected during clinical trials is very valuable to the organizations carrying out the trials to show the efficiency and harmlessness of their products or to (dis)prove a thesis. While the study register of the U.S. National Institute of Health contained approximately 23 500 clinical studies in 2006 [Bestehorn *et al.* (2006)], this number quadrupled (81 770) in November 2009. Especially the pharmaceutical industry and manufacturers of medical devices push the conduct of more and more studies. Therefore, rapid and efficient, but also accurate study planning, conduction and analysis of results are indispensable [Hanover and Julian (2004)]. The careful collection, handling and storage of data while obeying national and international regulations is a major task in clinical study management [Prokscha and Anisfeld (2006)].

Heterogeneous data sources are also a challenge in data management for clinical studies: device manufacturers often implement their own proprietary format, or several standards exist for the same kind of data [Fischer *et al.* (2003)]. Furthermore, the data format may change during the development of a medical device. Thus, flexible means to integrate data sources and their schemas are required. Many data integration architectures used in the medical domain facilitate an integrated schema and relational DBMSs as they provide efficient methods to store, query and analyze data [Prokscha and Anisfeld (2006)].

Despite the advantages of an integrated schema architecture, it also poses several problems. Such an architecture requires an immense up-front effort for design and implementation. Furthermore, the Extraction-Transformation-Loading (ETL) processes, including the mappings between the source schemas and the integrated schema, have to be created [Vassiliadis *et al.* (2001a)]. Hence, when a source schema has changed or new sources have to be added, mappings, ETL processes, and possibly the integrated schema have to be adapted as well. Especially in the medical domain, the definition of an integrated common schema is a major issue as there exists a plethora of synonyms, homonyms, and related terms [Gardner (2005)]. Today, a common means to deal with these lingual and domain-specific issues is the use of ontologies. In the medical field taxonomies and ontologies have already been used intensively and constitute an approved method to organize and structure knowledge [Hahn and Schulz (2004)]. However, purely knowledge-based systems lack the mature functionalities for storage, management, integration and analysis of huge amounts of data.

To overcome the described problems, we developed an ontology-based data integration system which is capable of creating executable ETL processes based on a mapping between a *core ontology* which contains a domains' vocabulary and separate *source ontologies*.

In this chapter, we describe the design and implementation of our system *OnTrIS* (Ontology-based Trial Information System), which supports the entire data integration process: the sources and the integrated schema are described by source ontologies and core ontology, respectively, and the integrated schema is created from a user-defined subset of the core ontology. Furthermore, mappings can be defined between core and source ontologies to enable the assembling of the integration process by ready-to-use data integration modules. Thus, we provide an end-to-end, ontology-based data integration solution which has not been shown in other approaches [Wache *et al.* (2001); Bellatreche *et al.* (2004); Skoutas and Simitsis (2006); Bergamaschi *et al.* (2009)]. The system has been evaluated in the field of clinical trials with a medical devices trial conducted in the My-Heart subproject Heart Failure Management (HFM) (http://www.hitech-projects.com/euprojects/myheart/). MyHeart aims at developing intelligent systems for the prevention and monitoring of cardiovascular diseases.

The remainder of the chapter is structured as follows: in the next section we briefly show the overall architecture of OnTrIS. Section 6.3 presents the core ontology of our approach and Section 6.4 explains the data integration approach. Section 6.5 details how we implemented the data integration processes. In Section 6.6, we present the evaluation results, which show the feasibility and usability of our approach. Section 6.7 discusses related work, before we conclude in the last section and point out future work.

6.2   System Architecture and Overview

Multidisciplinary teams in clinical trials include domain experts, such as medical professionals, physicians, chemists, or electrical engineers which are entrusted with the development of a medical product and responsible for the conduct of the trial. As these domain experts are usually not familiar with data management, we provide a comprehensible and fast approach to construct and deploy trial databases and corresponding data integration modules to import trial data from different sources. In this section, we will first describe the main constituents of OnTrIS and the basic steps to deploy a data management architecture for a clinical trial.

The architecture (see also Figure 6.1) contains first of all an extendable core ontology describing concepts and attributes of clinical trials called *Clinical Trial Data Management Ontology* (CTDMO). It is the basis for the clinical data management environment which will be created by OnTrIS. It is used to create new relational database schemas and data integration modules based on mappings between data source ontologies and concepts selected from the core ontology. To include trial specific concepts the user can extend the CTDMO using an ontology modeling tool (cf. Section 6.3). The *client application* enables the user to select concepts from the CTDMO which she wants to use in her database, to create a relational database schema on a dedicated database server, and to create mappings and corresponding data integration modules to import data from different data sources. Furthermore, the user can create and manage ETL packages.

A *web service* fulfils all complex tasks, such as the processing of the ontologies, the creation of the database schemas (directly on the DBMS or as SQL scripts), of the meta representation for the created databases and for the data sources, and of the integration modules. A web service has been used to make the system more modular and secure.

Finally, a *data integration tool* is responsible for executing the data integration modules. It accesses the data sources and extracts the data

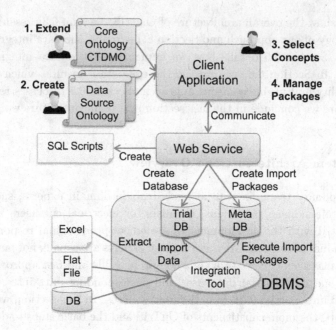

Fig. 6.1: The workflow in the OnTrIS architecture.

according to the specifications in the data integration modules.

We point out, that the OnTrIS architecture is not restricted to the CTDMO or the field of clinical trials. Any other domain ontology obeying the modeling principles described in Section 6.3 can be used as a basis for the architecture as well.

6.3 The CTDM Ontology

Ontologies have been identified as an approved method to model a domain of discourse on a highly abstracted and semantic level [Gruber (1993)]. Ontologies have been proven suitable for database design, automatic database generation and data integration [Calvanese *et al.* (2002); Wache *et al.* (2001); Zamboulis *et al.* (2008)]. The applicability in data sharing environments has already been pointed out in [Gruber (1993)] as an ontology is a *"a logical description of shared data, allowing application programs and databases to interoperate without having to share data structures."* Therefore, the basis for the OnTrIS data integration is a semantic description of clinical trials in form of an ontology, the Clinical Trial Data Management Ontology (CTDMO, the core ontology).

Several alternative methodologies exist, which can be used to develop ontologies, such as the Enterprise Model Approach, METHONTOLOGY or TOVE (see [Pinto and Martins (2004)] for a comprehensive survey of methods). Many of these methodologies have common steps, such as the definition of the purpose, the conceptualization, and the implementation (or formalization). The work of Noy and McGuinness [Noy and McGuinness (2001)] is a well known approach to manual ontology development and has been used in this work. The steps proposed by Noy and McGuinnness have been supplemented in our work by steps for ontology evaluation [Gomez-Perez (2004)]. As we focus on the data integration and creation of ETL processes in this chapter, we refer the interested reader to [Geisler *et al.* (2007)] for more details on the development. The core principles of the CTDMO are described in the following.

Eight core concepts have been identified to structure the CTDMO. The core concepts are shown as dark ellipses in Figure 6.2 and are described below. The example concepts in the figure have been adapted from the extended Heart Failure Management (HFM) trial ontology, which has been created during the evaluation of the system. There are two types of relationships: *isA*-relationships and object properties. *isA*-relationships represent an inheritance relationship and are illustrated with a thin line. If three dots follow the *isA* keyword, the inheritance relationship is deeper than it is shown, i.e., concepts between the two concepts in the hierarchy are hidden. Object properties are drawn as thick lines in the figure.

The root concepts comprise the following:

Activity subsumes all concepts which express some action executed during a clinical trial. An example is the concept *HFM_ECG_Measurement*.

Product is supposed to contain all things which are used to conduct an activity, e.g., *Composite_Card_Device*. Medical devices are medical products which are used and tested in a study.

Role describes all persons and roles involved in a clinical study, e.g., a *Patient*.

Information_Content contains all concepts which may represent data, e.g., *HFM_Card_Monitoring*, representing a cardiovascular measurement.

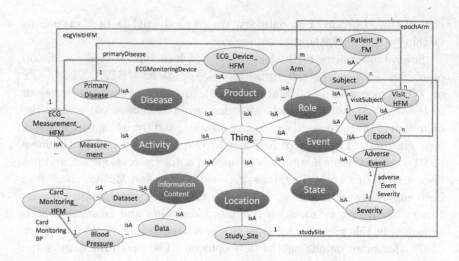

Fig. 6.2: Example concepts of the CTDMO.

Location   organizes spatial extents related to the study. The concept
Study Site is an example for a location.

Event   is an occurrence which is happening during a study and usually
having a start date. An example subconcept is a *Visit*, which subsumes all
information of one visit session.

Disease   is a parent concept for all disease concepts. *PrimaryDisease* is
a subconcept example.

State   is used to subsume concepts that describe a certain state of an
object, e.g., *Severity* of an adverse effect.

In the ontology development process we identified requirements for the
ontology, where the most important among them demand the ontology

(1) to be extendable, enabling the addition of concepts and properties describing data of new trials;
(2) to have a concise and user-friendly structure to enable fast orientation;
(3) to have a modular design (concepts can be reused to describe other
concepts), and
(4) to have a high quality regarding the consistency, documentation and
comprehensibility.

To fulfil the aforementioned requirements, we defined modeling principles. Remember that the CTDMO is a core ontology which will be extended by users for each trial to include new concepts and properties. The extensions are stored in the core ontology itself as they are expected to be reused in other trials which leads to a growth of the ontology. First we introduce the notion of *hot spots*. Hot spots are concepts that have to be refined in the core ontology by the users as they are too general to use.

An example for a hot spot is the concept *Subject*, which represents the persons participating in a study. Obviously, the data to be collected for a person varies in each study; therefore, refinement of this concept is necessary. The idea of hot spots accounts for the requirement of extensibility.

Furthermore, object properties have been used to model relationships between concepts and their individuals. To enable the mapping to relational schemas, constraints for object properties in the core ontology have been restricted to be 1:1 (defined as functional and inverse functional), 1:N (defined as functional) and N:M relationships (defined with no restrictions).

For modularity of the ontology and reusability of ontology elements, some terms have been represented as object properties and explicit concepts, which could also have been modeled as datatype properties and simple domains. Especially concepts that represent data units, such as *Blood Pressure* or *Weight*, can be of use for multiple concepts such as *Patient* or multiple measurement concepts. Therefore, these data units are not modeled as datatype properties of the specific concepts but as concepts on their own using inverse functional object properties to reference them.

Starting from scratch building a new ontology is admittedly a comparable or even higher upfront effort compared to other data integration systems. But if a suitable core ontology can be reused, only some adaptations, such as the correct modeling of object properties and the actual extensions for the required purpose have to be done. Once the core ontology has been agreed upon it can be reused and refined and is therefore suitable for long-term application, which is beneficial for recurring problems such as fast setup of clinical trial data management environments.

6.4 Ontology-based Data Integration of Study Relevant Information

An important feature of OnTrIS is, that the mappings between the sources and the integrated system are defined between ontologies on a semantic level. The mappings defined between ontologies are then translated into executable ETL processes which are able to extract the data from the sources and to load them into an integrated database. Figure 6.3 gives an overview of our ontology-based integration approach.

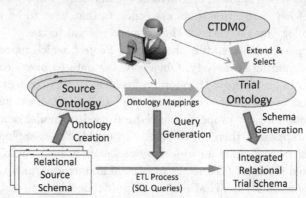

Fig. 6.3: Overview of the ontology-based integration approach.

To be able to define mappings between ontologies, these ontologies must be available. The *trial ontology* is created by the user by (i) extending the CTDMO with trial specific concepts and (ii) selecting relevant concepts which are included in the integrated database schema, i.e., the trial on-tology represents the integrated schema to be created. The selection is important as not all concepts of the extended ontology are required in the schema. As we follow a *multiple ontology approach* for data integration [Wache *et al.* (2001)], ontologies for each data source, including mappings to the trial ontology, also have to be defined. We use a semi-automatic ap-proach (according to [Bellatreche *et al.* (2004)]) in which the system assists the user in creating the data source ontologies by translating the source schema into an ontology automatically. Furthermore, the definition of the mappings is supported by an easy-to-use graphical user interface (see Fig-ure 6.4).

In addition, we follow an in-advance (or materialized) integration ap-proach, where the data is stored in an integrated database *in advance* to queries to this database. The in-advance integration facilitates fast query execution, especially with respect to data analysis and reporting. It also al-lows for auditing and metadata management, which are important features for clinical trial data management and which we implemented to adhere to legal regulations. Another important step in our approach is the trans-lation between the schemas (of the sources and the integrated schema)

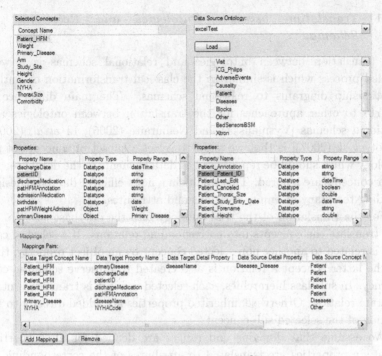

Fig. 6.4: The mapping editor.

and the corresponding ontologies. In OnTrIS, we support various types of data sources, including relational databases, flat files, and Excel sheets, which are common formats used in clinical trials. We assume, however, that the schemas of these sources can be represented in a relational way. The translation between ontologies and relational schemas has to be done in both directions, as indicated in Figure 6.3: the relational schemas of data sources are translated into source ontologies, and the trial ontology is translated into a relational schema for the integrated database. We will discuss the details of this translation in Section 6.4.1. Having defined the translation between ontologies and relational schemas, we are then able to specify how the ontology mappings should be translated into an executable query for the ETL process. The details of this query generation process will be discussed in Section Section 6.4.2.

6.4.1 *Translation between Ontologies and Relational Schemas*

The translation between ontologies and relational schemas is a well-studied process which is similar to the classical transformation of Entity-Relationship diagrams to relational schemas. The main difference of OnTrIS to other approaches for the translation between ontologies and relational schemas [Vysniauskas and Nemuraite (2006); Li *et al.* (2006); Cullot *et al.* (2007)] is that we allow to select a subset of concepts of the ontology which should be represented as data elements in the database. All other concepts are ignored. This results in a more efficient database design, avoiding too many or empty relations and attributes.

For the translation of the trial ontology into the database schema, we first translate the concepts into corresponding relations. If a selected concept is related to another non-selected concept by an object property, then for the latter concept a relation is also created to preserve semantic consistency. In subclass hierarchies, each selected concept is translated into a separate relation. Otherwise, inherited properties are added directly to the relation of the selected sub-concept.

We assume that domains and ranges are defined for all properties. Datatype properties are translated to attributes of the corresponding relation with appropriate data types. For object properties, we check the cardinalities: for a 1:1-relationship (functional and inverse functional property), we will add the attributes of the relation of the property range to the relation of the property domain, the relation for property range will be deleted; a 1:N-relationship will be translated into a foreign key constraint; an n:m-relationship will be represented by a separate relation with two foreign keys referencing the relations for the domain and range of the property.

If the ontology contains individuals, then they are translated into records of the corresponding relations.

The reverse translation of relational source schemas into ontologies is almost exactly inverse. However, object properties which are functional and inverse functional (1:1-relationships) will not be created as it is not possible to detect where concepts have been merged due to 1:1-relationships.

All transformations are logged in a metadatabase to identify the columns, tables and relationships to which concepts and properties have been translated to or stem from later. This information is used for the query generation as we will describe in the next section.

6.4.2 Mapping Creation and Query Generation

For the description of the mappings we use the following constituents of the OWL Lite language: the ontology is composed of a set of domain concepts C. The concepts are arranged in a concept hierarchy reflecting specialization relationships. Each concept defines a set of properties P (possibly the empty set). The set of properties consists of a set of object properties O and a set of datatype properties D, such that $P = D \cup O$. Each object property has a range concept C_r and a domain concept C_d. We assume $C_r \neq Thing$ and $C_d \neq Thing$, i.e., range and domain of a property must be defined. In the following, we denote concepts, properties and relations and attributes of a data source with the subscript S and concepts and properties of the integrated database (the target) with the subscript T, respectively. A relation R in the data source or data target is defined by a set of attributes $a_1, \ldots, a_n$, written $R = (a_1, \ldots, a_n)$.

A property in an ontology modeled according to the rules described in Section 6.3 can be one of the following kinds:

- a datatype property d
- an inverse functional and functional object property o_{if}, representing a 1:1-relationship
- a functional object property o_f, representing a 1:N-relationship
- an object property without restrictions o_w, representing a n:m-relationship

The query on the data source has to be assembled depending on the mapped properties of the data source ontology and the relations and attributes they represent. Hence, there are 16 possibilities to map properties between source and target (see Table 6.1). This also implies, that if properties representing columns of different data source tables are mapped to the same target table, joins between the data source tables have to be included in the query. Depending on the combination of mapped properties, there are different problems to overcome which we will address in the following subsections. We assume that a relational language is used for queries. OnTrIS implemented the query construction for SQL queries, but this does not influence the generality of our approach as it can also be adapted to other languages such as XQuery for XML documents.

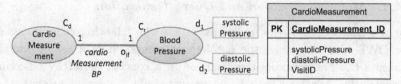

Fig. 6.5: Example for a 1:1-relationship mapping.

6.4.2.1 Mapping of Datatype Properties

Datatype properties are always transformed to simple relational attributes. If a datatype property d_S of the source ontology is mapped to a property p_T of the trial ontology, the attribute a_d corresponding to d_S has to be included into the assembled query by adding it with the respective relation $R_S = (a_1, \ldots, a_d, \ldots, a_n)$ to the projection clause (the SELECT-FROM part in SQL). Formalized in relational algebra:

$$\pi_{d_S}(R_S) \tag{6.1}$$

If a datatype property d_T is the target of a mapping, no further action has to be taken. The extracted data from the attribute a_p represented by a property p_S will be imported into the attribute represented by d_T (if their domains are compatible).

6.4.2.2 Mapping of Object Properties Representing 1:1-Relationships

The handling of 1:1-relationships differs for properties of the trial ontology and for properties of the source ontology. When an inverse functional object property o_{if_T} of the concepts of the trial ontology is translated using the procedure described in Section 6.4.1, the properties of its range C_r will be added as attributes to the relation representing the domain C_d and no relation will be created for the C_r. Therefore, a mapping involving a property o_{if_T} requires additional input by the user.

The example in Figure 6.5 details the problem. The concept *BloodPressure* contains two datatype properties *systolicPressure* and *diastolicPressure*. The concept *CardioMeasurement* defines an inverse functional object property *cardioMeasurementBP* with *BloodPressure* as range concept. During the translation, a relation *CardioMeasurement* is created which contains two columns *systolicPressure* and *diastolicPressure*. No relation *BloodPressure* is created. If the property o_{if_T} is now mapped, e.g., by a source datatype property d_S, it is not clear, if the data has to be imported into the *systolicPressure* attribute or the *diastolicPressure* attribute.

Source (S)	Target (T)	p_{detail_S}	p_{lookup_S}	p_{detail_T}	p_{lookup_T}
d	d				
d	o_{if}			✗	
d	o_f			✗	✗
d	o_w			✗	✗
o_{if}	d				
o_{if}	o_{if}	✗	✗	✗	
o_{if}	o_f	✗	✗	✗	✗
o_{if}	o_w	✗	✗	✗	✗
o_f	d	✗	✗		
o_f	o_{if}	✗	✗	✗	
o_f	o_f	✗	✗	✗	✗
o_f	o_w	✗	✗	✗	✗
o_w	d	✗	✗		
o_w	o_{if}	✗	✗	✗	
o_w	o_f	✗	✗	✗	✗
o_w	o_w	✗	✗	✗	✗

Table 6.1: The mapping matrix.

Therefore, the user additionally has to select a data target detail property d_{detail_T} to clarify the situation. The mapping between the source property p_S and d_{detail_T} is then included in the mappings.

If a source property o_{if_S} is mapped to any other property, it can be treated like an object property o_f representing a 1:N-relationship, because 1:1-relationships in the relational schema of the data source are considered as restricted 1:N-relationships. A summary of all mapping combinations and the required mapping components are listed in Table 6.1.

6.4.2.3 *Mapping of Object Properties Representing 1:N-relationships*

We represent 1:N-relationships as functional object properties o_f defined for the concept representing the side with cardinality N (or child side) of the relationship. A mapped property o_{f_T} representing a 1:N-relationship requires more than one attribute and relation to be added to the assembled relational query. First of all, the relations representing the domain concept C_d and the range concept C_r have to be added to the query. Then the attribute representing the foreign key and the primary key attribute of the referenced relation are added to the projection clause. Finally, a left outer join between the two relations is added. In relational algebra this is expressed as:

$$\pi_{a_{fk},a_{pk}}(R_d \bowtie R_r) \tag{6.2}$$

In case of nesting, i.e., if foreign key relationships have more than one level, this is also reflected in the assembled query. For example, a two level foreign key relationship would be expressed in relational algebra as follows:

$$\pi_{a_{fk},a_{pk},a_{fk1},a_{fk2}}((R_d \bowtie R_r) \bowtie R_{r2}) \tag{6.3}$$

Additionally, the user has to select a data source detail property $p_{detailS}$ for the mapping (which is also added to the projection clause of the statement), because the keys used in the data source relation referenced by the 1:N-relationship are not the same keys used in the target relation. Therefore, the relationships between record sets of the two relations have to be resolved in the data source and again established in the data target (if the target property is also a 1:N or N:M-relationship). This situation is exemplified in Figure 6.6 (a). The illustrated relationships are represented by the functional object properties in the respective ontologies. The detail property on the data source side, e.g., *Disease* in the relation *Disease_S*, is used to identify the correct record in the referenced target relation (*Disease_T* in the example) and to lookup the key of the desired record (note: $d_{detailS}$ does not necessarily have to be the primary key of the source relation). This key is then used as value for the foreign key attribute of the target relation R_T (*Primary_Disease_ID* in the relation *Patient_T* in the example) representing the domain concept of the respective object property.

In Figure 6.6 (b) the respective mappings are shown. On the left side the input attributes of the data source and on the right side the attributes of the lookup relation *Disease_T* are shown. The mapping is defined between *Disease* and *diseaseName*, where the former is an attribute of the relation *Disease_S*.

On the target side this implies that an additional step has to be done to lookup the respective key in the referenced relation. The lookup joins the two target relations on a specified attribute (the lookup attribute p_{lookup}) and produces an output attribute, which contains the keys of the rows looked up in the referenced relation. The respective mappings including the described 1:N-relationship mapped to a 1:N-relationship are illustrated in Figure 6.7.

If a datatype property d_S is mapped to a target object property o_{f_T} representing a 1:N-relationship, it is assumed, that d_S already represents

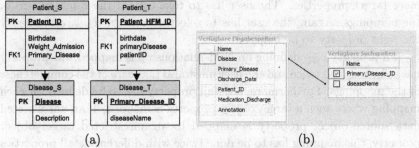

Fig. 6.6: Example for a 1:N-relationship mapping

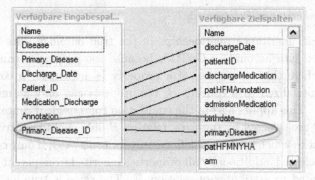

Fig. 6.7: Mapping of object properties representing 1:N-relationships.

the detail property field for the data source used for the join to get the respective key from the target relation R_T. On the other hand, if an object property o_{f_S} representing a 1:N-relationship is mapped to a property d_T, the data from the attribute representing the data source detail property is written to the respective target field.

6.4.2.4 *Mapping of Object Properties Representing n:m-relationships*

n:m-relationships are represented in relational schemas as intermediate relations which have foreign keys referencing each related relation. The set of foreign keys constitutes the primary key of the intermediate relation. Hence, N:M-relationships can be handled similar to 1:N-relationships. In this work N:M-relationships are modeled as unrestricted object properties o_w. Because an intermediate relation has more than one foreign key, the respective data source object property has to be mapped twice to one or more target properties. The user has to take care of the completeness of the mappings. Again, the user has to select a property $d_{details}$ to specify the right property to be mapped.

If a property o_{wT} defining an N:M-relationship is mapped, the property has to be mapped twice and the user must also take care of the completeness of the mappings. Furthermore, a detail property has to be defined for each mapping where such a target object property is mapped. If an unrestricted data source object property is mapped to an unrestricted target object property, this mapping has to be done twice with different detail properties on both sides.

6.4.2.5   *Inheritance Relationships*

The case of inheritance relationships in the trial ontology does not have to be taken into account in OnTrIS, because the properties can only be mapped where they occur, i.e., if a property is defined for a concept A, which is specialized by a concept B, the property can only be mapped at concept A. This applies also to the translation rules used: if concept A and concept B are selected by the user, relation B only contains attributes for the properties which have been defined only for concept B; if only concept B has been selected, additionally all properties inherited from parent concepts are translated to attributes of relation B. The same is true for the data source ontologies.

6.5   Assembly of ETL Processes Based on Ontology Mappings

Our approach for ontology-based data integration is a holistic approach which also includes the definition of ETL processes. ETL processes are crucial components of data warehouses and other integration architectures to integrate data from several sources into one global schema. With the information defined in the previous steps, the definition of ETL processes can be done almost automatically. Only administrative information, e.g., database connections or location of files, has to be specified by the user.

In general, an ETL process can roughly be divided into two main parts: the data flow and the control flow. The *data flow* describes the actual flow of data from the sources to the integrated schema, the data target. A wrapper extracts the required data from each source and "pumps" the data into the data flow.

The data flow can be viewed as a part of the *control flow*. In the control flow, organizational operations, such as copying of files or the execution of additional software, can be modeled. We used Microsoft SQL Server Integration Services (MS SSIS) to implement the ETL processes. There are also other commercial tools (see [Friedman *et al.* (2008)] for an overview), open source solutions (e.g. http://www.pentaho.com) and research prototypes (e.g., ARKTOS [Vassiliadis *et al.* (2005, 2001b)]), but the MS SSIS suited our needs best. They can access various types of data sources and targets, mappings and transformations can be defined easily, and there is not as much administrative overhead as with other integration solutions.

In MS SSIS, data and control flows are organized in integration modules (or packages). A module contains several *components*, each representing a specific "part" of the integration process, such as a data source component or an extraction component. For each data source a separate data integration module is created.

The integration modules in OnTrIS are able to access various source types, such as databases, Excel spreadsheets, and flat files. We provide a wizard to assist the user in creating integration modules.

Firstly, a wrapper for the target database has to be chosen and connection details have to be specified. Secondly, the order has to be determined, in which the data is extracted from the sources by data flow components and loaded into the integrated trial database. The order is important since some relations have to be filled before others, e.g., for lookup of key values or in case of foreign key constraints. Before the data flow components are created, all mapped relations of the target schema are retrieved from the user-defined mappings. Then, the tables are sorted according to their reference order. For example, if a relation *Patient* references a relation *Disease* by a foreign key constraint, the relation *Disease* has to be filled first.

The actual data extraction, transformation and loading is executed in the data flow components. For each relation of the target schema, a separate data flow component is assembled in which all mapped source attributes have to be retrieved from the sources using relational queries as described in Section 6.4. Based on the user defined mappings, foreign key relationships in the target schema are identified and a corresponding lookup component is created which matches a required key in the respective relation to resolve the relationship. Furthermore, it is checked whether a record is already existing in the database, also using a lookup component. Finally, the target component is created, which delivers the data to the target database.

6.6   Case Study and Evaluation

The architecture and its functional components have been evaluated with respect to several criteria in the course of a clinical pilot trial conducted by the Philips Research Europe Laboratories in Aachen.

In addition, the evaluation of the CTDMO with respect to the requirements and quality criteria we described in Section 6.3, we also evaluated the schema, mapping and integration module creation functionality according to usability and feasibility.

6.6.1   *The Heart Failure Management (HFM) Pilot Trial*

MyHeart is an FP6 Integrated Project, aiming to develop intelligent systems for the prevention and monitoring of cardiovascular diseases (CVD). The idea of the project is to develop smart devices for monitoring the health status of patients. Early diagnosis and guidance to a preventive lifestyle through electronic devices help to reduce the risk of CVD (http://www.hitech-projects.com/euprojects/myheart/).

The goal of the subproject Heart Failure Management (HFM) is to examine, how a decompensation of heart failure patients, i.e., a severe degradation of the state of health, can be predicted by collecting different vital signs using sensors and manual methods. Within the HFM project, a pilot study is conducted, which examines the quality and usability of special sensors to measure ECG, heart rate and other vital signs of an observed person. The pilot trial is conducted by the Philips research labs and the University Hospital in Aachen.

In addition to the sensor data, the physicians on site capture information gathered during measurements and findings in spreadsheets. There are different cycles of measurements during the trial. Some measurements are executed twice a day, some are running during night and some only take place at admission and discharge of the patients. The data is sent to the research labs once a day where statisticians analyze the data to get insights and to check the applicability. The data and files acquired during this trial have been used to evaluate the OnTrIS architecture. The first step has been the extension of the CTDMO with concepts required to fully describe the study.

6.6.2 Evaluation of the CTDMO

As described in Section 6.3, the CTDMO has already some concepts, which structure the ontology on a high abstraction level and that should help the user to easily add new concepts to the ontology.

The domain experts have been asked to extend the CTDMO with concepts and properties of the HFM study, in particular, representing the data which has been gathered by the physicians and scientists on-site.

A questionnaire has been elaborated, which is based on the suggestions for the evaluation of ontologies by Gomez-Perez [Gomez-Perez (2004)]. The questionnaire consists of five parts concerning the consistency, completeness, conciseness, extensibility and usability, and the documentation of the ontology.

Important outcomes according to usability were, that it is important for the users to get a personal introduction to ontologies, the editor, and the CTDMO structures. Due to the level of abstraction and the specific principles the CTDMO is based on, the inexperienced users had difficulties to extend the ontology only with the help of a written guideline.

After the instruction sessions the experts were able to model on their own, but still had some questions. They were, for example, unsure whether they had chosen the right way to model specific concepts and relationships. Their understanding of how to extend the ontology also improved a lot after they had seen the generated database schema. This indicates, that the modelling principles and goals are too strongly connected to the aim to convert the ontology into a relational schema.

6.6.3 Evaluation of the Mapping Definition and Integration Module Creation

The data integration part of this work has been evaluated according to two aspects. Firstly, the usability of this part of the application has been assessed. Furthermore, the feasibility of the data integration part is evaluated by discussing the challenges and issues while creating a data integration package for an example data source of the HFM pilot trial.

6.6.3.1 Evaluation of Usability

To assess the usability of the ontology-based data integration part of the application a questionnaire based on the ISO norm 9241 part 110 (cf. [ISO (1998)]) has been used. It turned out, that the users could easily generate a data source ontology and also had no problems with the creation of the mappings. The course of required steps were clear to them after a very short introduction. However, the learnability of the tool could still be improved as it required much time to understand the software. Nevertheless, we were satisfied with the results as the software tool is still a prototype, and it addresses a complex task which is hard to understand for non-database experts.

6.6.3.2 *Evaluation of Feasibility*

The data integration mechanism has been tested for the import of a complex Excel file, which is used in the HFM pilot trial to gather information about patients, findings,and the measurements conducted. The Excel file consists of 17 sheets, which are loosely related (relations are defined like in relational databases by keys, but without constraints, which are not supported by Excel). Therefore, this file format was a good example to test the mapping of simple datatype properties as well as mappings of object properties. To integrate the data from the example Excel source files in the database, 49 mappings have been defined. All possible cases (see Figure 6.1) have been tested, and all tests were successful. A typical issue, which occurred during mapping of the Excel data source ontology and the selected concepts, was the question on which level to map the properties. For example, if a concept *Subject* and its child concept *Patient_HFM* have been selected, and the user tries to map inherited properties on the *Patient_HFM* concept level, this will result in an error, because the corresponding table *Patient_HFM* does not contain the mapped property, but its parent table *Subject* does. This can be prevented in the mapping editor by hiding these inherited properties.

The algorithm to create the integration modules also ensures, that all values are inserted, as far as possible. If there is invalid data in an extracted data source row and the integration module cannot convert it implicitly, the row is ignored and redirected to an error log file. If one row is invalid, all other rows can be processed without stopping the ETL process. However, if records of other tables need to reference this record with a foreign key, the required record cannot be found and, thus, a NULL will be inserted instead of a correct ID. It has to be considered in daily use, if it is better to abort the ETL process, when an invalid row occurs, or to log the rows and go on with processing.

6.7 Related Work

Intensive efforts are made by commercial providers creating sophisticated ETL tools [Friedman *et al.* (2008)], which are also applied in the medical and pharmaceutical community [Gardner (2005)]. Nevertheless, ETL process creation based on metadata and holistic data integration approaches are still interesting topics in research. Especially, closing the gap between conceptual and logical ETL representations is still an active research area [Rizzi *et al.* (2006)].

Data Integration Based on Ontologies Ontology-based data integration approaches can be classified according to the number of ontologies used in the approach (single, multiple, and hybrid) and according to the degree of automation of the mapping definition (manual, semi-automatic, and automatic) [Bellatreche *et al.* (2004); Wache *et al.* (2001)].

Examples for single ontology approaches are SIMS [Arens *et al.* (1996)] and COIN [Madnick and Zhu (2005)], which both use a virtual mediator architecture. Other approaches, such as the OBSERVER system [Mena *et al.* (2000)], use multiple existing domain ontologies to describe the data repositories. The virtual integration architecture rewrites user queries based on relationships defined between the ontologies. Bellatreche *et al.* propose an automatic hybrid ontology architecture in which the ontologies for each data source are stored in an ontology-based database [Bellatreche *et al.* (2004)]. Furthermore, a global ontology is defined, which is referenced and can be extended by the local ontologies. The integration is made in two steps: first the ontologies are automatically integrated and subsequently the data.

Another hybrid but semi-automatic approach is MOMIS (Mediator Environment for Multiple Information Sources) [Beneventano *et al.* (2003)]. The system implements a Global-As-View approach. First, the source schemas are created by wrappers and annotated with terms from Word-Net. A common thesaurus is generated containing intra- and interschema relationships derived from the annotated source schemas. Based on the thesaurus and the source schemas, the global schema and mappings to the sources are automatically created.

Cruz and Xiao present a hybrid, virtual data integration approach [Cruz and Xiao (2009)], where users can issue queries to the global ontology and these are rewritten and send to ontologies describing the local schemas.

Creating ETL Processes Using Ontologies An early approach [Critchlow *et al.* (1998)] for creating ETL processes uses a single ontology to define the metadata for mediators on a high abstraction level. Concepts of the data sources and target database are mapped with each other by defining mappings inside the ontology. Another approach [Skoutas and Simitsis (2006)] automates the construction of ETL processes using a hybrid ontology principle. A common vocabulary is used to describe the data sources and the target database. Each data source is annotated with the vocabulary and notes for integration. This annotation constitutes the mapping for the data sources to the target database. An application ontology is created for each source according to the annotations. Based on this ontology, ETL processes can be automatically assembled using specifically defined transformation rules.

A current approach [Bergamaschi *et al.* (2009)] combines the data integration approach MOMIS described above with the clustering approach RELEVANT to create the mappings between the global schema and the data sources. They also provide a transformation function which enables the "semantic reconciliation of attribute values", i.e., values of source attributes mapped to an attribute in the global schema are merged to clusters including values with similar meaning. The cluster names are then used as values for the global schema attribute.

Discussion In contrast to the described systems, in this work an *end-to-end architecture* is offered to the user. The user can define the integrated schema as well as the mappings to the integrated schema in one system using an ontology-based approach. In addition, she can define a complete ETL process, which includes the mediator as well as the wrappers (the physical access to the data source). She can also define logistic tasks, such as file handling. Furthermore, the definition of the integrated schema by selecting concepts from the CTDMO, maintains the ontology as it is, hence, making it reusable for other applications. No metadata describing the target or the sources have to be added to the ontology which retains the ontology characteristic of describing domain knowledge.

6.8 Conclusion

Data management in clinical trials poses many challenges: several legal regulations and guidelines have to be obeyed while still providing an efficient and easy-to-use data management system. Furthermore, the users of such a system are often not data management and modeling experts, but they still have to manage the data of clinical trials efficiently such that reports and analyses based on the data can be done easily.

We have presented our ontology-based data integration system OnTrIS. It supports the modeling, management, and integration of data for a specific domain which we showed in a case study in clinical trials. The basis of the system is a core ontology; in the case study, the Clinical Trial Data Management Ontology (CTDMO), describing the field of clinical trials with medical devices. The CTDMO has been developed according to well-known guidelines for ontology development [Noy and McGuinness (2001)], and the evaluation has shown that the developed ontology is suitable for the given task. Modeling principles, such as modularity and structuring by the FDA device classification, have been rated useful within the evaluation.

The creation of the integrated database and the definition of mappings between sources and integrated schema is done on a conceptual level, using an ontology which is derived from the CTDMO by the user. This adaptation process requires additional effort by the user, but it is necessary for effective data management as each clinical trial has specific requirements for the data to be managed. In addition, by giving the user the ability to select a subset of the ontology as the basis for the integrated schema, we avoid unnecessarily complex database schemas and generate a schema which can be easily understood and efficiently queried.

The mappings are translated into executable, relational queries which are the basic building blocks of the ETL processes generated by OnTrIS. The ETL processes are implemented as data integration modules in MS SQL Server Integration Services.

During the usability testing it turned out, that the steps to create an integration module (define data sources, specify mappings etc.) are easily understandable to the users. Still, some users had problems with understanding and learning the mapping and integration functionality, because the full complexity of the integration process could not be completely hidden by our application.

The feasibility check using the HFM pilot trial, revealed strengths and weaknesses of the approach. The automatic creation of the packages and the easy execution is comfortable for the user. The handling of invalid rows of the data source is an issue, because skipping invalid rows can lead to inconsistencies in the data.

In a nutshell, we have shown that integration modules can be automatically created based on ontology mappings. In future extensions of the architecture further ETL tasks should be included, e.g., aggregation functions, the mapping of multiple source properties to one target property, or data type conversions. A generic metamodel [Kensche *et al.* (2007)] might enable the use of a wider range of modeling languages as source and target (e.g., XML Schema or object-oriented modeling languages). Schema matching [Rahm and Bernstein (2001); Quix *et al.* (2007)] can simplify the mapping process by providing candidate matches.

Acknowledgements: This work has been supported by the European research project *MyHeart* (http://www.hitech-projects.com/euprojects/myheart/) funded by the European Commission (6th framework, IST 507816) and by the DFG Research Cluster on Ultra High-Speed Mobile Information and Communication *UMIC* at RWTH Aachen University (http://www.umic.rwth-aachen.de).

Chapter 7

BIOBITS
A Study on Candidatus Glomeribacter Gigasporarum with a Data Warehouse

Francesca Cordero[1], Stefano Ghignone[2], Luisa Lanfranco[2], Giorgio Leonardi[3], Stefania Montani[3], Rosa Meo[1] and Luca Roversi[1]

[1] Università di Torino, Italy
[2] Università degli Studi di Torino, Italy
[3] Università del Piemonte Orientale, Italy

7.1 Introduction

Biotech is effectively changing the way the largest chemical companies do business, in which as demonstrated by pharmaceutical industries, DNA is used to create novel therapeutics. A crucial advance in this direction is coming from Metagenomics, the emerging science branch that has the potential to substantially impact industrial production, as shown by the company founded by Venter http://www.tigr.org/. Industries have different motivations to probe the enormous resource represented by uncultivated microbial diversity. Currently, there is a global political drive to promote biotechnologies as a central feature of the sustainable economic future of modern industrialized societies. This requires the development of novel enzymes, processes, products and applications.

Metagenomics is the branch of science that integrates biology and technology. Based on the genomic analysis of DNA, it has the power to solve problems in many different fields, from positively impacting human health to enabling a better understanding of the environment and agricultural systems as well as creating new biological sources of energy.

This chapter describes the on-going project BIOBITS[1] that aims to perform extensive comparative genomic studies in order to answer fundamental questions concerning the biology, ecology and evolutionary history.

The specific application field of these studies concerns the bacterial endosymbionts. These organisms are widespread in the animal kingdom, where they offer excellent models for investigating important biological events such as organelle evolution, genome reduction, and transfer of genetic information among host lineages [Moran *et al.* (2008)]. By contrast, examples of endobacteria living in fungi are limited [Lumini *et al.* (2006)] and those best investigated live in the cytoplasm of arbuscular mycorrhiza (AM) fungi [Bonfante and Anca (2009)]. AM fungi are themselves obligate symbionts since, to complete their life cycle, they must enter in association with the root of land plants. AM species, belonging to the family Gigasporaceae, have been grouped into a new taxon named Candidatus Glomeribacter gigasporarum [Bianciotto *et al.* (2003)]. The AM fungus and its endobacterium Ca. Glomeribacter gigasporarum are currently used as a model system to investigate endobacteria-AM fungi interactions.

The metagenomics focus of BIOBITS project is on studying the tripartite system: (i) endobacteria living in AM fungi, (ii) AM fungi living in plant roots, and (iii) plant roots, by the employment of a massive large-scale analysis and genomic comparison study of genomes belonging to phylogenetically related free-living bacteria. Moreover, the comparison with genomes of other endosymbionts species will provide insights about the reason of the strict endosymbiotic life style of this bacterium. Another aspect of metagenomics is the analysis of metabolic pathways. A strong reason of interest in this project is based on the assumption that the symbiotic consortia may lead to new metabolic pathways and to the appearance of molecules important for the development of novel therapies and other applications in biotech.

In this chapter we report specifically on a step of BIOBITS whose goal, roughly, is to develop a modular database which allows to import and store massive genomic data. Later in BIOBITS we will extensively develop computational genomic comparison (syntheny) focused on the above bacterium and fungi genomes. BIOBITS deploys a data warehouse that stores in a multi-dimensional model the interesting metagenomic components of the project. Such a metagenomic component should have the following char-

---

[1] BIOBITS is a project funded by Regione Piemonte under the Converging Technologies Call. BIOBITS involves Università di Torino, Università del Piemonte Orientale, CNR and the companies ISAGRO Ricerca s.r.l., GEOL Sas, Etica s.r.l.

acteristics: i) being able to store genomic data from multiple organisms, possibly taken from different public database sources; ii) annotating the genomic data making use of the alignment between the given sequences and the genomic sequences of other similar organisms; iii) annotating the genomic sequences and the protein transcript products by the full use of ontologies developed by the biology and bioinformatics communities; iv) comparing and visually presenting the results of the genomic alignment; iv) being able to cluster genomic or proteomic data coming from different organisms in order to easily find increasing levels of similarity and induce on one side the steps of the phylogenetic evolution and on the other side investigate on the metabolic pathways.

As a matter of fact, we wish to take advantage from the possibilities offered by computer science technology and its methodologies to analyse the genomic data the project will produce. The analysis of genomic data requires computing tools that allow to "navigate" flexibly data from arbitrary (at least in principle) user defined perspectives and under different degrees of approximation.

7.2 State-of-the-art of Metagenomics for Genomic Comparison

There is a wide variety of approaches in designing tools to analyze biological data. Experience suggests the best way to data analysis is to set up a database. An 'historical' example is ACeDB (A C.elegans Database), one of the first hierarchical, rather than relational, model organism databases. Another example is ArkDB [Hu J (2001)], a schema that was created to serve the needs for the subset of the model organism community interested in agriculturally important animals. ArkDB has been successfully used across different species by different communities, but is rarely used outside the agricultural community.

On "top" of databases a great variety of applications is available, from those ones for the annotation community to molecular pathway visualization, or from the workflow management to the comparative genome visualization.

Currently, there is a rich community and many available software tools built around GMOD(http://gmod.org/wiki/Main_Page) and MAGE (http://scgap.systemsbiology.net/standards/mage_miame.php).   GMOD stands for Generic Model Organism Database project (http://gmod.org), which brought to the development of a whole collection of software tools for creating and managing genome-scale biological databases, in the forthcoming description. In the BIOBITS project GMOD and its database Chado have been selected as the data elaboration and management center.

7.2.1   GMOD *and* Chado *Database*

The BIOBITS software architecture is built upon a layer provided by GMOD system. The design and implementation of database applications is time consuming and labor-intensive. When database applications are constructed to work with a particular schema, changes to the database schema require in turn changes to the software. Unfortunately, these changes are frequent in real projects due to changes in requirements. In particular they are frequent in bioinformatics. Most critical are the changes in the nature of the underlying data, which follow the current understanding of the natural world. Additional requirements are placed by the rapid technological changes in experimental methods and materials. Finally, the wide variety of biological properties in the organisms species always has made difficult to create a unique model schema valid for all the species.

All the above outlined motivations led to the design of Chado database model which is a generic and extensible model, whose software is available under an open source delivery policy. Chado schema can be employed as the core schema of any model organism data repository. This common schema increases interoperability between software modules that operate on it.

Chado data population is driven by *ontologies*, also known as *controlled vocabularies*. Ontologies give a typing to the entities with the result of partitioning the whole schema into *subschemas*, called *modules*. Each *module* encapsulates a different biological domain and uses an appropriate ontology. An ontology characterizes the different types of entities that exist in a world under consideration by means of primitive relations. These primitives are easy to understand and to use, are expressive and consitently allow the reasoning about the concepts under representation. Typical examples of ontological relations are: (i) *is_a* which expresses when a class of entities is a subclass of another class, and (ii) *part_of* which expresses when a component constitutes a composite. Many others are discussed in [Eilbeck and Lewis (2004)].

Concerning the schema of Chado it is worth remarking *feature* and *sequence* entities. *feature* allow both data and meta data. *feature* can be populated by instances each determining the type of every other instance in the schema, in accordance with the ontology SO [Eilbeck and Lewis (2004)]. *sequence* contains biological sequence features, that include genetically encoded entities like genes, their products, exons, regulatory regions, *etc. feature* and *sequence* are further described by properties.

7.3   BIOBITS System Architecture

Here we deepen the description of the system which is designed to manage all the information and all the in-silico activities in the context of the project BIOBITS. This system is implemented through a modular architecture, described in detail in Section 7.3.2. The system architecture permits (1) to store and access locally all the information regarding the organisms to be studied, and (2) to provide algorithms and user interfaces to support the researchers' activities like: (i) searching and retrieving genomes, (ii) comparing and aligning with a genome of reference, (iii) investigating syntenies and (iv) locally storing potentially new annotations.

The system architecture has been engineered exploiting the standard modules and interfaces offered by the GMOD project (http://gmod.org/wiki/Main_Page), and completed with custom modules to provide new functionalities. The main module of the system contains the database which provides all the data needed to perform the in-silico activities related to the project.

Thanks to the adoption of Chado database schema we take advantage for its support in controlled vocabularies and ontologies. Furthermore, Chado is the standard database for most of the GMOD modules; therefore we can reuse these modules to support the main activities of the project and extend the system incrementally as the researchers needs evolve. An example, is the possibility to use BioMart Chado's module which helps the user to identify the relevant dimensions of the problem, their hierarchies and to transform and import input data in the data warehouse conforming them in a typical star schema.

The database stores and provides in a multidimensional schema all the information about the organisms to be studied (i.e. bacteria), their genomes, their known annotations, their proteins and metabolic pathways, and the newly discovered annotations, which can be stored and managed locally until they are confirmed and published.

7.3.1   *Star Schema in* BIOBITS *Data Mart*

Essential in the data warehouse is the logical star schema of the stored data. The star schema defines the dimensions of the problem. Often, each dimension of the star schema can be viewed at different abstraction levels. The levels are organized in a hierarchy. Finally, the central entity in the star schema collects the main facts or events of interest. In the case of BIOBITS project, there are two star schemas.

(1) The star built around the *genome composition* facts. It represents the composition of each genome in terms of genes and chromosoms and with reference to the belonging organism.
(2) The star schema around *protein* facts. It describes the proteins in terms of PROSITE domains and with respect to the dimensions of phylogenetic classification and metabolic pathways.

The genes and proteins facts are linked by the relationship representing the enconding.

For most of the dimensions, such as genes and phylogenetic classification, the scientific literature already has provided an ontology (e.g. GO) and controlled vocabularies (e.g. COG) that are available in public domain databases and are imported in the system. Another example of available hierarchy on the genes and proteins are the family organizations.

In the following we describe the BIOBITS Data Mart schema (shown in Figure 7.1) in detail.

Genome composition: It includes all the relevant information about a genome fragment. Considering a fragment view of the genome, genome composition includes all the known fragments composing a genome: it reports the precise boundaries of the fragments (which depend on the user experience and discoveries), the start position and the fragment order w.r.t to the genome, its nucleotide sequence and strand.

Chromosome/Plasmid DNA: It specifies the localization of the fragment expressed by the number or the name of the corresponding chromosome/plasmid location. Indeed, the genome could be inserted either in a chromosome sequence or in a plasmid sequence.

Organism: It specifies both endosymbiotic and ectosymbiotic bacteria. Extensive comparative genomics studies of many organisms are needed. It represents the identifier, the organism scientific name and its classifications in the taxonomy database.

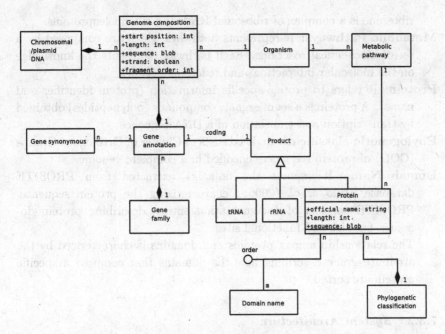

Fig. 7.1: Star schema of BIOBITS data mart.

Gene annotation: It consists in a short report of gene-specific information (identifier and name), comprehensive of a brief description of gene products using both the information reported in Gene Ontology and the main reference stored in Pubmed.

Gene synonymous: It contains all the synonymous names associated to each gene. Genes and proteins are often associated to multiple names; additional names are included as new functional or structural information is discovered. Since authors often alternate between synonyms, computational analysis benefits from collecting synonymous names.

Gene family: Following the gene classification into families, consistent to the genes biochemical similarity, it reports the family identifiers.

Product: It is a class of the products that genes codify. Products are categorized into in three classes: transfer RNA (tRNA), ribosomal RNA (rRNA) and proteins. Moreover it reports a pseudogene indication if the gene has lost its coding ability.

tRNA: Transfer RNA is a small RNA molecule that transfers a specific active amino acid to a growing polypeptide chain.

rRNA: Ribosomal RNA is the central component of the ribosome. The ribosome is a complex of ribosomal RNA and ribonucleoproteins.

Metabolic Pathways: It represents pathways which are composed by a set of biochemical reactions. Each pathway represents the knowledge on the molecular interactions and reactions network.

Protein: It refers to protein-specific information (protein identifier and name). A protein is a set of organic compounds (polypeptides) obtained by transcription and translation of a DNA sequence.

Phylogenetic classification: It consists of Cluster of Ortologous Groups (COG) of protein sequences encoded in a complete genome.

Domain Name: It reports the domains extracted from PROSITE database [Hulo *et al.* (2006)], characterizing the protein sequence. PROSITE consists of documentation entries describing protein domains, families and functional sites.

The relationship among proteins and domains is characterized by the attribute *order* describing how the domains that compose a specific protein are sorted.

7.3.2 *System Architecture*

Figure 7.2 summarizes the main architecture of **BIOBITS** system. In the following we focus on objectives and features of **BIOBITS** system.

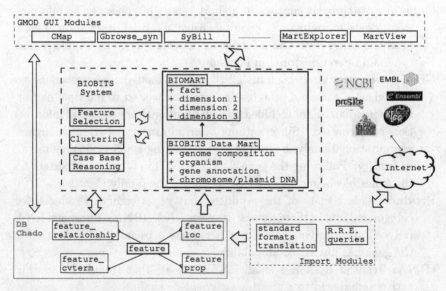

Fig. 7.2: The architecture of **BIOBITS** system.

Local and global access to data.   The instance of Chado we want to set up will contain both data on genome we shall explicitly produce as part of the project BIOBITS and data retrieved from the biological databases accessible through the Internet. The Import modules in Figure 7.2 will accomplish such a requirements. Concerning the retrival from Internet, *RRE - Queries* is a GUI wizard, built on the basis of a previously published tool [Lazzarato *et al.* (2004)], able to query different biological databases like, for example GenBank (http://www.ncbi.nlm.nih.gov/Genbank/), converting the results of the queries into standard formats. Alternatively, we can convert the format of data retrieved from Internet thanks to the scripts available as part of the GMOD project. A remarkable example are those scripts that convert GenBank genes annotations into the Generic Feature Format (GFF), adopted as a standard in the GMOD project. Of course, once data have been retrieved, *Import Modules* update Chado, either on-demand, or automatically, possibly on a regular basis.

An On Line Architecture Mining architecture.   One of the advantages of a data warehouse is the ready availability of clean, integrated and consolidated data represented by a multiplicity of dimensions. Once that data are stored in the data warehouse, elementary statistics can be computed on the available facts and aggregation of measures and frequencies of facts can be immediately computed. The results can be browsed and compared by OLAP primitives and tools. Finally, on these statistics the power of data mining algorithms can be further exploited. This is the On Line Architecture Mining (OLAM) view of a software architecture [Han and Kamber (2001)]. OLAM is composed by a suite of data mining algorithms that receive from the client a query for a knowledge discovery task. The request can be answered by the predictive and semi-automatic capabilities of data mining algorithms that work on the results of an underlying OLAP server that receives the input data from the underlying data warehouse.

For the transformation of the data stored in Chado into the star schema of Figure 7.1 we exploit BioMart (http://www.biomart.org/), which is a software package available inside GMOD.

7.3.2.1   *Services on Chado and the Star Schema*

In Figure 7.2, associated to both the Chado instance and to the BIOBITS data mart we plan to offer two types of services. One type is implemented on the basis of existing modules of GMOD. Figure 7.2 highlights them in the uppermost dashed box, named GMOD GUI Modules. The second type of services are internal to the real BIOBITS system: they are shown in Figure 7.2 inside the central dashed box, named BIOBITS system. Now, we discuss the latter components in more detail, putting much emphasis, of course, on the features of the software modules that we specifically develop to support the realization of the goals of the BIOBITS project.

GMOD Graphical User Interface Modules. These modules exploit the available GMOD modules using Chado database to provide the researchers with the tools for comparative genomics needed by the BIOBITS project. GUI modules have also a graphical user interface and allow the user to interact with the system. In particular,

- CMap allows users to explore comparisons of genetic and physical maps. The package also includes tools for maintaining map data;
- GBrowse is a genome viewer, and also permits the manipulation and the display of annotations on genomes;
- GBrowse_syn is a GBrowse-based synteny browser designed to display multiple genomes, with a central reference species compared to two or more additional species;
- Sybil is a system for comparative genomics visualizations;
- MartExplorer and MartView are two user interfaces allowing the user to explore and visualize the stored experimental results and the database content.

BIOBITS system specific modules. Their goal is to allow data analysis under two perspectives that should each other complement and validate.

The first perspective is the one offered by the *Case Base Reasoning* module. It supports efficient retrieval strategies in the context of the search for genomic similarity and syntenies, directly operating on our implementation of the star schema inside BioMart.

The other perspective will exploit tools from Data Mining. We shall use them to perform advanced elaboration on the genomic data. Among the data mining modules we foresee modules for classification, for feature selection and clustering. The latter will be discussed in more detail in this chapter, since it will be the first to be integrated into the BIOBITS system. Indeed, one of the main goal of the whole BIOBITS project is to provide the results of fragment alignment tools (syntheny). Since, clustering provides a specifically useful service for the exploration and elaboration of the similarities among genes and proteins, its results could provide to the syntheny tools additional information that would enhance the fragment elaboration.

As a concluding remark, the plan is to develop BIOBITS system specific modules as web-based GUI to gain user-friendliness, similar to current GMOD modules and will be able to connect to other modules by standard interfaces. Moreover, we do not exclude some work will be required to customize current GMOD modules to the usage requirements of biologists involved in the BIOBITS project. Of course we shall adhere to the open source philosophy. So, any BIOBITS system specific module will be available as part of the whole project GMOD.

7.4   Software Modules to Support Researchers' Activities

The following section will describe the details of the new modules introduced in the BIOBITS system.

7.4.1   *Case-based Reasoning*

Within the BIOBITS architecture, we are currently working at the design and implementation of an *intelligent retrieval* module, which implements the *retrieval* step of the Case-Based Reasoning (CBR) [Aamodt and Plaza (1994)] cycle. CBR is a reasoning paradigm that exploits the knowledge collected on previously experienced situations, known as *cases*. The CBR cycle operates by (1) *retrieving* past cases that are similar to the current one and by (2) *reusing* past successful solutions; (3) if necessary, past solutions are properly *adapted* to the new context in which are used; (4) the current case can then be *retained* and put into the system knowledge base, called the *case base*. *Purely retrieval* systems, leaving to the user the completion of the reasoning cycle (steps 2 to 4), are very valuable decision support tools [Watson (1997)], especially when automated adaptation strategies can hardly be identified, as in biology and medicine [Montani (2008)].

Our retrieval module is meant to support comparative genomic studies that represent a key instrument to: (i) discover or validate phylogenetic relationships, (ii) give insights on genome evolution, and (iii) infer metabolic functions of a particular organism.

7.4.1.1   *Multiple Abstractions on the Genome*

In our module, cases are genomes as sequences of nucleotides, each one taken from a different organism, and properly aligned with the same reference organism. For each nucleotide, a percentage of similarity with the aligned nucleotide in the reference organism is also provided. However, depending on the type of analysis which is required, a "view" of the genomes at the nucleotide level may not always be the most appropriate: sometimes, a "higher level" view, abstracting the available data at the level of genes, regions, or even complete chromosomes, would be more helpful. Our tool supports this need, by allowing the retrieval of the available cases at any level of detail, according to a taxonomy of granularities, which is depicted in figure 7.3.

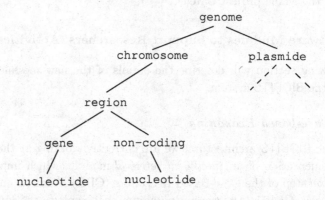

Fig. 7.3: A taxonomy of sequence granularities.

Moreover, a sequence of consecutive granules, sharing the same *qualitative level* (e.g. low, medium, high) of similarity with respect to the reference organism, can be abstracted into a single interval, labeled with the qualitative level of similarity itself: such an abstraction process is very similar to the Temporal Abstractions (TA) methodology, described in [Shahar (1997); Bellazzi *et al.* (1998)], even if in our domain the independent variable is the granules sequence instead of time. As in TA, in fact, we move from a *point-based* to an *interval-based* representation of the data, where the input points are the granules, and the output intervals (*episodes*) aggregate adjacent points sharing a common behavior, persistent over the sequence. In particular, we rely on *state* abstractions [Bellazzi *et al.* (1998)], to extract episodes associated with qualitative levels of similarity with the reference organism, where the mapping between qualitative abstractions and quantitative values (percentages) of similarity can be parametrized on the basis of domain knowledge.

Different levels of abstraction can be further exploited both to reduce space occupancy in the database and to allow the user to focus on a different level of detail.

In synthesis, our retrieval framework allows for *multi-level abstractions*, according to two *dimensions*, namely a taxonomy of state abstraction symbols, and a variety of sequence granularities. In particular, we allow for *flexible querying*, where queries can be expressed at any level of detail in both dimensions, also in an *interactive* fashion, progressively refining the retrieval set.

7.4.1.2 *Multi-dimensional Index Structures*

Moreover, our framework takes advantage of *multi-dimensional orthogonal index structures*, which make retrieval faster, allowing for early pruning and focusing. Technical details of the query answering algorithms can be found in [Montani *et al.* (2009)]. Indexes can be defined and grow on demand, depending on the types of queries issued so far. An example multi-dimensional index, rooted in the H symbol, is represented in figure 7.4.

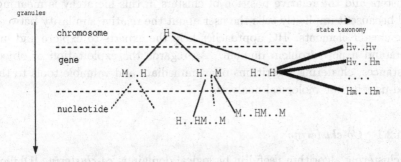

Fig. 7.4: An example multi-dimensional orthogonal index. Note that indexes may be incomplete with respect to the taxonomies: here, for instance, the *region* level is missing in the granularity dimension.

7.4.2 *Clustering Modules*

In this chapter we do not go in detail in describing all the predictive and exploratory capabilities offered by data mining algorithms. The aim of this section is to depict a portray built on a single example: *clustering*.

It offers the possibility to show the benefits in terms of interoperability, extendability and flexibility offered by a modular system built upon a data warehouse in which a multi-dimensional representation of a ground set of facts is stored. On these data, whenever it is needed, a query can be issued by the user in order to retrieve from the data warehouse the values of the interesting subset of dimensions. On this initial set of values multi-level reasoning is possible exploiting the relationships between facts in the knowledge network.

One of the classical aims of clustering is to provide a description of the data by means of an abstraction process. In many applications, the end-user is used to study natural phenomena by the relative proximity relationships existing among the analyzed objects. For instance, he/she compares organisms by means of the relative similarity in terms of the common features with respect to a same referential example. Many Hierarchical Clustering (HC) algorithms have the advantage that are able to produce a dendrogram which stores the history of the merge operations (or split) between clusters. Moreover, the dendrogram produced by a hierarchical clustering algorithm constitutes a useful, immediate and semantic-rich conceptual organization of the object space. As a result HC algorithms produce a hierarchy of clusters and the relative position of clusters in this hierarchy is meaningful because it implicitly tells the user about the relative similarity between the cluster elements. HC approaches help the experts to explore and understand a new problem domain. As regards the exploitation of object distances, clustering algorithms offer immediate and valuable tools to the end-user for the biological analysis.

7.4.2.1 *Co-clustering*

A clustering algorithm useful in biological domain is *co-clustering* [Dhillon *et al.* (2003)] whose solution provides contemporaneously a clustering of the objects and a clustering of the attributes. Further, often co-clustering algorithms exploit similarity measures on the clusters in the other dimension of the problem: that is, clusters of objects are evaluated by means of the clusters on the features and vice versa. They simultaneously produce a hierarchical organization in two of the problem dimensions: the objects and the features that describe the objects themselves. In many applications both hierarchies are extremely useful and are searched for.

An appealing algorithm based on co-clustering has been obtained by the introduction of *constraints*. Constraints are very effective in many applications, including gene expression analysis [Pensa et al. (2010)] and sequence analysis [Cordero et al. (2009)], since the user can express which type of biological knowledge leads to the association among gene clusters and biological condition clusters. The sequence analysis was directed into the discovery of gene motifs or protein domains. It relies on two main ideas: exhaustive search and automatic association of motifs with protein subfamilies. The same idea can be also applied on genome sequence in order to discover regularity associated to specific portions of the nucleotide sequence.

Sebat and co-authors report in [Sebat et al. (2003)] the importance of expression profile data in metagenomics. Indeed, the use of microarrays to profile metagenome libraries offers an effective approach to characterizing many organisms rapidly. As a consequence, in the future, microarray data could be integrated into the proposed star schema making possible this kind of analysis in our system. Constrained co-clustering algorithms will allow us to identify groups of genes that show similar activity patterns under a specific subset of the experimental conditions by measuring the similarity in expression within these groups. Under this view point, constraints are effective because take into account the similarity/dissimilarity between pairs of genes.

7.4.2.2   Proximity Measures

The majority of clustering algorithms are driven by distances between objects. In our multi-dimensional problem distances may be computed in different ways according to the dimension. Moreover distances can take into account the hierarchy on the dimension itself. Notice in fact, that for the main dimensions in the star schema of Section 7.3.1 (gene annotations, proteins, etc) a hierarchical ontology is defined (GO and orthology) starting from the available knowledge on the biological domain. Therefore, the hierarchies can be exploited to define a distance between two facts. Later these distances could be used for distance-based classification and clustering algorithms.

A distance measure d_i on a single dimension X_i can be integrated in the standard distance function (like the euclidean one) in an m-dimensional space. In the computation of the distance between two objects o_k and o_j, we can combine the distances between the values of any dimension in the two objects. The result of this combination is the following:

$$dist(o_k, o_j) = \sqrt{\sum_i d_i(o_k[X_i], o_j[X_i])^2}$$

where o_k and o_j represent two facts stored in the data warehouse fact table, X_i denotes i-th dimension in the star schema and finally $o_k[X_i]$ and $o_j[X_i]$ are the values of the dimension i for the two facts. $d_i(o_k[X_i], o_j[X_i])$ represents the computed distance measure between two facts with respect to the i-th dimension. Whenever, $o_k[X_i]$ and $o_j[X_i]$ represent two values of the dimension X_i in two different positions of the X_i hierarchy, a measure that takes into account the different position in the hierarchy can be adopted. We mention here [Wang *et al.* (2007)] in which such a measure has been proposed and frequently adopted for the gene ontology.

7.5 Conclusion

In this chapter we reported on BIOBITS project whose goal is to extensively develop a computational genomic comparison (known as syntheny) focused on the Ca. Glomeribacter gigasporarum bacterium and arbuscular mycorrhiza (AM) fungi genome.

We presented the software architecture essentially developed over an existing software layer provided by GMOD Community. GMOD system offers powerful data visualization and analysis tools, data warehouse modules, such as BioMart and the possibility to exploit import modules for the inclusion of data from the external, public resources. Furthermore, it contains the Chado database which presents an extensible and flexible model for any organism species built upon the generic concept of feature which can be customized by the use of types and ontologies.

We presented the logical data representation of the genomic and proteomic components of the biological problem: it has the form of a double star schema - the first one centered around the genetic fragments composing the genome and the second one on the proteins encoded by the genes.

Finally we presented the main software blocks of BIOBITS system: a Case-Based Reasoning module and a clustering module - first of a series of data mining modules that will be integrated in the future - which allow the user to retrieve and analyse in a flexible and intelligent way the data coming from the multidimensional star schema.

Both these modules complement each other. Case-Based Reasoning and temporal analysis retrieve the information at different abstraction levels, as needed by the analyst. Clustering provides a novel annotation to genetic sequences based on computational data mining algorithms. The annotation occurs on the basis of proximity measures defined by the analyst. Notice, however, that proximity could be defined on the genome fragments viewed at the desired abstraction level by the former Case-Based Reasoning module.

Chapter 8

Quality of Medical Data: A Case Study

Matteo Bertoni[1], Giuliano Furlini[2], Gianluca Gozzoli[1], Maria Paola Landini[2], Matteo Magnani[1], Antonio Messina[1], Danilo Montesi[1]

[1] *Università di Bologna Mura Anteo Zamboni, Bologna, Italy*
[2] *Azienda Ospedaliero-Universitaria di Bologna Policlinico S.Orsola-Malpighi, Bologna, Italy*

Daily hospital activities generate a very large amount of data, which are often stored inside information systems to enable their persistence and searchability and to increase their effectiveness. While these data are potentially very valuable, not only for direct patient care but also for statistical analysis, collecting a large amount of *low quality* data can be useless.

Quality, according to the International Organization for Standardization (ISO), is *the totality of features and characteristics of an entity that bears on its ability to satisfy stated and implied needs* [ISO95] and *the degree to which a set of inherent characteristics fulfils requirements* [ISO05]. This general concept can be applied to the data stored in hospital databases, in which case we speak of *data quality*. It is worth noticing that data quality is one aspect of a more general problem, not treated in this chapter, concerning the *quality of information processing in medical information systems*. This last problem regards additional aspects, e.g., paper archives, that do not directly concern data stored in digital database systems.

Storing low quality data may have negative consequences, and this is especially relevant in the context of medical databases, where wrong actions may determine irreversible events. As an example concerning the hospital under analysis in the second part of this chapter, in 2007 two kidney x-rays taken from two distinct people with the same surname were attributed to a single (healthy) person. As a consequence, a woman had a kidney unnecessarily removed and died after post-surgery complications[1].

Unfortunately, this is only one example of low data quality and of its implications, concerning the usage of an identifier (surname) corresponding to more than one person. In general, data quality is a complex concept, which can be split into many *dimensions* and should be verified and improved following a well defined methodology.

In this chapter, which extends our previous work [Bertoni *et al.* (2009)], we provide an introduction to the problem of data quality in the context of medical databases. In the next section we introduce the general problem of data quality, and discuss its specificities when applied to a medical context. In particular, we identify a set of quality dimensions which are particularly relevant in this context and can be used to simplify and organize the analysis of the quality of a working database. We also describe a methodology, i.e., a sequence of steps to be performed to assess these dimensions. In Section 8.2 we apply these concepts to a real database, and present a case study concerning a large medical database containing clinical and administrative data from hospitals and private clinics in the Bologna district area, in Italy. Finally, in Section 8.3 we discuss how to summarize the information collected using our data quality dimensions. We conclude with a summary of the results of the case study and of the main concepts presented in this chapter.

8.1   Introduction

Data quality has been defined as *fitness for use* by the US Census Bureau [Tupek (2006)]. Therefore, every data quality process must consider the intended application of the data itself. If the data have been collected for patient care, as it is usually the case for hospital digital archives, it may be unusable for other activities, e.g., epidemiological studies. As an example, consider a database field containing ZIP codes of birthplaces. Even if a significant percentage of this data is missing or erroneous, this will not have any consequences on therapy. However, it would definitely affect the result of a study correlating birthplaces with specific diseases. In general, the existence of poor quality data is an important problem with relevant consequences on everyday life.

---

[1]Appeared on the principal Italian newspapers, and available on line (in Italian) at: http://bologna.repubblica.it/dettaglio/santorsola-il-giallo-delle-lastre/1375658 (judicial proceeding under course).

In addition to being dependent on the context, data quality is a *multi-dimensional concept*. In order to fully characterize the quality of a dataset, this should be evaluated according to the quality of the **data** itself, the quality of the description of the data, also called **meta-data**, and the quality of the **system** used to manipulate it. Each of these criteria concerns many aspects, e.g., accuracy, completeness and interpretability, that depend themselves on the peculiar features of the data under consideration.

Finally, the analysis of the quality of data is influenced by its **structure** and **time validity**. Medical data are usually stored inside *relational databases*, that can be seen as collections of tables. A table is a set of *records*, or *rows*, each representing a real world entity — for example, a biological specimen analysis, or a patient's personal data. Columns contain specific attributes of each entity, e.g., a telephone number, name or ZIP code. In addition to this kind of data, which are usually called *structured*, hospital databases contain large amounts of *unstructured* data, e.g., x-ray images. Finally, from the point of view of time validity, medical databases mainly contain *stable data*, which are unlikely to change (e.g., test results), and *long-term-changing data*, having a low update rate (e.g., personal information).

8.1.1   *Quality and Medical Data*

Hospital databases may constitute a valuable source of information to conduct epidemiological research, when the data is representative of the population to be studied, and also to improve business processes, e.g., to identify and cut unnecessary and costly procedures [Gordis (2008)]. Moreover, such databases could be considered important after some studies on inappropriate laboratory use, in light of methodological criteria [van Walraven and Naylor (1998)] and with reference to an academic medical department [Miyakis *et al.* (2006)]. Therefore, these databases should be designed not just for immediate diagnosis, but also to support further analyses and to evaluate the suitability of the required tests. However, low quality data may negatively affect the result of these analyses.

Unfortunately, despite the relevance of their content, medical databases are not free from quality issues, as highlighted by the case study presented in the second part of this chapter, and consistently with the literature. As an example, in 1997 a study compared the encoding of cancer reports, processed by the South West Cancer Intelligence Service, with the physicians' original reports [Moss *et al.* (1997)]. A nine digit alphanumeric code was used to translate information about topography, behaviour and morphology of neoplasms into a database compliant format. Approximately two thirds of all coded pathology reports turned out to contain some error, and one out of four errors could distort incidence statistics, especially regarding rare cancers. In 2004, another study verified if diagnoses stored in administrative data sets corresponded to the correct written diagnoses, made by physicians during 348 unannounced visits on 45 standardized patients. The intent of this study was to obtain measures and localizations of errors during the complete management flow of medical data, and it turned out that the correct primary diagnosis was recorded for only 57% of visits [Peabody *et al.* (2004)].

8.1.2   *Features of Medical Data*

In the medical context, data present a set of absolutely unique features: they are **privacy-sensitive**, **heterogeneous** with regard to their type, format and source, and they are often **produced by different information systems**. Moreover, these data are primarily **directed at patient-care** activities, and data collections reflect this purpose.

Information concerning individuals' health is obviously highly sensitive, because of its intrinsic social and economic implications. As a consequence, the entire process of medical information management has to be strictly regulated and supervised in order to avoid improper uses. Furthermore, the ownership of medical records and aggregated data produced for statistical analysis is often unclear. As a result, accessing medical data not for patient-care activities can be very difficult.

Clinical data can be extremely heterogeneous with regard to type, format and source: the same kind of information can be sometimes stored as numerical values, images, videos or text. Data is often meaningful only when coupled with physicians' interpretation, expressed in unstructured natural languages (e.g., English, or Italian). The underlying meta-data, e.g., the description of the kinds of values that are acceptable inside a given column, is poorly characterized mathematically and the concept of *canonical form*[2] is almost absent. Each medical facility often has its own terminology and notations, making data comparison difficult, and different instruments or different information systems can produce incompatible data formats. As a consequence, medical data may be difficult to standardize, aggregate and analyze.

---

[2]A preferred notation encapsulating all equivalent forms of the same concept.

Finally, as we have aforementioned, medical data are usually produced, structured, stored and manipulated only to support patient care. Technical aspects and good practices of data production and storage are thus under-considered. For example, constraining the structure or format of the data can be unnecessary to practical activities related to patient care, but fundamental for statistical analysis. Therefore, one should expect poor impact from these data as far as statistical analysis is concerned.

8.1.3 *A Quality Methodology for Medical Data*

The Total Data Quality Methodology considers four steps in a data quality activity: *definition* of the data quality dimensions, *measurement* of metrics, *analysis* of the results to identify the sources of error, and *improvement* [Shankaranarayanan *et al.* (2000)]. Basically, there is a first phase in which data quality dimensions are selected and measured (steps 1 and 2), and a second phase where these measures are used to improve the quality of the data (steps 3 and 4). In the case study presented in the following we focus on the first phase. More in detail, the main steps performed during our analysis are the following, adapted from the abstract methodology presented in [Batini and Scannapieco (2006)]:

- *Data analysis*, to acquire knowledge on the schema and the semantics of the data.
- *Identification of critical areas.*
- *Extraction and exploration* of a sample of the critical data.
- *Choice of a set of quality dimensions.*
- *Extraction* of the complete data set to be analyzed.
- *Measurement.*

While data extraction may be technically challenging, the most important step of this methodology is certainly the definition of the dimensions of analysis. In fact, while this methodology can be applied to generic data quality problems, for each application there is a set of specific relevant dimensions. We conclude this general discussion of the data quality problem by presenting the main dimensions that can be found in real medical data quality activities, and that we will later use to perform our case study.

8.1.4   *Dimensions of Analysis*

The quality of medical information management is evidently a very important asset, that can be evaluated according to several *dimensions*. In its pioneering work, Donabedian defines three main dimensions of hospital information processing quality: *structure* (i.e., resources), *processes* and *outcome* [Donabedian (1980)]. When we speak of *data* quality we usually refer to a very specific *structural* aspect. In addition, we address this problem from the point of view of data analysis, and not as part of an assessment of the quality of the hospital information system.

Similarly, [Ammenwerth *et al.* (2007)] define six quality criteria for the evaluation of the outcome of hospital information processing:

- Q1 Availability.
- Q2 Correctness and completeness.
- Q3 Readability.
- Q4 Usability for statistical analysis.
- Q5 Fulfilment of legal regulations.
- Q6 Time needed.

All our dimensions can be seen as a detailed specification of Q4: usability for statistical analysis. Although some of the other quality criteria may seem related to our dimensions (e.g., completeness) they refer to different domains. In particular, these criteria measure how well information processing tools support clinical and administrative workflows, while we focus on the support to data analysis. In addition, we deal with digital data, while in [Ammenwerth *et al.* (2007)] the authors consider all kinds of information, including paper data. Therefore, as we mentioned in the introduction, our work can be seen as an in-depth investigation of a specific aspect of a more general assessment process.

The following quality dimensions have been selected after the analysis of a large medical database, presented in the second part of the chapter, among the ones discussed in the literature [Wang and Strong (1996); Wand and Wang (1996); Redman (1997)], and can be classified into *data-related*, *meta-data related* and *system-related* dimensions.

8.1.4.1   *Data-related Dimensions*

Data-related dimensions regard the *content* of the tables stored in the medical database. In this section we briefly present the following: accuracy, completeness, consistency, interpretability, representation consistency, precision consistency and trustability.

Inaccuracy implies that the information system represents a real world state different from the one that should have been represented [Wand and Wang (1996)]. Therefore, accuracy provides a measure of erroneous data. There are two relevant kinds of accuracy: syntactic (if the value does not belong to the expected domain) and semantic (if the value belongs to the expected domain but is wrong). An example of syntactic inaccuracy is the time 25.12, because 25 is outside the domain of valid hours, i.e., [0–23]. Clearly, these inaccuracies are easy to identify. Then, there can be semantic inaccuracies, like 11.30 (in case the hour is wrong). These are very difficult to identify in general, and they can be usually verified only if the database contains functional dependencies[3] (in which case inaccuracies may generate inconsistencies) or if external information is available.

Incompleteness indicates that some data is missing. A first case of incompleteness regards missing rows. A second case regards missing values inside existing rows. In this case, values can be replaced by NULL values, making completeness check very easy, or they can be represented using special values, like empty strings or the value 0.

Inconsistency is a state in which semantic rules, defined over the rows of the tables, are violated. The majority of consistency errors are determined by missing integrity constraints: missing domain constraints[4], missing key constraints (more than one entity corresponding to the same identifier), missing functional dependencies.

Representation **consistency** refers to the fact that different instances of the same values are always represented in the same way [Loshin (2001)]. For example. we have representation inconsistency if a negative outcome of a test is stored sometimes as NEGATIVE and sometimes as N. This is often due to the absence of domain constraints — therefore, this dimension can be seen as a specific kind of data consistency. In addition, we may also find that similar values are expressed using varying degrees of **precision**, e.g., 615 ± 10 or 615 ± 100.

Data **interpretability** regards the documentation and information

---

[3]A functional dependency imposes that the values contained in some columns are determined by the values stored in other columns. An example is the name of a city which is determined by the ZIP code. When a value is wrong, dependencies may no longer be satisfied.

[4]A domain constraint specifies which values are allowed inside a column. As an example, a date (Nov. 30, 2009) can be represented inside a database as a date or as a generic sequence of characters. Only in the first case the value Nov. 35, 2009 would be identified as an error, and automatically rejected by the system.

sources that can be used to interpret the meaning of the data. For example, the value 615 cannot be interpreted without a unit of measure or some meta-data describing it.

Finally, in [Wang and Strong (1996)] **trustability** of a data source corresponds to three dimensions: believability (how much the data can be regarded as true), reputation of the information source, and objectivity, which measures the impartiality of the source.

8.1.4.2   *Meta-data-related Dimensions*

Meta data-related dimensions regard the *header* of the tables stored in the medical database, and all the additional information regarding the data that is considered valid for each column. This information in its entirety is often called *schema*, and its main dimensions are interpretability, normalization, minimization, pertinence and completeness.

Schema **interpretability** regards the documentation and information sources that can be used to interpret the meaning of the schema: names and meaning of tables and columns, and relations between them.

A **normalized** schema can be seen as set of tables that cannot contain redundant data. Normalization is very important, because whenever we duplicate some data it is possible that only one of its copies is later modified, creating an inconsistency. In fact, data inconsistency may be an expression of an unnormalized schema. A related dimension is **minimality**, which is verified when there are no redundant columns — for example, if we store admission and discharge dates, it is not necessary to keep an additional column to store the duration of hospitalization.

Minimality concerns the presence of columns containing relevant data which are already stored, sometimes implicitly, inside other columns. On the contrary, **pertinence** refers to columns or tables containing data which are relevant to the expected use of the database. Therefore, we may have one or more columns containing data which are not redundant, but of no interest — in which case we will have a low level of pertinence. Finally, a schema is **complete** if all the data of interest can be stored inside the database, i.e., there is at least one column for each attribute of the data we would like to represent. Obviously, this notion is not absolute but depends on the requirements of the users.

8.1.4.3 *System-related Dimensions*

Databases are useful only when a system is available to store and extract information into and from them. Therefore, in evaluating the quality of a database it is also important to consider some features of the systems used to manage it.

Accessibility measures the ability of users to access the data, with regard to the technology they can use and their knowledge of the data. **Access security** provides a measure of the quality of data access processes and tools, to verify if only authorized people can retrieve specific portions of the data.

8.2 Case Study

In this section we evaluate the data quality of a medical database containing clinical and administrative data from hospitals and private clinics in the Bologna district area (Italy). In particular, we focus on the data processed by microbiology laboratories. The objective of this case study is to determine to which extent this data could be used to perform a data analysis activity, and in particular to identify the relationships between hepatitides, personal information (age, gender, place of residence, nationality) and test number and type.

8.2.1 *Description and Extraction of the Data*

The source database is stored on an Oracle 10g system and is part of a complex clinical information system located at University Hospital "S. Orsola–Malpighi" and shared between all public hospitals in the Bologna district area. The database contains 1,352 tables, has a size on the order of several ten million records, and stores both administrative and clinical data used to partially automate daily workflows in clinical laboratories.

Through interviews with the staff of the Microbiology Unit, we acquired a preliminary knowledge of the content of the relevant portion of the database, which is illustrated in Figure 8.1. The database stores requests of tests, each associated to a single patient. The result of each biological specimen analysis is stored in a dedicated column, and a medical report is then produced, containing all the available results. Requests for analyses can be submitted by hospital physicians, departments, private clinics, or by specialized Unified Booking Centers (CUP[5]).

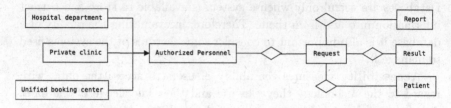

Fig. 8.1: Conceptual diagram of the analyzed portion of the database.

In the relational database, all the concepts illustrated in Figure 8.1 are logically and physically stored partitioning the data into three sets of tables with the same attributes (columns), where records are accommodated by time. As shown in Figure 8.2, the first set of tables stores daily data, the second one is filled at night with the records of the previous day, and the third one is used to archive older records. In addition, all tables containing personal data have a corresponding companion table (indicated by the prefix MODIFIED) to keep the history of address changes and other updates.

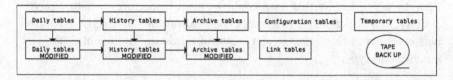

Fig. 8.2: Physical organization of the database, and life cycle of the data
— arrows indicate that records are moved from one partition to another after a predefined amount of time, or when they are modified.

From these tables, we have first extracted a random sample of 23,946 tests executed from year 2006 to 2008 on 5,618 distinct patients, to explore the data and identify the dimensions of data quality to be later evaluated on a larger data set. Then, we have extracted all the data pertaining requests for analyses from April 2007 to June 2008, to evaluate and measure these dimensions. This data set contained 3,096,268 tests and about 1,243,000 distinct patients. This activity is known as ETL (Extract, Transform and Loading) process [Kimball and Ross (2002)].

As a technical note, after a first attempt to extract the data using MS

---

[5]http://www.cup2000.it

Access as an interface over the Oracle database (the only tool to which we had access at the beginning) and the open source ETL tools Pentaho[6] and JasperETL[7], we asked to have access to Oracle clients for performance reasons. Tables containing test results were processed using Oracle Export scripts, performing partial extractions of data not to affect system performance — this because the database is active 24/7 and shared between hundreds of final users. These dump files were later loaded into an Oracle Express Edition database management system and exported as a single CSV file.

Moreover, tables with personal data were anonymized as follows:

- We removed names, surnames, telephone and fax numbers, and email addresses.
- We kept only ZIP codes and cities from the addresses.
- We removed the first 6 digits from national identification numbers, representing part of name and surname (the remaining ten characters encode place and date of birth).

While these steps do not necessarily produce a k-anonymous data set for a given k [Sweeney (2002b)], they can be performed without practically affecting the computational complexity of the extraction process. In addition, all the results of our study have been reported in aggregate form or without reference to single record identifiers. As these operations require the expression of SQL queries, not allowed by the Oracle Export utility, we used Oracle SQL*Plus to create the CSV files. This approach, even though simple, proved to be even faster than Oracle Export, extracting data at a speed in the order of ten thousand records per second. At the end of this process we had all the data in CSV format, ready to be imported in the target SQLServer 2008 database.

The ETL activity resulted in two different tables dedicated respectively to personal information and test results. Data were subsequently joined into a single table, to enable efficient analysis.

8.2.2 *Quality Assessment*

We started our analysis by identifying all sources of the data, to highlight potential inconsistencies due to disparate sources. In our case, we worked on a single database, so we did not have heterogeneity problems regarding its

---

[6]http://kettle.pentaho.org/
[7]http://www.jaspersoft.com/JasperSoft_JasperETL.html

schema, e.g., tables or columns with different names containing semantically related data. However, the database was filled by several organizations, therefore we had to look for heterogeneity at the data level. Data entry was performed by different entities such as hospitals' administrative offices and national health points of booking. Each of these structures applied different methodologies, from both an administrative and clinical point of view, and we will see that this has been reflected on the data.

8.2.2.1 *Data*

In the database, we identified about 500 syntactic **inaccuracies** regarding years of birth, following different patterns:

- Missing century, e.g., 0081 instead of 1981.
- Swapped digits, e.g., 1697 instead of 1967.
- Wrong century, e.g., 0181, 0981, 1081 instead of 1981.

Similar syntactic inaccuracies concerned ZIP codes: they should be 5 digit long, but we identified about 800 shorter values. It is worth noticing that some ZIP fields contained two-character city codes (e.g., BO for Bologna), which could be used to repair the corresponding tuples.

With regard to other significant attributes, about 3,500 records contained the value N instead of M or F on the gender column, and about 8,500 contained invalid national identification numbers. Finally, more than 2% of the tests were of uncertain attribution. Other inaccuracies that can be classified more specifically, like completeness and inconsistency, are treated in the following sections.

With regard to data **completeness**, we could not identify missing tuples from the analysis of the data, because there were no dangling references — however, this does not exclude the existence of missing tuples. On the contrary, we could verify a significant number of missing values (not represented using NULLs, but empty strings or the value 0). 45% of the fields in the table with personal data were empty. Among these, 29% of the patients lacked at least one of the two ZIP codes (temporary and permanent addresses), and in particular 27% lacked the one regarding temporary address and 21% lacked the other. About 67,000 patient records (5%) lacked the national identification number.

The majority of **consistency** errors were determined by missing integrity constraints:

(1) *Missing domain constraints*: all columns except the ones containing

dates had a `VARCHAR` type. Therefore, their content was not constrained. This is typical in medical databases, where users want to be free to write everything, and the database is seen as an extension of paper reports.

(2) *Missing key constraints*: the data with personal information contained two identifiers: a patient ID and the national identification number. However, the correspondence was not one-to-one: on average, each national identification number was associated to 1.2 IDs on average (up to about 90), and in one case the same patient ID had two distinct national identification numbers. The first fact, which shows that the table does not contain one single record for each real person, highlights a problem in the process of registering new patients. Notice that these values can be overestimated, because after anonymization there may no longer be a one-to-one relationship between national identification number and individuals.

(3) *Missing functional dependencies*: The relationship between ZIP code and municipalities should have been one-to-one but the average number of different codes linked with each municipality was 2.19 (up to 54 values for the city of Casalecchio di Reno, and excluding Bologna which regularly has more than one ZIP code), and 14% of the patients with temporary and permanent address in the same town have different ZIP codes.

With regard to **interpretability**, in the database the results of several tests are expressed using abbreviated codes, and from an interview with the responsible of the database and of the Microbiology Unit it appeared that not all the codes were meaningful. The cause of this problem can be found in the multiple sources populating the database, and the absence of standard codes.

Being unconstrained, columns storing the result of tests do not contain a single kind of values. Analyzing the data we noticed that more than 58,000 ($\sim$1.9%) results did not have an accurate numerical value but an approximation (i.e. ≥ 250). For example, if we consider the QHCV (Quantitative Hepatitis C Virus) test, results are expressed in terms of intervals, e.g, <600, in terms of point values, e.g., 1,048, and using symbolic values, e.g., N. While this is easily understandable by a doctor, it poses difficulties when we want to analyze the data, which must be preprocessed to obtain a consistent representation (for example, by clustering the results into two classes `POSITIVE` and `NEGATIVE`).

Similarly, even when only symbolic values are used, there may be alternative representations of the same result (e.g., NEGATIVO (negative) and N). A similar problem concerned the extensive use of abbreviations: there were 1,153 non-numeric different values indicating test results, many of them with the same meaning: boolean results such as Negative/Positive had about 90 synonyms.

The two values <600 and NEGATIVE mentioned in the previous paragraphs constitute a problem of **inconsistent representation** of the data (two ways of representing the same concept), but their **precision** is the same. However, we have also identified the contemporary presence of values at different levels of precision, e.g., <600 and 323.

As we have aforementioned, **trustability** and its sub-dimensions *believability, reputation* and *objectivity* can be used to define the quality of the data sources. In our analysis, other dimensions (accuracy and consistency) already provide an assessment of *believability*. With regard to reputation and objectivity, we notice that the database can be filled only by hospital departments, recognized private clinics, and booking centers, and all updates are logged, allowing traceability.

8.2.2.2   *Meta-data*

Before performing our analysis, we expected a good schema (metadata) quality, both because the database is relational, i.e., structured, and because the same schema is in use in other hospitals, being provided by an external specialized company. However, as we will see, also the schema suffered from quality problems.

The names of the columns are concatenations of strings indicating the type of the column and its actual name. While this is not a good practice, after having understood the convention it is easy to read the column names, expressing the meaning of their data. While the names can be easily *interpreted*, it is more difficult to *understand* their meaning without the help of a domain expert with some knowledge of the medical procedures. While we may assume that this knowledge is owned by the users of the database, some documentation would certainly increase its understandability.

However, the main problem regarding schema **interpretability** concerns the semantics of the several partitions described in Section 8.2.1. These partitions are used to store data during different phases of their life cycle, but we have found records with dates not compatible with the description of the tables.

Now, we focus on schema normalization, minimization, pertinence and completeness, i.e., those dimensions to be used to check if the tables and columns contained in the database match exactly the information we would like to represent.

The schema is not **normalized**, as already indicated while discussing the consistency of the data. The missing functional dependencies regarding ZIP codes are in fact the cause of inconsistent values in ZIP codes and cities. Similarly, there should be a dependency between patient identifier and national identification number, which does not seem to be present. Schema **minimization** has been manually checked, and no redundant attributes have been identified. Many attributes seem not to be **pertinent**, and this is shown by the fact that they are never or rarely used. Using a threshold of 99.5% empty fields to consider a column as empty, 4 columns out of 27 for personal data and 6 columns out of 66 for test data were empty, and thus practically useless.

Finally, the database schema appears to be **complete**, because the system administrator has not notified any data that could not be stored inside the database — obviously, this notion is not absolute but depends on the requirements of the users. However, the N indicated in some records on the gender attribute may be interpreted as a flag — we could not verify this hypothesis, but it was suggested by some internal users. In this case, this would indicate the existence of a missing attribute/column, replaced using the gender, and thus a schema incompleteness. Anyway, this is certainly a case of poor documentation.

8.2.2.3 *System*

Accessibility measures the ability of users to access the data, with regard to the technology he/she can use and his/her knowledge of the data. We remind the reader that the database is mainly used for patient care, and to support this activity it has an application interface that enables the personnel to interact with it. However, we have not analyzed this interface, as this is not object of our analysis. To manipulate the data, hospital workstations use MS Access as an interface over the Oracle database, which is not adequate both from an usability point of view (tables must be manually linked because the tool does not import schema constraints) and for efficiency reasons (it is practically impossible to manage queries with only a few join tables or retrieving hundreds of thousand tuples). As previously said, when it became evident that this program was not adequate to manage the required volume of data, we switched to Oracle shell and clients to perform our study.

The database was accessible only from inside the hospital intranet, through time-limited individual passwords with varying access privileges created by the local administrators. It is worth noticing that this dimension has been evaluated only with regard to the operations performed to make our data quality analysis. An extensive study of the security of the whole information system was outside the scope of our contribution.

8.3 Generation of a Summary Table

The figures presented in the previous section may be difficult to be used to define quality improvement activities. The fact that 8,500 national identification numbers are syntactically wrong does not constitute a problem of data quality in itself, but only if it is considered as such. Therefore, to make these measurements usable we need to provide an interpretation. In particular, to obtain a clean summary of the data analysis activity, we have defined three classes of quality[8] (Low – Average – High).

As the judgement of a statistical figure is an expression of personal opinion, asking several people to map the results of data analysis to these degrees of quality may increase the value of the outcome. In fact, someone could identify an area of criticality not perceived by others. Several techniques can be used to aggregate the opinions of different experts. While aggregation of judgements may be difficult, and majority voting can produce inconsistent results in general, majority voting can be used without negative consequences when the simple aggregation of alternative choices is involved [List and Puppe (2009)]. Alternatively, we may interpret single judgements as preferences, and merge them using operators like *min*, which result in highlighting the fact that someone is considering a given dimension as critical [Benferhat *et al.* (2006)]. Alternatively, if we want to keep all opinions and there is a satisfactory degree of agreement, we may indicate the *union* of all judgements. While other aggregation rules may be used, it seems that no additional efforts should be put into this activity, considering the simple aim of this summarization step.

The result of this summarization, as performed by the members of our research group, is indicated in Table 8.1. This table provides an ordering

---

[8]The choice of the number of classes is evidently arbitrary, the only requirement is to provide an intuitive summarization.

Table 8.1: Dimensions of data quality and their qualitative evaluation. All members of the research group assigned a degree of quality (L: low quality, A: average quality, H: high quality) to each analyzed dimension. For each dimension we indicate the most frequent degree, also called majority voting (maj.), the lowest degree, to emphasize potential criticalities (min.), and the set of all assigned degrees (union)

Dimension	Maj.	Min.	Union
Data			
accuracy	A	A	A
completeness	L	L	L
consistency	L	L	L/A
interpretability	L	L	L/A
representation consistency	L	L	L
precision consistency	L	L	L/A
trustability	H	H	H
Schema			
interpretability	A	A	A/H
normalization	A	L	L/A
minimization	H	H	H
pertinence	L	L	L/A
completeness	H	H	H
System			
accessibility	L	L	L/A
access security	H	H	H

with respect to the priority concerning the analyzed dimensions. For example, data completeness and data representation consistency turn out to be the most important aspects to be improved.

8.4 Conclusion

In this chapter we have provided an introduction to the problem of data quality in the context of medical databases. In particular, we have shown that data quality is a context-dependent and multidimensional concept. Therefore, we have selected some criteria and dimensions resulting from the analysis of the quality of a large medical database.

The application of these dimensions presented in the case study allowed us to identify a number of data quality issues that can be summarized as follows: wrong dates, wrong ZIP codes, wrong genders, a large amount of missing data, absence of domain, key and functional constraints, difficult interpretability of some test results, inconsistent representation of values (intervals, point values and abbreviations), synonyms, different precisions in the representation of test results, un-normalized tables without a well understood semantics, and useless columns. Many of these problems regard data entry, this suggesting low motivation and training of personnel, as well as the adoption of an interface allowing to introduce wrong data and a database with missing constraints.

While designing a hospital database, it would be important to consider its usefulness to support data analysis, which may have a greater impact on National Health Services than the management of each single test. The findings of this work provide an experimental validation of the idea that before using hospital data to perform data analysis it is fundamental not only to verify if the selectivity in hospital admissions may bias the result of the analysis, but also if the quality of the data is adequate. The detailed dimensions of quality used in our work can be then used as a guideline to identify the sources of errors and define appropriate improvement procedures.

Chapter 9

Efficient EMD-based Similarity Search in Medical Image Databases

Marc Wichterich[1], Philipp Kranen[1], Ira Assent[2] and Thomas Seidl[1]

[1] *RWTH Aachen University, Germany*
[2] *Aalborg University, Denmark*

9.1 Introduction

Over the past few decades, advances in digital imaging have led to widespread use of image data in medicine and the life sciences and to the creation of large image databases. Diagnoses and scientific research and analysis can be aided by the retrieval of similar images within these databases. For example, an image similar to one taken for a medical case under investigation might support the validation of a diagnostic hypothesis.

Similarity search requires effective distance measures to separate relevant images from the majority of the database. The Earth Mover's Distance (EMD) has been shown to provide excellent classification and retrieval performance [Puzicha *et al.* (1999)] and has been successfully used in medical and other applications. Moreover, it is robust with respect to errors that might originate from measuring inaccuracies, quantization effects, or artifacts of medical imaging processes, to name a few examples.

The retrieval performance however comes at a price in terms of computational cost. The EMD is defined as the minimal amount of changes required to transfer one image feature representation into another. To compute the EMD, a linear optimization has to be solved, which can be achieved using the simplex method for transportation problems [Hillier and Lieberman (1990)].

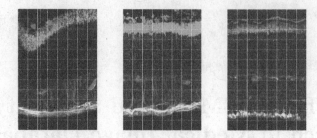

Fig. 9.1: RETINA: Images from the UCSB Bio-image Database [Ljoså *et al.*
(2006)], (http://www.bioimage.ucsb.edu).

Due to the complexity of the underlying optimization problem, filter
and refine approaches have been proposed in the literature that reduce the
number of costly EMD computations. This reduces the necessary time to
answer a query, which is crucial for doctors or scientists who cannot be
expected to tolerate long waits when working with the data.

In contrast to arbitrary image databases as found on home PCs or on
the web, medical databases often contain many similar images since they
stem from a domain-specific application. Moreover, the differences in their
feature representation are also likely to exhibit certain similarities due to
the underlying task. This chapter describes an approach from [Wichterich
et al. (2008)], which is especially suitable for such domain-specific image
databases in medicine or life sciences. The goal is to speed up EMD-based
similarity search on medical image data to enable medical personnel to
profit from the excellent retrieval performance of the EMD in a reasonable
amount of time. For this purpose, we provide a dimensionality reduction
technique for the EMD that takes the characteristics of the application data
into account and that guarantees completeness of the result. To achieve this
goal we formally define dimensionality reduction for the EMD in Section
9.2.1 and prove an optimal reduced cost matrix that is used in the EMD in
Section 9.2.2. We argue that finding the optimal reduction is infeasible due
to the time complexity, hence good heuristic solutions are required. We
present a data-dependent approach in Section 9.2.3 along with a detailed
discussion and helpful pseudo codes for the main parts of the algorithm.
Further advantages of the approach are the flexibility in choosing the degree
of reduction through the number of reduced dimensions and the possibility
of combining the described filter with existing EMD filtering techniques.

We show the efficiency of the approach on medical image data from

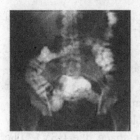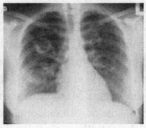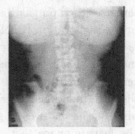

Fig. 9.2: IRMA: Image Retrieval in Medical Applications project [Lehmann *et al.* (2004); Deselaers *et al.* (2005)], (http://www.irma-project.org/datasets_en.php).

the UCSB Bio-image Database (http://www.bioimage.ucsb.edu) of feline retina scans labeled with various antibodies. Example images are shown in Fig. 9.1. Efficiency is also demonstrated on data from the Image Retrieval in Medical Applications project (http://www.irma-project.org/datasets_en.php), which contains radiography images from medicine as depicted in Fig. 9.2.

Before detailing the proposed approach, we review related work, formally introduce the Earth Mover's Distance, and detail the multi-step filter-and-refine querying process.

9.1.1 *Related Work*

The EMD is an adaptable distance function that was developed in computer vision as a perceptually meaningful dissimilarity measure [Rubner *et al.* (1998)]. It has been successfully used in a number of application areas as diverse as physics [Lavin *et al.* (1998)] and musicology [Typke *et al.* (2003)] and also in a number of medical and life science applications. For example, the EMD is used to discern personal characteristics from common search patterns in a recent study of cognitive processes associated with visual search [Dempere-Marco *et al.* (2006)]. Leff *et al.* use manifold embedding and the EMD to quantify cortical patterns of surgical expertise in functional near infrared spectroscopy data [Leff *et al.* (2007)]. It is employed to assess the change in CT scans in order to measure disease progression in advanced cancers [Nwogu and Corso (2008)]. In [Saalbach *et al.* (2005)], dynamic contrast-enhanced MRI similarities are assessed using the EMD. The EMD has also been found to be an effective distance measure for clinical decision-making based on gastroscopic images [Wu and Tai (2009)] and for medical image registration [Chefd'hotel and Bousquet (2007)].

To increase the efficiency of EMD-based retrieval processes in multi-media databases, a number of techniques have been developed. The approaches in [Rubner *et al.* (1998)] and [Assent *et al.* (2006)] devise filter distance functions other than the EMD and are limited by the dimensionality of the features (e.g. 64 in 64-dimensional color histograms) and by the feature space (e.g. 3 in a 3-dimensional color space like HSV). The filter proposed in [Ljoså *et al.* (2006)] allows for variability regarding the dimensionality of the feature representations in fixed hierarchical steps of factor 4. For a filter to ensure completeness of the result in a multi-step filter-and-refine querying process (cf. Section 9.1.3), it has to be a lower bound of the original distance [Korn *et al.* (1996); Seidl and Kriegel (1998)]. Other approaches perform approximate similarity search, i.e. they do not guarantee completeness of the retrieval process. In [Indyk and Thaper (2003); Grauman and Darrell (2004)] the EMD is embedded into a high-dimensional L_1 space with an upper bound for the distortion. In [Klein and Veltkamp (2005)] upper bounds for the minimum of the EMD over families of transforms on the input are presented. None of these approaches takes the characteristics of the database into account, i.e. they are all data independent approaches. For fast and complete similarity search in domain-specific medical image databases we describe a lower-bounding filter based on dimensionality reduction for the EMD that takes the characteristics of the application data into account.

9.1.2 *Formal Definition of the Earth Mover's Distance*

Unlike bin-by-bin distance measures commonly employed in similarity search, the EMD is a so-called cross-bin distance measure. Given widely used feature histograms of vector form $x = (x_i, \ldots, x_d) \in \mathbb{R}^d$ as a representation of the feature distribution of data objects to be compared, bin-by-bin distance measures such as L_p norms ($L_p(x, y) = \sqrt[p]{\sum_{i=1}^{d} |x_i - y_i|^p}$) compute histogram distances by comparing one histograms bin at a time. The correlation between differing bins is ignored. For example, if similarity is defined based on colors occurring in the images, then the feature distribution is extracted as the number of image pixels that belong to each bin x_i (represents a certain range of colors in the color space). Small changes in color may lead to large distances when two similar colors are assigned to differing bins. This contrasts with human perception, where the overall

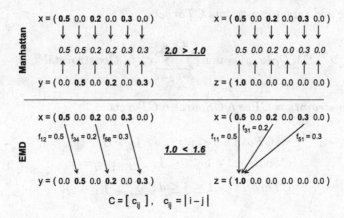

Fig. 9.3: The Earth Mover's Distance as a cross-bin approach reflects the perceived similarity better than more simple bin-by-bin approaches.

color distribution outweighs small color changes. An example is given in Figure 9.3 (top): a slight shift in color might lead to the depicted color histograms x and y for otherwise identical images. An unrelated image might lead to a very different histogram z. According to the Manhattan distance L_1, x would be more similar to z than to y ($1.0 < 1.6$). This is in stark contrast to human perception.

The EMD is based on a cross-bin approach, taking the overall distribution of the histogram entries into account. It measures the minimal amount of work necessary to transform ("move") one histogram distribution ("earth" or "mass") into the other. The movement of the mass is referred to as "flow". To determine the EMD, each flow is multiplied with the corresponding ground distance in the feature space that represents the dissimilarity of the according histogram bins. The total amount of work is the sum of these weighted flows. Finally, the EMD is the minimum over all cost-weighted flows that solve the problem.

We formally define the EMD for non-negative vectors of normalized total mass:

Definition 9.1. Earth Mover's Distance (EMD). For two d-dimensional vectors $x = (x_1, \ldots, x_d)$ and $y = (y_1, \ldots, y_d)$, $\forall 1 \leq i \leq d$: $x_i, y_i \geq 0$ of normalized total mass $\sum_{i=1}^{d} x_i = \sum_{i=1}^{d} y_i = 1$ and a cost matrix $C = [c_{ij}] \in \mathbb{R}^{d \times d}$, the EMD is defined as a minimization over all possible flows $F = [f_{ij}]$ under positivity constraints $CPos$, source constraints

CSource and target constraints *CTarget*:

$$EMD_C(x,y) = \min_F \{\sum_{i=1}^{d} \sum_{j=1}^{d} c_{ij} f_{ij} | Constraints\} \qquad (9.1)$$

with *Constraints* = *CPos* ∧ *CSource* ∧ *CTarget* :

$$CPos : \forall\, 1 \leq i,j \leq d : f_{ij} \geq 0 \qquad (9.2)$$
$$CSource : \ \forall\, 1 \leq i \leq d : \ \textstyle\sum_{j=1}^{d} f_{ij} = x_i \qquad (9.3)$$
$$CTarget : \ \forall\, 1 \leq j \leq d : \ \textstyle\sum_{i=1}^{d} f_{ij} = y_j \qquad (9.4)$$

The ground distance in feature space is reflected in the cost matrix C, where c_{ij} denotes the cost of moving one unit of mass from bin i to bin j. The constraint *CPos* ensures that only non-negative flows are considered. *CSource* restricts flows from bin i to the amount of mass available in the "source" bin x_i. Likewise, *CTarget* requires flows to bin j to equal the mass in the "target" bin y_j. Referring back to the example in Figure 9.3, Manhattan ground distance yields the cost matrix entries c_{ij}. The optimal EMD flow is depicted by the arrows. The EMD between x and y is $c_{12} * f_{12} + c_{34} * f_{34} + c_{56} * f_{56} = 1 * 0.5 + 1 * 0.2 + 1 * 0.3 = 1$, for x and z it is $c_{11} * f_{11} + c_{31} * f_{31} + c_{51} * f_{51} = 0 * 0.5 + 2 * 0.2 + 4 * 0.3 = 1.6$. Thus, the cross-bin computation of the EMD results in a more intuitive assessment of the dissimilarities of image pairs (x, y) and (x, z).

The EMD is a special linear program that searches for matrix F of flows such that all constraints are adhered to and such that the transformation work is minimized. It can be solved using the simplex method from operations research. In this optimization algorithm, an initial feasible solution for F such as Vogel's approximation is iteratively improved by updating F until a global optimum has been found [Hillier and Lieberman (1990)]. The theoretical worst case complexity of the simplex method is exponential in the dimensionality. In practical applications, however, the typical runtime is about cubic [Rubner and Tomasi (2001)]. As the optimization is over quadratic matrices in the size of the histograms, the complexity is at least quadratic. For large medical databases or fine resolution features, this is infeasible. In [Rubner and Tomasi (2001)], the authors state that coarse histograms are typically inadequate as bins are too large to benefit from cross-bin dissimilarity assessment while for fine histograms run-times are too slow.

9.1.3   Multi-Step Query Processing and the EMD

From a database perspective, efficiency can be improved by multi-step filter-and-refine architectures. A filter that is **(1) efficient, (2) lower-bounding** and **(3) selective** generates a set of candidates that is refined using the original distance function (cf. Figure 9.4 left). The following benefits are obtained from such a setting:

(1) Efficient filter computation is necessary to obtain a speedup compared to original distance computations.
(2) A lower-bounding filter guarantees that the original distance is never overestimated. For multi-step algorithms such as *G*eneric *M*ultimedia *I*ndexing (GEMINI) or *K* *N*earest neighbor *O*ptimal *P*rocessing (KNOP), underestimating asserts completeness, i.e. no false dismissals. (For proofs see [Korn *et al.* (1996); Seidl and Kriegel (1998)]).
(3) Selectivity of a filter refers to the tightness of a lower bound. The tighter the filter approximates the original distance, the smaller the set of candidates. Hence, fewer refinements and lower runtimes.

For the Earth Mover's distance, specialized lower bounds have been suggested [Rubner *et al.* (1998); Assent *et al.* (2006); Ljoså *et al.* (2006)]. These include averages in feature space, weighted L_p norms and dimension-wise optimization of EMD-components. The filter presented in [Rubner *et al.* (1998)] is limited by the dimensionality of the underlying feature space, the ones from [Assent *et al.* (2006)] by the original dimensionality, and [Ljoså *et al.* (2006)] only allows for limited flexibility regarding the reduced dimensionality. Neither filter makes use of the data characteristics to improve filter selectivity. Section 9.4 shows that incorporating knowledge on the data can significantly improve the retrieval performance in medical image databases.

Dimensionality reduction does not rely on separate classes of filter functions. Instead, the original type of distance function is used, yet on a smaller representation of the features. This is especially helpful for distance functions with superlinear complexity, like the Earth Mover's Distance. For smaller dimensionalities, distance calculations can be performed in reasonable time. Moreover, dimensionality reduction can be *chained* with existing filter functions for the EMD, i.e an existing filter can additionally be applied to the reduced data as the result of the dimensionality reduction is again an EMD.

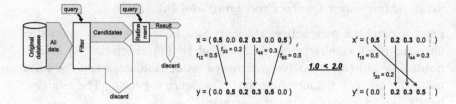

Fig. 9.4: Left: Schematic view of multi-step query processing. Right: Discarding of dimensions in the EMD can lead to violations of the lower-bounding property.

For most bin-by-bin distances like L_p norms, simple dimensionality reduction is straightforward. By discarding histogram dimensions, only non-negative addends are dropped, thus the resulting distance is guaranteed to be a lower bound. For the EMD, discarding dimensions can result in larger distances, as the resulting match might be worse than the original one. Consider the example on the far right of Figure 9.4: Removing two dimensions results in a larger EMD distance. Recall that all mass has to be moved from histogram x to the other histogram y. If "cheap" dimensions two and six are removed, the EMD between the reduced x' and y' grows accordingly. Consequently, to avoid false dismissals (not reported true query results), simply discarding is not a valid option for the Earth Mover's Distance.

9.2 Dimensionality Reduction for the EMD

Before describing the data-dependent reduction approach for medical image databases we define general dimensionality reduction and discuss optimal reduction for the EMD. The Earth Mover's Distance of two d-dimensional vectors is defined using a cost matrix C that reflects the feature space ground distance. Any dimensionality reduction technique thus has to specify a rule on how dimensions of the vectors are reduced and a rule on how entries in the cost matrix are aggregated. In section 9.2.1, we formalize the dimensionality reduction of the EMD. The optimal cost matrix reduction given a reduction of the vector dimensions is detailed in section 9.2.2.1. In section 9.2.3 we then concentrate on finding a data-dependent reduction for the dimensions of the vectors.

9.2.1   *Dimensionality Reduction*

Formally, a linear dimensionality reduction of vectors can be described via a reduction matrix. Multiplication of the original higher dimensional histogram vectors with this reduction matrix then results in a lower dimensional representation.

Definition 9.2. General linear dimensionality reduction. A general linear dimensionality reduction from dimensionality d to d' is characterized by a reduction matrix $R = [r_{ij}] \in \mathbb{R}^{d \times d'}$. The reduction of a d-dimensional vector
$x = (x_1, \ldots, x_d)$ to a d'-dimensional vector $x' = (x'_1, \ldots, x'_{d'})$ is defined as:

$$x' = x \cdot R \tag{9.5}$$

A subtype of linear dimensionality reductions especially useful for the reduction of the EMD are those reductions that combine original dimensions to form one reduced dimension.

Definition 9.3. Combining dimensionality reduction. The set $\Re_{d,d'} \subset \mathbb{R}^{d \times d'}$ of linear dimensionality reduction matrices that reduce the data dimensionality from d to d' by combining original dimensions to form reduced dimensions is defined by:

$$R \in \Re_{d,d'} \Leftrightarrow \forall 1 \leq i \leq d \ \ \forall 1 \leq j \leq d' : r_{ij} \in \{0,1\} \tag{9.6}$$

$$\wedge \forall 1 \leq i \leq d \qquad : \textstyle\sum_j^{d'} r_{ij} = 1 \tag{9.7}$$

$$\wedge \forall 1 \leq j \leq d' \qquad : \textstyle\sum_i^{d} r_{ij} \geq 1 \tag{9.8}$$

Constraints (9.6) and (9.7) together assert that each original dimension is assigned to exactly one reduced dimension, i.e. the disjoint union $\bigcup_{i'=1}^{d'} \{i | r_{ii'} = 1\}$ equals $\underline{d} = \{1, \ldots, d\}$ and $(i' \neq j') \Rightarrow (\{i | r_{ii'} = 1\} \cap \{j | r_{jj'} = 1\} = \emptyset)$. The set $\{i | r_{ii'} = 1\}$ represents dimensions i that are combined to reduced dimension i'. Additionally, restriction (9.7) induces the reduced vector to be of equal total mass as the original vector, which complies with Definition 9.1. Restriction (9.8) ensures that every reduced dimension is assigned at least one original dimension.

A reduced Earth Mover's Distance is defined via a reduction for the query vector and a reduction for the database vectors. Both reductions are used to compute a reduced cost matrix (cf. Figure 9.5).

Definition 9.4. Reduced Earth Mover's Distance. For two d-dimensional vectors x, y and a cost matrix C according to Definition 9.1 and

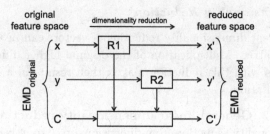

Fig. 9.5: Reduction matrices $R1$ and $R2$ of the query object x and a data base object y yield the reduced cost matrix C'.

for two reduction matrices $R1 \in \Re_{d,d1}$ and $R2 \in \Re_{d,d2}$, the lower-bounding reduced EMD is defined as:

$$EMD_C^{R1,R2}(x,y) = EMD_{C'}(x \cdot R1, y \cdot R2) \qquad (9.9)$$

where $C' \in \mathbb{R}^{d1 \times d2}$ is a lower-bounding reduced cost matrix.

Please note that this general definition allows reducing database feature vectors independently from the query feature vector given a more general EMD definition (e.g. in [Rubner and Tomasi (2001)]).

We formally introduce a lower-bounding reduced cost matrix C' for the EMD in the following.

9.2.2 *Optimal Dimensionality Reduction*

We define optimality of dimensionality reduction with respect to the efficiency of similarity search as the effectiveness is not affected in the lower-bounding filter framework. During multi-step query processing, dimensionality reduction is used to generate a set of candidates that is refined using the original dimensionality (cf. Figure 9.4). Smaller candidate sets induce fewer refinement computations and thus result in less computation time in the refinement step. For given target dimensionalities $d1$ and $d2$, the optimal dimensionality reduction is therefore the reduction that yields the smallest candidate sets during query processing.

9.2.2.1 *Optimal Cost Reduction*

Any reduction of the dimensionality of the Earth Mover's Distance requires specification of a corresponding reduced cost matrix. This cost matrix provides the ground distance in the new reduced feature space. Consequently, the reduced cost matrix depends on the reduction matrices of Definition 9.3. The optimal cost matrix with respect to given reduction matrices is the one that provides the largest lower bound to the EMD in the original dimensionality (e.g., it should lose as little cost information as possible without violating the lower-bounding property). As we will prove, the best possible reduced cost matrix consists of minima over the original cost entries.

To illustrate why those minima have to be chosen, we give an example of the worst case that leads to this condition: To ensure the lower bound property, the true distance has to be underestimated. In the worst case, original mass was transfered at minimum cost. Consider $x = (0, 1, 0, 0)$ and $y = (0, 0, 1, 0)$ and Manhattan ground distance (as e.g. in the cost matrix in Figure 9.3). Their Earth Mover's Distance is then simply 1 (moving one unit of mass from dimension x_2 to y_3 at ground distance 1: $1 * 1 = 1$). Combining the first two and the last two dimensions, the reduced features are $x' = (1, 0)$ and $y' = (0, 1)$. The minimum cost entry from the original dimensions x_1 and x_2 to dimensions y_3 or y_4 is the cost from x_2 to y_3, which is indeed the 1 that was used in the original EMD. If this value were to be exceeded, the lower bound property would be lost.

The lower-bounding reduced cost matrix C' in Definition 9.5 is based on this worst-case assumption to guarantee the lower-bounding property for the filter step. The sparse combining reduction matrices according to Definition 9.3 limit the worst cases that can occur (cf. section 9.2.2.1) when compared to dimensionality reduction techniques such as PCA, ICA and Random Projection where $r_{ij} \in \mathbb{R}$. Our tests with alternative dimensionality reduction techniques such as PCA (amended by an extra dimension to preserve the total mass) resulted in very poor retrieval efficiency due to the concessions that had to be made for the reduced cost matrix in order to guarantee the lower-bounding property.

We formalize the concept of the optimal reduced cost matrix.

Definition 9.5. Optimal Reduced Cost Matrix.   For two d-dimensional vectors x, y and a cost matrix C according to definition 9.1 and for a reduced $EMD_C^{R1,R2}$ according to definition 9.4, the optimal reduced cost matrix $C' = [c'_{i'j'}]$ is defined by:

$$c'_{i'j'} = \min\{c_{ij} | r1_{ii'} = 1 \wedge r2_{jj'} = 1\} \qquad (9.10)$$

In case of $R1 = R2 \in \Re_{d,d'}$, the reduced cost matrix C' defined by (9.10) is equivalent to the lower-bounding cost matrix of [Ljoså *et al.* (2006)]. The lower-bounding property also holds for $R1 \neq R2$.

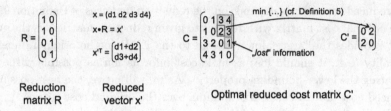

| Reduction matrix R | Reduced vector x' | Optimal reduced cost matrix C' |

Fig. 9.6: Dimensionality reduction based on a single reduction matrix R: reduced vector x' and optimal reduced cost matrix C'.

Theorem 9.1. *Lower bound.* *Given two reduction matrices $R1 \in \Re_{d,d1}$ and $R2 \in \Re_{d,d2}$ and a cost matrix $C \in \mathbb{R}^{d \times d}$, the reduced cost matrix C' according to (9.10) provides a lower bound:*

$$\forall x, y \in \mathbb{R}^d : EMD_{C'}(x \cdot R1, y \cdot R2) \leq EMD_C(x, y)$$

Proof. The proof is a generalization of the proof in [Ljoså *et al.* (2006)] and can be found in [Wichterich *et al.* (2008)].   □

Figure 9.6 gives an example for a reduction from $d = 4$ to $d' = 2$. The original dimensions $d1$ and $d2$ are combined to the reduced dimension $d1'$ while $d3$ and $d4$ are reduced to $d2'$. In this case, the lost distance information within $d1'$ is $c_{12} = c_{21} = 1$ and within $d2'$ it is $c_{34} = c_{43} = 1$. The distance that is preserved between $d1'$ and $d2'$ is $c_{23} = c_{32} = 2$, which is the minimum according to Definition 9.5.

We state that the reduced cost matrix chosen according to Definition 9.5 results in a greatest lower bound for given reduction matrices $R1$ and $R2$. There is no better reduced cost matrix for given reduction matrices $R1$ and $R2$, i.e. C' according to definition 9.5 is optimal.

Theorem 9.2. *Optimality.* *Given a cost matrix $C \in \mathbb{R}^{d \times d}$ and two reduction matrices $R1 \in \Re_{d,d1}$ and $R2 \in \Re_{d,d2}$, there is no greater lower bound than the one provided by C' according to (9.10):*

$$\neg \exists C'' \in \mathbb{R}^{d1 \times d2} \; \forall x, y \in \mathbb{R}^d : Tighter \wedge LB \wedge (C'' \neq C')$$

where

$$LB : EMD_{C''}(x \cdot R1, y \cdot R2) \leq EMD_C(x, y)$$

$$Tighter : EMD_{C'}(x \cdot R1, y \cdot R2) \leq EMD_{C''}(x \cdot R1, y \cdot R2)$$

This is due to a monotony property of the EMD. The quality of lower-bounding dimensionality reduction increases if the values in the cost matrix increase (i.e., the reduced EMDs are tighter with respect to the original EMDs).

Theorem 9.3. *Monotony of the EMD.* *Given two cost matrices* $C1, C2 \in \mathbb{R}^{d \times d}$ *it holds:*

$$C_1 \leq C_2 \;\; \Leftrightarrow \;\; \forall x, y: \; EMD_{C1}(x, y) \leq EMD_{C2}(x, y)$$

where

$$C1 \leq C2 \Leftrightarrow (C1 = C2) \vee (\forall i, j \in \underline{d}: c1_{ij} \leq c2_{ij} \wedge \exists i, j \in \underline{d}: c1_{ij} < c2_{ij})$$

Proofs for theorems 9.2 and 9.3 are given in [Wichterich *et al.* (2008)].

With Theorem 9.2 we have that the reduction of a cost matrix C to C' according to definition 9.5 leads to an optimal lower bound for given reduction matrices $R1$ and $R2$. Therefore, we now focus on how to find good reduction matrices. For this, the monotony property will prove useful. To simplify the discussion, we assume $R1 = R2$ and write $EMD_C^R(x, y) := EMD_C^{R,R}(x, y)$. However, the described reduction methods can be extended to different simultaneous reductions in a straightforward manner.

9.2.2.2 *Optimal Flow Reduction*

As discussed above, optimal reduction of the cost matrix in the Earth Mover's Distance depends entirely on the reduction matrices. Consequently, the efficiency of any EMD reduction according to Definition 9.4 depends solely on the choice of R. We define what would constitute an optimal choice of R. As that R is not attainable in practice, we then introduce approximations that are found to result in efficient reductions as shown in our evaluation on medical data sets in Section 9.4.

Given a d-dimensional query point x and a query distance ϵ, the optimal reduction $R \in \Re_{d,d'}$ to dimensionality d' can be defined in terms of the number of refinements required to answer an ϵ-range query for a database DB:

$$R = \arg\min_{R' \in \Re_{d,d'}} |\{y \in DB | EMD_C^{R'}(x, y) \leq \epsilon\}|$$

Due to the lower-bounding property, only elements in the above set can potentially still have a refined distance below ϵ. Since this optimality is only concerned with one single query x, one typically chooses a workload w

representative of the expected queries and defines optimality with respect to said workload.

Definition 9.6. Optimal EMD reduction. Given a workload $w = \{(x_1, \epsilon_1), \ldots, (x_t, \epsilon_t)\}$, where x_i is a query vector and ϵ_i the corresponding range threshold, the optimal reduction $R \in \Re_{d,d'}$ for w is:

$$R = \arg\min_{R' \in \Re_{d,d'}} \sum_{(x,\epsilon) \in w} |\{y \in DB | EMD_C^{R'}(x,y) \leq \epsilon\}|$$

Thus, the optimal reduction matrix R' is the one where the sum over the cardinalities of the candidate sets in the workload is minimal.

While this equation describes the desired optimal reduction, the search space for the optimization is immense even for small databases and small dimensionalities. Due to the size of the combining reduction matrix, a $(d \cdot d')$-variable 0-1 integer optimization problem with restrictions according to Definition 9.3 has to be solved. Summing over the workload, the objective function consists of $|w| \cdot |DB|$ individual $(d' \cdot d')$-variable linear optimization problems. Exhaustive enumeration of all possible reductions requires the computation of a total of $d'^{(d-d')} \cdot |w| \cdot |DB|$ reduced EMDs. Even for a reduction from 16 to 8 dimensions of a database of size 1000 and a workload of size 100, this requires over $1.67 \cdot 10^{12}$ EMD computations. As this is practically infeasible, we discuss heuristics that result in efficient reductions as shown in the experimental evaluation on medical databases in Section 9.4.

9.2.3   *Flow-based Reduction*

We call the data-dependent methods for dimensionality reduction flow-based reductions (FB reductions). The algorithms incorporate knowledge on the underlying data set to generate a reduction that leads to a selective filter for the EMD. Information about the flows of unreduced EMD computations is collected to guide the process of generating tighter reduction matrices. At first, computing unreduced EMDs to later approximate them in a second step might sound paradoxical as this preprocessing step requires additional effort. However, this investment is more than justified through faster search times during query processing, i.e. the preprocessing is done once and positively affects the response times for many queries.

The unreduced EMD is a sum of terms $c_{ij} \cdot f_{ij}$. For a tight lower bound, we want to achieve large reduced terms $c'_{i'j'} \cdot f'_{i'j'}$. Since we can

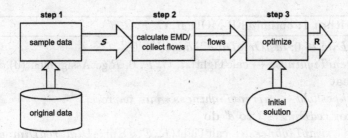

Fig. 9.7: Flow-based reduction uses the flows occurring in the original EMD to optimize the reduction matrix with respect to the underlying database.

derive an optimal reduced cost matrix $[c'_{i'j'}]$ by applying Theorem 9.2, we have to increase the reduced flows with respect to $c'_{i'j'}$. This way, the reduced EMD increases and with it the tightness of the lower bound. The information we incorporate is the average flow matrix $F^{\mathcal{S}} = [f^{\mathcal{S}}_{ij}]$ with $f^{\mathcal{S}}_{ij} = \frac{1}{|\mathcal{S}|^2} \sum_{x,y \in \mathcal{S}} \hat{f}_{ij}(x,y)$ over a sample $\mathcal{S}$ of the database. We approximate the flows occurring in a reduced EMD with the average original flows aggregated according to the respective reduction matrix.

$$aggrFlow(F, R, i', j') = \sum_{\{i|r_{ii'}=1\}} \sum_{\{j|r_{jj'}=1\}} f_{ij} \qquad (9.11)$$

The aggregated flow from the reduced dimension i' to j' is based on original flows f_{ij} between dimensions i and j that the reduction matrix R combined to i' and j' respectively.

We measure the approximate tightness of a reduction R as the sum of the aggregated sampled flows $F^{\mathcal{S}}$ weighted by the cost matrix C' optimally reduced according to R:

$$\sum_{i'=1}^{d'} \sum_{j'=1}^{d'} aggrFlow(F^{\mathcal{S}}, R, i', j') \cdot c'_{i'j'} \qquad (9.12)$$

The global optimization of this term requires computing all possible reductions, which is infeasible (cf. Section 9.2.2.2). Therefore, in the presented algorithms, one original dimension is reassigned to another reduced dimension at a time to iteratively improve the reduction matrix.

Figure 9.7 illustrates the steps taken to create a reduction matrix with the flow-based heuristics. In the first step a sample $\mathcal{S}$ is drawn from the

---

Algorithm 1: optimizeFB-MOD(R, C, F, d, d')

1    $origDim \leftarrow 0$; $lastOrigDimChanged \leftarrow 0$;
2    $currentTightness \leftarrow$ calcTight(R, C, F, 0, R.getAssignment(0),d');
3   **repeat**
4       $threshold \leftarrow currentTightness * min\_improve$;
5   **for** $redDim \leftarrow 1$ **to** d' **do**
6         $swapTighness \leftarrow$ caltTight(R, C, F, $origDim$, $redDim$, d');
7   **if** *($swapTighness - currentTightness > threshold$)* **then**
8           $currentTightness \leftarrow swapTighness$;
9   R.reassign($origDim$, $redDim$);
10           $lastOrigDimChanged \leftarrow origDim$;
11   **break**;
12   **end if**
13   **end for**
14       $origDim \leftarrow (origDim + 1)$ mod d;
15   **until** *($origDim = lastOrigDimChanged$)*;
16   **return** R;

---

database. In the second step the EMD (original dimensionality) is calculated on the sample, i.e. the distances for each pair of histograms in S. While doing this, the EMD flow matrices $\widehat{F}$ of the histograms pairs are summed up to obtain the average flows F^S. Starting from an initial reduction matrix, the third and main step of the approach finds a local maximum of the expected lower bound tightness (Equation 9.12) by utilizing the aggregated flow information.

We describe two variants of an algorithm that solve step 3. Algorithm 1 shows a pseudo code for the first variant, which we named FB-Mod (flow-based reduction - modulo). The algorithm takes the current reduction matrix, starts at the first original dimension, and changes its assignment. To this end, it iteratively assesses the assignment of the original dimension to each reduced dimension (line 6). If the quality of the resulting reduction matrix is better than the current solution, the change is made persistent (line 9) and the algorithm continues with the next original dimension. Once it reaches the last original dimension it starts over at the first one (line 14) until it visits the same original dimension twice without any changes in assignments.

The expected tightness of a reduction matrix is calculated via Algo-

---

Algorithm 2: calcTight(R, C, F, $origDim$, $newRedDim$, d')

---

1 $result \leftarrow 0$;
2 $R' \leftarrow R$;
3 R'.reassign($origDim$, $newRedDim$);
4 $C' \leftarrow C$.reduce(R');
5 **for** $i' \leftarrow 1$ **to** d' **do**
6   **for** $j' \leftarrow 1$ **to** d' **do**
7 | $result \leftarrow result + $ aggrFlow(F, R, i', j') $*$ $C'[i'][j']$;
8   **end for**
9 **end for**
10 **return** $result$;

---

rithm 2 (*calcTight*). It consists of three steps.

(1) Change the assignment of the given original dimension from its current assignment to the given reduced dimension (line 3).
(2) Reduce the original cost matrix according to the resulting reduction matrix (line 4).
(3) Sum up the products of the reduced costs and the aggregated flows according to (9.12) (line 7).

The second variant of the algorithm does not necessarily apply the first reassignment that yields a better solution. Instead, it evaluates all possibilities before choosing a single reassignment that results in the best reduction matrix. It then starts the next iteration until no further improvement is achieved. We therefore call it FB-All.

Both algorithms take an initial reduction matrix as a parameter. For the experiments we use a $k-medoid$ clustering of the original dimensions where the cost matrix of the EMD defines the distance between the dimensions to be clustered. Clustering is an approach from the data mining field, which automatically groups the data (here: into k cluster groups) such that elements within a cluster are similar to one another, whereas elements in different clusters are dissimilar. Our clustering-based reduction matrix can be seen as a generalization of the grid-approach in [Ljoså *et al.* (2006)]. It can not only be used as an initialization for the flow-based algorithms but also as a reduction of its own (denoted as *kMedoids* in our evaluation). Details for the *kMedoids* reduction and alternative initializations can be found in [Wichterich *et al.* (2008)].

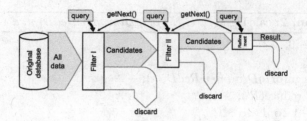

Fig. 9.8: Multi-step setup for query processing using two chained filters.

9.3   Query Processing Algorithm

In this section, we describe query processing for k nearest neighbor queries. K nearest neighbor queries return the k most similar images to the query image. Processing of k nearest neighbor queries extends to range queries (returning all images within a similarity range) in a straightforward manner. While in knn-queries the value for ε is not known a priori, the distance of the kth nearest neighbor corresponds to an ε value for a range query with the same result set.

The dimensionality reduction techniques presented can be flexibly combined. As the reduced distance function again is an EMD computation, existing filters for the EMD can be used on the reduced dimensionality. This chaining of lower-bounding filters, widely used in multi-step query processing, allows for efficient query processing as our experiments show. The LB_{IM} technique introduced in [Assent *et al.* (2006)] is such a lower bound with respect to the Earth Mover's Distance.

In our evaluation, we use the chaining multi-step setup illustrated in Figure 9.8. A combination of three different distance functions is employed to determine the final result. LB_{IM} on dimensionality-reduced features (Red-IM) forms the first filter followed by the EMD on reduced features (Red-EMD, filter 2). The refinement step computes the final result set using the EMD on unreduced features. The two filters and the refinement step are not run sequentially but in an interlinked manner. Whenever a filter has found the next best object in the database according to its distance, the object is passed on to the next filter (or the refinement step). The process stops when the refinement step is able to determine that it found the final result set. This is the case when the highest refinement distance in the candidate result set is smaller than the filter distance of the next object being passed to the refinement step by the filter. Each of the filter functions in the chain is a lower bound to the next one, which

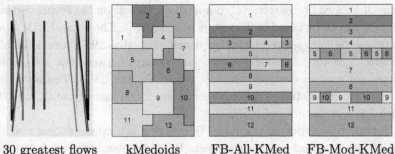

30 greatest flows   kMedoids   FB-All-KMed   FB-Mod-KMed

Fig. 9.9: Left: Greatest flows within the feature space of a sample of
RETINA2-All. 2nd: kMedoids partitioning as used for initialization. Other: Partitioning of the feature space into 12 dimensions
via the flow-based reduction approaches.

guarantees completeness in multi-step query processing as proven in [Korn
et al. (1996); Seidl and Kriegel (1998)]. A more detailed discussion of the
algorithms may be found in [Wichterich *et al.* (2008)].

9.4   Evaluation on Medical Data Sets

Data sets. We evaluate the flow-based approach on real world medical
data sets. The RETINA image data set (cf. Fig. 9.1) from the UCSB Bio-
image Database (http://www.bioimage.ucsb.edu) consists of 3,932 feline
retina scans labeled with various antibodies and was used in experiments
on EMD lower bounds in [Ljoså *et al.* (2006)]. For each image, twelve 96-
dimensional histograms reflecting a tile-based spatial distribution of twelve
MPEG-7 color layout descriptor measures were computed by the authors of
[Ljoså *et al.* (2006)]. We select the first three dimensions for the following
experiments, and denote the normalized histograms (sum of 1) for each
dimension as RETINA1-All to RETINA3-All. We divide each of them
into query sets of size 100 and database sets of size 3,832. We calculate
reduction matrices based on sample sets of size 383 (roughly 10%).

Our IRMA image data set (cf. Fig. 9.2) consists of 10,000 radiography images from the Image Retrieval in Medical Applications
project (http://www.irma-project.org/datasets_en.php) and [Lehmann
et al. (2004); Deselaers *et al.* (2005)]. The raw data set is available from
(http://www.irma-project.org/datasets_en.php) and was part of the 2005

ImageCLEFmed image retrieval competition. Details on the feature extraction process can be found in [Deselaers *et al.* (2005)]. The dataset IRMA-All comprises the image-wise cluster frequencies stored as 199-dimensional histograms. The 40-dimensional Euclidean distances between the 199 cluster centers are used to compute the cost matrix for the EMD. The reduction matrices are calculated on a sample set of size 1,000 taken from IRMA-DB, which has a cardinality of 9,900.

Setup. The reported results in this section are averages over a workload of 100 k-nearest neighbor queries. Each complete data set (-All) was divided into a query set (-Q), containing the 100 query objects, and the database (-DB), containing the remaining objects. From the database we then drew a sample set, on which we calculate the flow-based reduction matrices (cf. Figure 9.7). We use the terminology (-All, -Q, -DB) for both data sets throughout this section. All experiments were executed on Pentium 4 2.4GHz work stations with 1GB of RAM running Windows XP.

We compare the following approaches using the architecture from Figure 9.8: The flow-based dimensionality reduction variants (FB-All-KMed, FB-Mod-KMed), the clustering-based dimensionality reduction (kMedoids) and (for the RETINA data set) the 24-dimensional filter from [Ljoså *et al.* (2006)] (Ljosa), which effectively is a lower resolution 6 × 4 grid imposed on Figure 9.1. For the IRMA database, Ljosa is not applicable as the 40-dimensional feature space is not organized in a grid-like fashion. In addition to the aforementioned four approaches, we run the weighted averaging filter from [Rubner *et al.* (1998)] (Rubner) in a direct filter-and-refine set-up. Since the averaging filter requires an explicit ground distance function while the reductions deliver a reduced cost matrix, Rubner can only be applied to the original EMD. To complete the set of competing approaches, we also evaluate the Independent Minimization filter from [Assent *et al.* (2006)] for non-reduced EMDs in a direct filter-and-refine architecture. All EMD computations are based on Euclidean ground distance.

RETINA experiments. At the far left of Figure 9.9 we see for twelve reduced dimensions that the greatest averaged original "flow × cost" components in RETINA2 occur in a vertical direction roughly between the two bands of antibody labels that can be seen in Figure 9.1. The flow-based reductions keep dimensions separate that induce great "flow × cost" components in the original EMD while combining those that do not. As can be seen in Figure 9.9, both variants adapt to the largely vertical flows by assigning different rows to different reduced dimensions. This also keeps the reduced costs between the new dimensions high compared to the kMe-

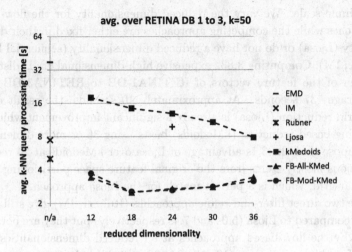

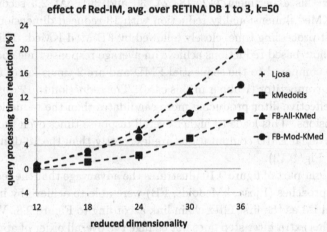

Fig. 9.10: Top: Computation time vs. reduced dimensionality (avg. over RETINA1 to RETINA3). Bottom: Relative speedup gained through applying Red-IM as the first filter chain link.

doids reduction where each dimension has between 3 and 6 neighboring reduced dimensions with distance 1. Both the FB-All-KMed and the FB-Mod-KMed approach show a balanced distribution of the new dimensions and adapt well to the vertical flows.

The left part of figure 9.10 shows the 50-nearest neighbor query processing time averaged over datasets RETINA1-DB to RETINA3-DB on a logarithmic scale. We vary the reduced dimensionality for the flow-based approaches while the competing approaches are either fixed in their dimensionality (Ljosa) or do not have a reduced dimensionality (sequential EMD, Rubner, IM). Computing 3,832 expensive high-dimensional EMD distances for each of the feature vectors of RETINA1-DB to RETINA3-DB takes on average 37 seconds. At approximately 10 seconds, the result of the fixed grid reduction (Ljosa) is already a significant improvement which the clustering-based reduction (kMedoids) beats using 36 or more dimensions. We suppose that the 3.1s advantage of Ljosa over kMedoids at 24 reduced dimensions mostly stems from the original feature space partitioning being a regular grid, which is a perfect match for the Ljosa approach.

The two direct filter-and-refine approaches (Rubner, IM) give still faster results compared to Ljosa (5.0s and 7.4s respectively) but they are both surpassed by the flow-based approaches at all reduced dimensionalities evaluated for this experiment (12, 18, 24, 30 and 36). At 2.5 seconds, the FB-All-KMed dimensionality reduction with 18 reduced dimensions shows the lowest processing time, closely followed by FB-Mod-KMed. This means that the flow-based reductions achieve an average response time speedup of factor 15 compared to the sequential EMD and are 2 times faster than the next best competitor (Rubner in this case). The reduction to 12 dimensions is a less effective filter producing more candidates than the reduction using 18 dimensions. This leads to higher overall response times even though the 12-dimensional EMD computations are less costly than the 18-dimensional ones (cf. Fig. 9.12).

The right part of figure 9.10 illustrates the advantage that the reduction-based approaches (Ljosa, kMedoids, FB) were able to achieve by including a reduced IM as the first filter chain link according to Figure 9.8. While removing this extra filter step does not change the overall order of approaches seen in Figure 9.10, it is favorable to have this option as it reduces absolute processing times in almost all cases we studied. The higher the reduced dimensionality, the more it is worth to apply the filter. When varying the parameter k of nearest neighbors to retrieve (Figure 9.11), the observed order of relative speed remains stable but for one exception. The IM filter performance improves when reducing k. It is consistently faster than Rubner at $k \leq 15$ but matches the flow-based reductions only for $k = 1$. This means that IM was particularly good at approximating distances of very similar histograms. IM returns the nearest neighbor in 0.74s for $k = 1$ where the approaches show response times between 0.81s and 1.06s. Even for k as small as 5, both flow-based dimensionality reductions outperform

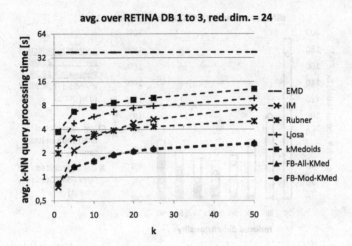

Fig. 9.11: Computation time vs. number of nearest neighbors (RETINA2).

all competitors.

IRMA experiments. Figure 9.12 (left) shows the trade-off between the decreasing selectivity and rising processing time of the filter step with increasing dimensionality d'. For the larger IRMA data set with 199 original dimensions, the required number of expensive EMD refinements drops to 2% at a reduced dimensionality of 80 when using FB-All-KMed. At the same time, the superlinear complexity of the EMD causes the share of time spent on the filter step to decrease rapidly for low reduced dimensionalities. The optimum for finding 50 nearest neighbors is achieved at a reduced dimensionality of 60 where roughly 36% of the time is spent on filtering and the remainder of the time is spent on computing high-dimensional EMD refinements for 3.2% of the data. For the same setting, the average filter selectivity of IM is at 21% and at 18.1% for Rubner.

Due to the larger number of vectors and the higher dimensionality, overall query processing times are higher for the IRMA set than for the RETINA sets. This holds for all evaluated approaches. A complete sequential scan of the database using the EMD requires approximately 17 minutes, which is not tolerable in typical retrieval of medical imagery for analysis or diagnosis. For 50 nearest neighbors, Figure 9.12 (right) shows that the two approaches that do not rely on a dimensionality reduction (Rubner and IM) decrease the response times to between 3 and 4 minutes. This is in line with the selectivity values stated above. kMedoids performs similarly well

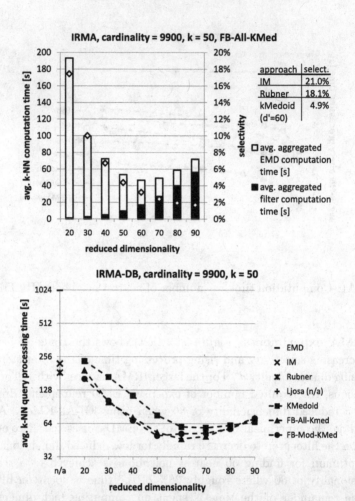

Fig. 9.12: Top: Computation time shares and selectivity of the filter step (IRMA). Bottom: Computation time vs. reduced dimensionality (IRMA).

when reducing the dimensionality to between 10% and 15% of the original dimensionality and reaches its optimum of just below 1 minute around dimensionality 60. This value is beaten by both flow-based reductions, where FB-All-KMed gives the fastest response time at 46.5 seconds. Compared to the 17 minutes of the sequential scan and to the 3 minutes of the next best competing approach (Rubner), this equates to a speedup of factor close to

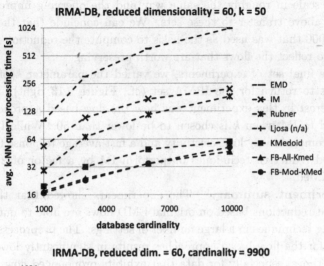

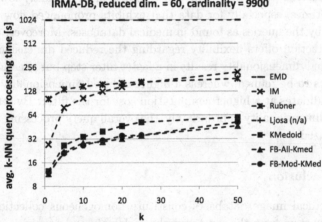

Fig. 9.13: Computation time (logarithmic scale) vs. cardinality (left) and vs. the number of nearest neighbors (right) for the IRMA data set.

22 and close to 4 for the flow-based techniques.

We subsampled the IRMA-DB data set in three steps to assess the efficiency of the flow-based approaches over a range of database cardinalities. Each of the smaller databases includes the sample that was taken from IRMA-DB during preprocessing time to compute the flows for the flow-based dimensionality reductions. As Figure 9.13 (left) depicts, all approaches scale in roughly the same way and the querying improvements reported above transfer to these sets. We can conclude that the sample size of 1,000 that was used as the basis to compute the reduction matrices sufficed to reflect the flows that are worth preserving.

In the final set of experiments, we varied the parameter k of nearest neighbors to return for the IRMA set (cf. Figure 9.13 right). Of foremost interest in this experiment was how the flow-based approaches fare compared to IM when k is chosen to be lower than 50. While IM again shows a comparatively low selectivity and a fast average response time, the flow-based reduction techniques outperform IM by a factor of 2.35 with FB-All-KMed.

Experiment summary. The experiments showed that the data-dependent reductions based on original EMD flows are able to outperform competing techniques in a large number of settings. The preprocessing step required for the flow-based approaches results in significantly lower query response times, especially for data that exhibits pronounced flow patterns matched by the queries as found in medical databases. Moreover, the flow-based reduction offers flexibility regarding the reduced dimensionality. A low reduced dimensionality results in a faster filter step but generates more candidates to be refined, whereas a higher reduced dimensionality leads to fewer candidates at a higher computation cost for the filter. By setting the reduced dimensionality appropriately, the overall query processing time can be optimized.

9.5 Conclusion

Many medical image databases constitute homogeneous collections since the images stem from the same underlying domain and acquisition process. Identifying the most similar images to a query supports diagnostic and analytical processes in medicine or life sciences. For image retrieval, the Earth Mover's Distance is known to show excellent performance, yet at high computational cost. To enable the use of the EMD on medical image databases in reasonable time we described a specialized lower-bounding filter based on dimensionality reduction that takes the characteristics of the underlying database into account (flow-based reduction). We showed on real world medical image data sets that flow-based reduction outperforms all competing filter techniques in a large number of settings. The described approach enables the efficient use of the EMD for effective image retrieval in medical databases.

Acknowledgments: We thank V. Ljosa, T.M. Deserno, and T. Deselaers for providing us with data sets. This work was partially funded by DFG grants EXC89 and SE1039/1-3.

Chapter 10

Fast Multimedia Querying for Medical Applications

Andreas Wichert and Pedro Santos

Technical University of Lisboa, Portugal

10.1 Introduction

The clinical record is a key element for assisting the delivery of health care to a patient. It is a dynamic informational entity that continuously monitors/the evolution of the health status of a patient. The major advantages of electronic health record over their paper-based counterparts (besides the more commonly known provided by the electronic management of data) is that all diagnostic tests, especially medical imagery, become attached to the patients profile and available on electronic format. Most of those tests consist of unstructured media formats, like the images. This fact complicates the search and retrieval of information since its semantic structure is not directly interpretable. This type of data cannot be searched by conventional queries of a relational database as any normal text field, unless the corresponding data files are annotated with external descriptors containing metadata describing and qualifying their content (such as MPEG7 files for the videos) [Dunckley (2003)]. The problem with this solution is the construction of those annotations, namely the extraction of image features and the assignment of a semantic value. Moreover, the resulting descriptors usually have a very specific and limited use, and their classification is subjective to human interpretation [Dunckley (2003)]. For instance, the diagnosis using radiological imagery may not be uniform. An alternative to high-level descriptors is the search through the low-level structural features of the image (like texture, color, shape), through a process called CBIR (Content Based Image Retrieval). These characteristics are easily retrievable, and if properly combined in sets (through standardized patterns), they can translate into a high semantic value and therefore become directly usable in a given context [Dunckley (2003)]. Content-based image retrieval (CBIR) is a technique for retrieving images on the basis of automatically-derived features. An image or some drawn user input serves as a query example, and all similar images should be retrieved as results. An image query is performed through the generation of a weighted combination of features, and through its direct comparison with the features stored in the database. A similarity metric (e.g. the Euclidean distance) is then used to find the nearest neighbors of the query example in the feature vector space. Feature extraction is the crucial step in content-based image retrieval. Traditional fast multimedia queering leads to dilemma. Either the number of features has to be reduced and the quality of the results in unsatisfactory, or approximate queries are preformed leading to a relative error during retrieval. In the medical domain both approaches are not acceptable. Subspace-tree propose a solution to this dilemma. It works in extreme high dimensional space (order of several thousands) and performs fast exact queries. We demonstrate its power by integration into an electronic health record (see Figure 10.1).

Beside the CBIR the most typical functionalities provided by electronic health record system for Public Primary Health Care Center were implemented. Our system supports searching, browsing and managing patient data sheets; registration of consultations, new patients and doctors; upload of medical tests and other documents; definition of personal system settings; among others.

The patient data masks are based on the official standard patient record forms (in paper), being used in the Public Primary Health Care Center (see Figure 10.2). The Figure 10.3 shows part of the patient data stored in the system. The system is a web based client-server (thin client) application composed by three layers (presentation, logic and data) developed in Java and WebObjects. It consists on a central server where the application is deployed, as well as the database with the patient information (we use MySql 5) and the file systems where the stored medical tests are kept. It can be deployed on any operating system (e.g. Solaris, Linux, Windows, OS X) since the basic technology is Java and a relational database.

The subspace-tree was implemented in java. Instead of dividing the space itself as most metric trees do [Böhm *et al.* (2001)], the subspace

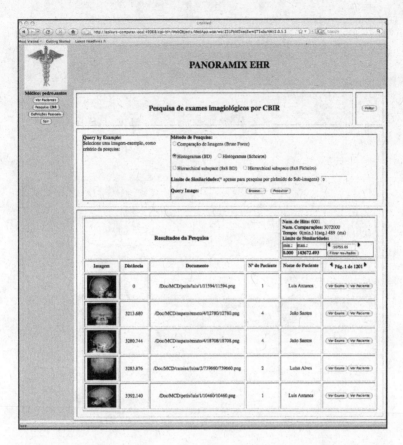

Fig. 10.1: Mask of the electronic health record with CBIR search.

trees divide the distances between the subspaces [Wichert (2008)] [Wichert *et al.* (2009)]. These distances correspond to the values represented by the difference between the mean distance of all the objects in one space and a corresponding mean distance of the objects in a subspace. The number of nodes of such a tree does not represent the multimedia objects but the dimension of the subspace in the hierarchy in which the multimedia objects are projected [Wichert *et al.* (2009)] . The costs are equivalent to the search costs in a tree plus the additional costs of dimension of the feature vector. It means that we have a logarithmic growth in the number of elements and their dimension as shown in [Wichert (2008)], [Wichert *et al.* (2009)].

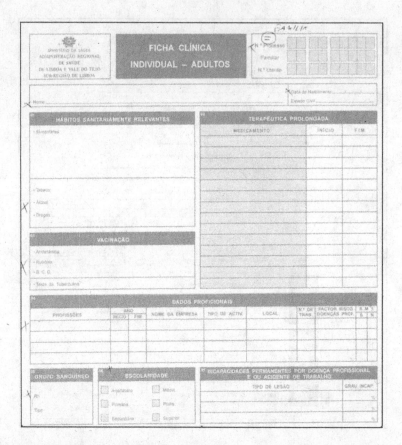

Fig. 10.2: Official form of the Portuguese Public Primary Health Care
Center.

10.2   Related Work

The application of the CBIR concept in Medicine is relatively new. Most
applications depend on the imaging modalities [Zhou *et al.* (2008)]. However, there are some academic studies and projects including non modality-
specific studies of CBIR in medicine: IRMA [Lehmann *et al.* (2004)], I2C
[Orphanoudakis *et al.* (1994)], KMed [Chu *et al.* (1994)], [Muller *et al.*
(2005)]. However, there still is not any integrated application fully functional in the real clinical practice. Fast queries relay on the use of indexing
methods.

Traditional indexing trees can be described by two classes, trees derived

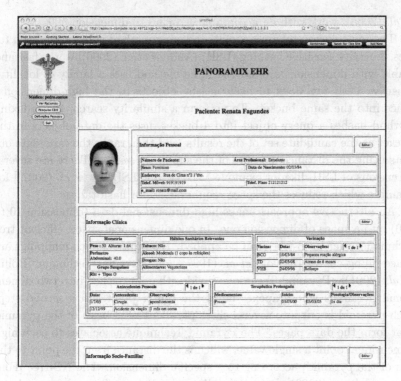

Fig. 10.3: Patient main information page based in the official form.

from the kd-tree and the trees composed by derivatives of the R-tree. Trees in the first class divides the data space along predefined hyper-planes regardless of data distribution. The resulting regions are mutually disjoint and most of them do not represent any objects. In fact with the growing dimension of space we would require exponential many objects to fill the space. The second class tries to overcome this problem by dividing the data space according to the data distribution into overlapping regions, as described in the second section. An example of the second class is the M-tree [Paolo Ciaccia (1997)]. It performs exact retrieval with 10 dimensions. However its performance deteriorates in high dimensional spaces.

A solution to this problem consists of approximate queries which allow a relative error during retrieval. M-tree [Ciaccia and Patella (2002)] and A-tree [Sakurai *et al.* (2002)] with approximate queries perform retrieval in dimensions of several hundreds. A-tree uses approximated MBR instead of a the MBR of the R-tree. Approximate metric trees like NV-trees [Olafsson *et al.* (2008)] work with an acceptable error up to dimension 500.

The most successful approximate indexing method is based on hash tables. Locality sensitive hashing (LSH) [Andoni *et al.* (2006)] works fast and stable with dimensions around 700. The method uses a family of locality-sensitive hash functions to hash nearby objects in the high-dimensional space into the same bucket. To perform a similarity search, the indexing method hashes a query object into a bucket, uses the data objects in the bucket as the candidate set of the results, and then ranks the candidate objects using the distance measure of the similarity search. There are several extensions of LSH, like for example Multi-Probe LSH [Lv *et al.* (2007)] for example which reduces the space requirements for hash tables.

An alternative approach maps high dimensional data (dimension 10 to 270) into a space of dimension one. In one dimensional space, efficient tree techniques such as B-trees can be applied. Examples of such mappings are space filling curves [Zaniolo *et al.* (1997)] and Pyramid Technique [Böhm *et al.* (2001)]. Pyramid Technique divides the data space into two dimensional pyramids whose apexes lie at the center point. In a second step, each pyramid is cut into several slices parallel to the basis of the pyramid that form the data pages. The Pyramid Technique associates to each high dimensional point a single value, which is the distance from the point to the top of the pyramid, according to a specific dimension. The NB-tree [Fonseca and Jorge (2003)] maps the d dimensional space into a hyper-cube of the same dimension with edges of length one. In the next step the length of the corresponding points is determined, so that the objects can be ordered and represented by a simple B-tree.

A limitation of all these methods is the dimension of the data, which is limited to the order of several hundreds. Because of this constraint neither of those techniques can be compared with a subspace tree, simply because they do not work in such a extreme high dimensional space (order of several thousands) performing exact queries.

10.3   Subspace Tree

The idea behind the generic multimedia indexing (GEMINI) [Faloutsos *et al.* (1994)],[Faloutsos (1999)] approaches is to find a feature extraction function that maps the high dimensional objects into a low dimensional space. In this low dimensional space, a so-called 'quick-and-dirty' test can discard the non-qualifying objects. Objects that are very dissimilar in the subspace are expected to be very dissimilar in the original space. (see Figure 10.4). The size of the collection in the feature space depends on ϵ and the proportion between both spaces may reach the size of the entire database if the feature space is not carefully chosen. In the GEMINI approach the feature space does not need to be a subspace. In our approach map the computed metric distance between objects in the f-dimensional subspace U into the m-dimensional space V which contains the subspace U.

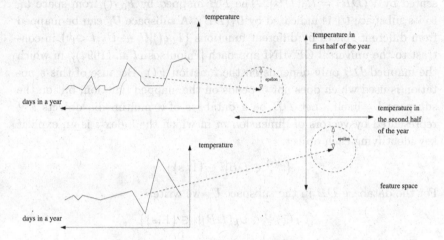

Fig. 10.4: $F()$ maps the high dimensional objects from the space V into a low dimensional subspace U. The temperature in a city measured in days is mapped into the temperature of the first half of the year and the second half of the year. The distance between similar objects should be smaller or equal to ϵ. This tolerance is represented by a sphere with radius ϵ in the subspace.

The lower bounding postulate [Faloutsos *et al.* (1994)] which guarantees that no objects will be missed in the subspace space is expressed mathematically as follows:

Let O_1 and O_2 be two objects ; $F()$, the mapping of objects into f dimensional subspace U should satisfy the following formula for all objects, where d is the Euclidian distance function $d = l_2$ in the space V and d_U is the Euclidian distance function $d = l_2$ in the subspace U:

$$d_U(F(O_1), F(O_2)) \leq d(F(O_1), F(O_2)) \leq d(O_1, O_2). \qquad (10.1)$$

We can define a sequence of subspaces $U_0, U_1, U_2, \ldots, U_n$ with $V = U_0$ in which each subspace is a subspace of another space

$$U_0 \supset U_1 \supset U_2 \supset \ldots \supset U_n$$

and

$$dim(U_0) > dim(U_1) \ldots > dim(U_n).$$

All s multimedia objects of DB are in space $V = U_0$, which is represented by $V(DB) = U_0(DB)$. The DB mapped by $F_{0,1}()$ from space U_0 to its subspace U_1 is indicated by $U_1(DB)$. A subspace U_k can be mapped from different spaces by different functions $\{F_{l,k}()|U_l \to U_k, l < k\}$ in contrast to the universal GEMINI approach [Faloutsos *et al.* (1994)], in which the mapped DB only depends on the function $F()$. Because of this a notation is used which does not depends on the mapped function, but on the subspace U_k itself. Let DB be a database of s multimedia objects $\vec{x}^{(i)}$ represented by vectors of dimension m in which the index i is an explicit key identifying each object,

$$\{\vec{x}^{(i)} \in DB | i \in \{1..s\}\}.$$

For the database DB in the subspace U_k we write:

$$\{U_k(\vec{x})^{(i)} \in U_k(DB) | i \in \{1..s\}\}$$

The set DB can be ordered according to a given multimedia object $\vec{y}$ using the Euclidean distance function d in the space U_k. This is done by a monotone increasing sequence corresponding to the increasing distance of $\vec{y}$ to $\vec{x}^{(i)}$ in the subspace U_k with an explicit key that identifies each object indicated by the index i,

$$d[U_k(y)]_n := \{d(U_k(x^{(i)}), U_k(y)) \mid \forall n \in \{1..s\} : d[U_k(y)]_n \leq d[U_k(y)]_{n+1}\}. \tag{10.2}$$

If $\vec{y} \in DB$, then $d[y]_1 := 0$. The set of similar multimedia objects in correspondence to $\vec{y}$, $DB[y]_\epsilon$, is the subset of DB, $DB[y]_\epsilon \subseteq DB$ with size $\sigma = |DB[y]_\epsilon|$, $\sigma \leq s$. $DB[y]_\epsilon$ can be as well represented in the subspace U_k:

$$U_k(DB[y])_\epsilon := \{U_k(x)_n^{(i)} \in U_k(DB) \mid d[U_k(y)]_n = d(U_k(x)^{(i)}, U_k(y)) \leq \epsilon\}, \tag{10.3}$$

with the size $U_k(\sigma) = |U_k(DB[y]_\epsilon)|$ and $U_0(\sigma) < U_1(\sigma) < \ldots < U_{(n)}(\sigma) < s$.

Let be $dim(U_0) := m$, the computing costs of the linear subspace sequence method are

$$\sum_{t=1}^{n} U_t(\sigma) \cdot dim(U_{(t-1)}) + s \cdot dim(U_n). \qquad (10.4)$$

The computing cost corresponds to the area defined by the sigma value and the preceding dimension $U_t(\sigma) \cdot dim(U_{t-1})$. To minimize the computing costs, the corresponding sum of areas has to be minimized. The costs are equivalent to the search costs in a tree plus the additional costs of $ln(dim(U_0))$. It means that we have a logarithmic growth in the number of elements and their dimension. The temporal complexity depends on the dimension and the number of data points. It does not suffer from the curse of dimensionality as traditional tree-based spatial access methods. For more information, consult [Wichert (2008)], [Wichert *et al.* (2009)].

10.3.1 *Orthogonal Projection and the Mean Value*

We propose a linear mapping $F()$ that meets all the required properties, namely the orthogonal projection which corresponds to the computation of the mean value of the projected points (projection on the bisecting line). In first step we show that the orthogonal projection satisfies the lower bounding postulate:

Let O_1 and O_2 be two vectors; if $V = \mathbf{R}^m$ is a vector space and U is an f-dimensional subspace obtained by a projection and an Euclidian distance function $d = l_2$, then

$$d_U(U((O_1), U(O_2)) \leq d(U(O_1), U(O_2)) \leq d(O_1, O_2). \qquad (10.5)$$

Furthermore, we can map the computed metric distance d_U between objects in the f-dimensional orthogonal subspace U into the m-dimensional space V which contains the orthogonal subspace U by just multiplying the distance d_u by a constant $c = \sqrt{\frac{m}{f}}$,

$$d(U(O_1), U(O_2)) = \sqrt{\frac{m}{f}} \cdot d_U(U((O_1), U(O_2)). \qquad (10.6)$$

Proof. An orthogonal projection P onto U is a mapping $P : \mathbf{R}^m \to U$. It orders every vector $\vec{x} \in \mathbf{R}^m$ a vector $P(\vec{x})$ with the shortest distance to $\vec{x} \in \mathbf{R}^m$. If $(w^{(1)}, w^{(2)}, \ldots, w^{(m)})$ is the orthonormalbasis of $\mathbf{R}^m$, and

$(w^{(1)}, w^{(2)}, \ldots, w^{(f)})$ is the orthonormalbasis of U, then $\vec{x}$ can be represented by the unique decomposition

$$\vec{x} = \sum_{i=1}^{f} < \vec{x}, w^{(i)} > \cdot w^{(i)} + \sum_{i=f+1}^{m} < \vec{x}, w^{(i)} > \cdot w^{(i)}$$

and the orthogonal projection of $\vec{x}$ onto U can be represented by

$$P(\vec{x}) = \sum_{i=1}^{f} < \vec{x}, w^{(i)} > \cdot w^{(i)}$$

$$O(\vec{x})^{\perp} = \sum_{i=f+1}^{m} < \vec{x}, w^{(i)} > \cdot w^{(i)}$$

An orthogonal basis can be decomposed, for example, through the classical method named 'Gram-Schmidt orthogonalization' process. According to the Pythagorean theorem, $||\vec{x}||^2 = ||P(\vec{x})||^2 + ||O(\vec{x})^{\perp}||^2$; consequently, $||\vec{x}|| \geq ||P(\vec{x})||$, from which the lower bound lemma results [Lang (1970)], [Jedrzejek C. (1995)].

For the second part of the theorem, we indicate that such an orthogonal projection exists. It is the mean value of the projected points, or the projection on the bisecting line. Suppose that we have a vector $\vec{a} = (a_1, a_2, .. a_k, .., a_m)$ with $a_1 = a_2 = \ldots = a_k = \ldots = a_m$ which represents the mean value of the projected points in m dimensional space. The length of this vector in Euclidian space of the dimension m is $\sqrt{m} \cdot a$. The length of $\vec{a} = a_1$ in one dimensional space is just a. The length of $\vec{a} = (a_1, a_2, .., a_k, .., a_f)$ with $a_1 = a_2 = \ldots a_k = \ldots = a_f$ in dimension f is $\sqrt{f} \cdot a$, so the division of the length between the two Euclidian spaces is $\sqrt{\frac{m}{f}}$.

If we compute several mean values (as done in the image pyramid), for example we compute a mean value of a m dimensional vector $\vec{y}$ in a window of size w. We get a new reduced vector $\vec{z}$ of the dimension f with $f = \frac{m}{w}$. The length of the vector $\vec{z}$ is $l = ||z||_2$ and the length of the projected vector in m dimensional space is $\sqrt{w} \cdot l = \sqrt{\frac{m}{f}} \cdot l$.

Why is the orthogonal projection and the mean value a good choice for evenly distributed data and the Euclidian distance function? To a given vector $\vec{x}$ of a dimension m we determine the closest vector $\vec{a} = (a_1, a_2, .. a_k, .., a_m)$ with $a_1 = a_2 = \ldots = a_k = \ldots = a_m = \alpha$ according to the Euclidian distance function. Each component is equal in vector $\vec{a}$. How do we chose the value of α? We want to minimize the distance $d(\vec{x}, \vec{a})$

$$\min_{\alpha} \left(\sqrt{(x_1 - \alpha)^2 + (x_2 - \alpha)^2 + ... + (x_k - \alpha)^2 + ... + (x_m - \alpha)^2} \right)$$

$$0 = \frac{\partial d(\vec{x}, \vec{a})}{\partial \alpha} = \frac{m \cdot \alpha - (\sum_{i=1}^{m} x_i)}{\sqrt{m \cdot \alpha^2 + \sum_{i=1}^{m} x_i^2 - 2 \cdot \alpha \cdot (\sum_{i=1}^{m} x_i)}}$$

with the solution

$$\alpha = \frac{\sum_{i=1}^{m} x_i}{m}$$

which is the mean value of the vector $\vec{x}$.

We indicate an example: The first example is an intuitive demonstration of the relation ship between the Pythagorean theorem and the orthogonal projection on the bisecting line. The orthogonal projection of points $\vec{x} = (x_1, x_2) \in \mathbf{R}^2$ on the bisecting line $U = \{(x_1, x_2) \in \mathbf{R}^2 | x_1 = x_2\} = \{(x_1, x_1) = \mathbf{R}^1\}$ corresponds to the mean value of the projected points. The orthonormalbasis of U is $x^{(1)} = (\frac{1}{\sqrt{2}}, \frac{1}{\sqrt{2}})$. The point $\vec{a} = (2, 4)$ is mapped into $P(\vec{a}) = 3$, and $\vec{b} = (7, 5)$ into $P(\vec{b}) = 6$. The distance in U is $d_u(P(\vec{a}), P(\vec{b})) = \sqrt{|6 - 3|^2}$, $c = \sqrt{2}$, so the distance in $\mathbf{R}^2$ is $d(P(\vec{a}), P(\vec{b})) = 3 \cdot \sqrt{2} \leq d(\vec{a}, \vec{b}) = \sqrt{26}$ (see Figure 10.5).

10.3.2 *Image Pyramid - A Subspace Tree*

We combine the gray information and its spatial distribution through simple image matching in high-dimensional space. We scale the digital images to a fixed size. With this transformation, we are able to represent the images as vectors and to compute the Euclidian distance between any pair at the pixel-level. Our naive features are the scaled images themselves representing the autocorrelogram and layout information. This naive features are seldom used in CBIR, due to their extremely high dimension. Two images $\vec{x}$ and $\vec{y}$ are similar if their distance is smaller or equal to ϵ, $d(\vec{x}, \vec{y}) \leq \epsilon$. The result of a range query computed by this method is a set of images that have spatial color characteristics that are similar to the query image.

We use the subspace tree method to speed up the search considerably. The search starts in the subspace with the lowest resolution of the images. In this subspace the set of all possible similar images is determined. In the next subspace additional metric information corresponding to a higher resolution is used to reduce this set. This procedure is repeated until the similar images can be extracted after elimination of the false candidates.

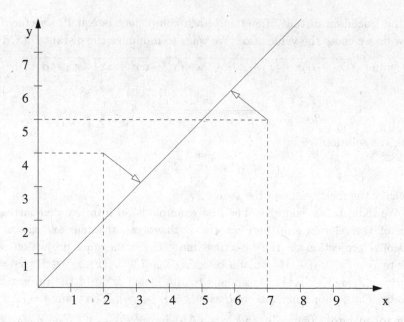

Fig. 10.5: For example, the orthogonal projection of points $\vec{x} = (x_1, x_2) \in$ $\mathbf{R}^2$ on the bisecting line $U = \{(x_1, x_2) \in \mathbf{R}^2 | x_1 = x_2\} =$ $\{(x_1, x_1) = \mathbf{R}^1\}$ corresponds to the mean value of the projected points. $\vec{a} = (2, 4)$ is mapped into $P(\vec{a}) = 3$, and $\vec{b} = (7, 5)$ into $P(\vec{b}) = 6$.

A lower resolution of an image corresponds to an orthogonal projection in rectangular windows, which define sub-images of an image. The image is tiled with rectangular windows W of size $j \times k$ in which the mean value is computed (averaging filter). The arithmetic mean value computation in a window corresponds to an orthogonal projection of these values onto a bisecting line. Because of this, the different resolutions of an image correspond to a sequence of subspaces that satisfy the lower bounding postulate. The representation of images in several resolutions corresponds to a structure which is called image pyramid in digital image processing [Burt and Adelson (1983)]. The base of the pyramid contains an image with a high resolution, its apex being the low-resolution approximation of the image.

10.4 Experiments

We applied the subspace tree for medical CBIR. The dataset was composed of 12 000 gray X-ray images (size $256 \cdot 256$). The images came from 116 different categories (different views of x-rayed body parts), belonging to persons of different genders, various ages and different diseases. We used the following down-sampling function $F_{a,b}()$ from space U_a to space U_b; $F_{0,1}() := \{mean\ over\ W | W\ with\ size\ 4 \times 4\}$, $F_{1,2}() := \{mean\ over\ W | W\ with\ size\ 4 \times 4\}$, $F_{2,3}() := \{mean\ over\ W | W\ with\ size\ 2 \times 2\}$, see Figure 10.6. The dimensions of the subspaces are

$$dim(U_0) = 65536 > dim(U_1) = 4096 > dim(U_2) = 256 > dim(U_3) = 64.$$

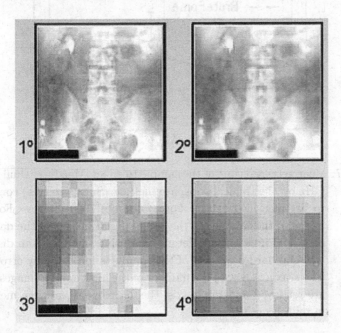

Fig. 10.6: (1) Image with the size 256×256. (2) Image resolution 64×64. (3) Image resolution 16×16. (4) Image resolution 8×8.

For testing purposes, a sample of 600 query images was randomly selected from the original dataset. For each image of the sample set the most similar images of the database of 12 000 images were determined using the

Euclidian distance. The actual retrieval time on a computer differs from the theoretical computing cost of the subspace tree according to the Equation 10.4. In Figure 10.7, we relate the actual mean retrieval time of the most similar images on an iMac Intel Dual Core 2.0 GHz measured in milliseconds, in Figure 10.8 the computing cost according to the Equation 10.4, see as well Table 10.1.

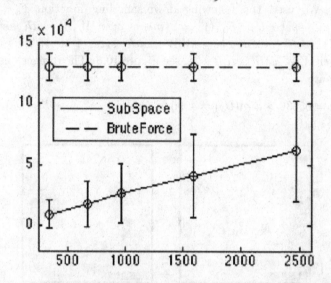

Fig. 10.7: Mean retrieval time of the sample to on an iMac Intel Dual Core 2 GHz by hierarchical subspace method (Subspace tree) compared to list matching (Brute Force) out of 12000 images. For each image of the sample set the most similar images of the database of 12 000 images were determined using the Euclidian distance. The standard deviation of the sample is indicated by error bars. The x-axis indicates the number of the most similar images which are retrieved and the y-axis, the actual retrieval time measured in milliseconds.

The actual retrieval costs depend on the implementation of the system. For the list matching we read one sequential file representing the whole collection of images and compare it to the query image. The time to read of the sequential file is fast but varies due to large size of the file and the used operating system OS X, which does not guarantee constant execution time (real time). For the subspace tree method it is required that

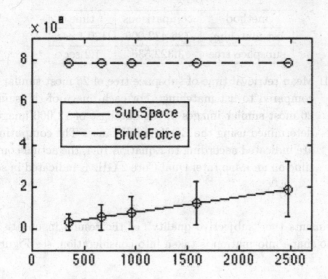

Fig. 10.8: Mean computing costs according to the Equation 10.4 of the sample by hierarchical subspace method (Subspace tree) compared to list matching (Brute Force) out of 12000 images. For each image of the sample set the most similar images of the database of 12 000 images were determined using the Euclidian distance. The standard deviation of the sample is indicated by error bars. The x-axis indicates the number of the most similar images which are retrieved and the y-axis, the number of comparisons.

each image is represented in a separated file which increase the computing time.

We introduced and demonstrated the subspace tree by CBIR examples. Without the subspace tree multimedia indexing are constrained by the dimension of the extracted features, as for example the histogram method. The histogram method consists in the comparison of the histograms of images. The histogram of a medical X-ray image gives the pixels count of the same gray value. For each gray value there is a corresponding bin. We used histograms with 256 bins, hence capable of counting 256 different shades of grey. This means we have 256 comparisons per image. Since we are using 12 000 images, the number of total comparisons per query is only $256 \cdot 12000 = 3.072.000$ which requires only 1 sec on a iMac Intel Dual Core 2 GHz without any indexing method. However compared with the previ-

method	comparisons	time
list matching	786.432.000	130.1 sec
subspace tree	3.322.536	1.2 sec

Table 10.1: Mean retrieval time of subspace tree of 26 most similar images compared to list matching. For each image of the sample set 26 most similar images of the database of 12 000 images were determined using the Euclidian distance. The computing steps are indicated according to Equation 10.4, the actual computing time on an iMac Intel Dual Core 2 GHz is indicated in seconds.

ous experiments the "subjective quality" of the results in unsatisfactory, because no shape information is taken into consideration, see Figure 10.9.

10.5 Conclusion

We built an electronic health record, incorporating a "Content-addressable" multimedia database, through a fast CBIR search methods. A prototype system was successfully deployed. The system consists of a web application, accessible from any device with Internet connection and a Web browser.

For a fast CBIR we used the subspace-tree. It works in extreme high dimensional space (order of several thousands) and performs fast exact queries. A limitation of other indexing methods is the dimension of the data. They do not work in such a extreme high dimensional space (order of several thousands) performing exact queries. As a consequence the images are described by lower dimensional feature vectors, as in the histogram method.

Subspace trees divide the distance between the subspaces, and not the space itself. The search in such a structure starts in the subspace with the lowest dimension. In this subspace, the set of all possible similar vectors is determined. In the next subspace, additional metric information, corresponding to a higher dimension, is used to reduce this set. We performed experiments with a new indexing technique on a dataset of 12 000 images in shades of grey resulting from several X-rays randomly collected from 116 different categories. Each image is described by an extremely high dimensional feature vector of dimension 65536. To retrieve the 26 most similar images out of 12 000, our system took, on average, 1.2 sec.

Histogramas		Hierarchical Subspace	
Imagem	Distância	Imagem	Distância
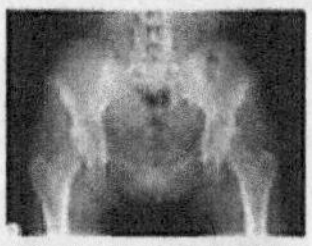	0	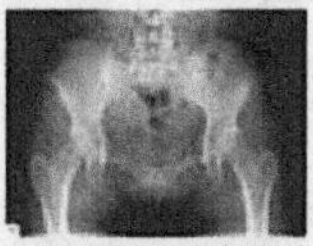	0
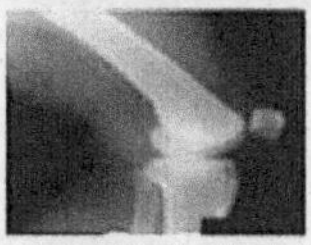	6848.892	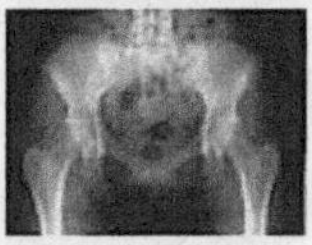	477904061.977
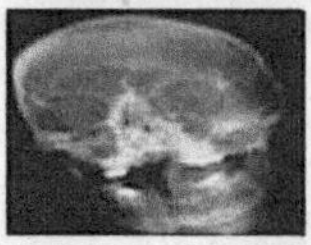	8418.711	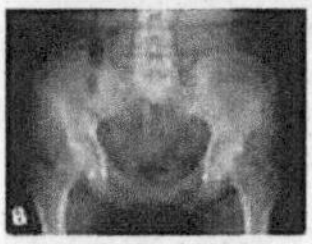	532367453.218
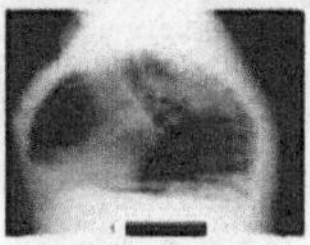	8425.311	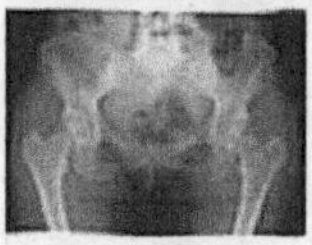	555600385.971
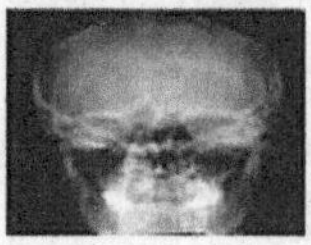	8656.168	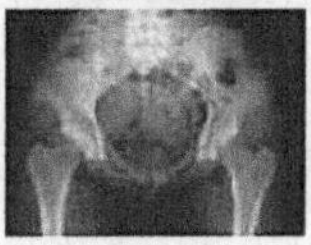	579158566.285

Fig. 10.9: The histograms method is not very effective in finding similar images. In the subspace tree - hierarchical subspace method (or list matching) the pixels compared have equivalent spatial positions. On the left side the results of the histogram method are shown, on the right side those of the subspace tree. The first image is the query image. Beside the image the distance to the query image is shown, the bigger the distance, the more dissimilar the images are. The distances of the hierarchical subspace method are bigger, because more information is taken into account. An extension to the proposed method would be a sub-pattern matching based on the subspace tree. The query would correspond to a template sub-pattern (for example, a tumor), and would allow to answer the following question: *How does my patient's tumor compare to other similar cases?*

Acknowledgments

The author would like to thank for the permission to use the data set for experimental tests purposes to TM Deserno, Dept. of Medical Informatics, RWTH Aachen, Germany.

Chapter 11

Ensemble Feature Selection in Biomedical Applications

Michael Netzer and Christian Baumgartner

University for Health Sciences, Medical Informatics and Technology (UMIT), Hall in Tirol, Austria

Recent technologically significant advances in the area of life sciences research are resulting in the rapid production of massive amounts of data. Mass spectrometry (MS), for instance, has become an important tool to measure the abundance of compounds such as metabolites, lipids or proteins in body fluids or tissue. Microarray technologies and their complementary techniques are proving to be powerful tools for probing genetic sequences and their transcriptional manifestations. Data from these analytical techniques are key components of a full spectrum of biochemical analyses (genomic, proteomic, lipidomic, metabolomic, etc.) that is collectively referred to as the "omics". In combination with clinical assessments and other medical information, omics data can potentially provide very useful insight into a wide variety of different biomedical issues such as disease causation, phenotype characterization and therapeutic response evaluation. In general however, omics data is characterized by high complexity and dimensionality. Sophisticated data mining approaches are required to discover biomarkers that are specific for a pathogenic processes, or pharmacologic responses to a therapeutic intervention. The success of data mining algorithms strongly depends on factors such as which information is irrelevant or redundant. Feature selection algorithms use different measures, e.g. statistical- or entropy-based, to select relevant features. However, it has been recently shown that the combination (ensemble) of feature selection approaches produces favorable results compared to single approaches (Netzer *et al.*, 2009). The idea behind ensemble feature selection is to consult several "experts" before making a final decision. The search for an optimal feature subset using ensemble techniques is basically built into a two-step procedure, (1) creating a set of different feature selectors, and (2) aggregating the results to a consensus set.

In this chapter we give a survey on the combination of feature selection methods. Section 11.1 reviews several popular feature selection approaches. Section 11.2 describes the evaluation of feature selection approaches. In Sec. 11.3 we introduce a novel approach for the combination of feature selection methods. From Sec. 11.4 on we give a biomedical example for the application of ensemble feature selection to identify potential liver disease marker candidates in breath gas samples.

11.1   Introduction

Supervised feature selection methods reduce the number of features of a data set to a smaller set, anticipating superior discriminatory and predictive power. Thus, the benefits of feature selection are lower computational costs due to reduction of dimensionality, improved interpretability, and higher classification accuracy due to reduction of noise (Osl *et al.*, 2009). Therefore, feature selection is an important step before classification. In general, feature selection methods can be classified into filters, wrappers and more advanced methods like ensemble-based approaches. Filter methods rank features based on their quality to discriminate between two or more predefined classes [Baumgartner and Graber (2007)]. Popular filters are the information gain [Quinlan (1993)], the reliefF [Kononenko (1994)], the biomarker identifier (Baumgartner and Baumgartner, 2006) or statistical hypothesis testing. Examples for statistical null-hypothesis testing include the χ^2 statistics, the Student t-test or Welch test (parametric tests), or the Wilcoxon rank sum test as an example for a nonparametric test, respectively.

11.1.1   *Statistical Hypothesis Testing*

In biomedical research, statistical analyses are mostly used to compare groups of individuals, different procedures or treatments. The corresponding numerical value as a result of this comparison of interest is called "effect". The hypothesis stating, that the effect is zero is called the null hypothesis (e.g., there is no significant difference in the average of serum cholesterol in men and women). The null hypothesis is the negation of the research hypothesis, which is also termed the alternative hypothesis. This hypothesis states, that the effect of interest is not zero. The probability that the observed data was obtained when the null hypothesis was true is called the P-Value [Altman (1991)]. The smaller this value the more implausible the null hypothesis is. The P-Value can be calculated employing a test statistic, which compares the observed value (estimate of interest such as difference in mean serum cholesterol) to what we would expect if the null hypothesis was true. The test statistic is given by

$$test\ statistics = \frac{observed\ value - hypothesized\ value}{standard\ error\ of\ observed\ value} \tag{11.1}$$

A popular parametric hypothesis test for two independent groups is the two sample Student's t test (also referred to as t test), which is given by

$$t = \frac{\bar{x}_1 - \bar{x}_2}{se(\bar{x}_1 - \bar{x}_2)} \tag{11.2}$$

where $\bar{x}_1$ and $\bar{x}_2$ denote the means of the two samples and se is the standard error defined as

$$se(\bar{x}_1 - \bar{x}_2) = s \times \sqrt{\frac{1}{n_1} + \frac{1}{n_2}} \tag{11.3}$$

where s is the pooled standard deviation of the two groups of sizes n_1 and n_2.

If, however, the assumption of normality is reasonable for the two groups, but having unequal population variances, the Welch test (Welch, 1947) should be used. The Welch test is a modification of the t test, which treats the two sample variances separately rather than taking a pooled average of two sample variances. The Wilcoxon rank sum test is the non-parametric alternative to the t test. It ranks all observations as if they were from a single sample and calculates a statistic based on the difference between the sums of the ranks of two groups (Mann and Whitney, 1947).

11.1.2 *Information Gain*

The information gain (IG) [Quinlan (1993)] computes the discriminatory ability of every feature by computing how well a given feature separates data by expecting a reduction of entropy, a measure of the purity within the data. The expected reduction of entropy caused by partitioning the data according to feature f_i can be calculated and further be used for feature

ranking (Osl *et al.*, 2008). More formally the IG in feature F with relation
to class C is the mutual information between F and C (Nelson, 2005):

$$I(C, F) = H(C) - H(C|F), \text{ where} \qquad (11.4)$$

$$H(C) = \sum_{c_i} P(c_i) \times \log_2 \frac{1}{P(c_i)}, \text{ the initial entropy in C} \qquad (11.5)$$

$$H(C|F) = \sum_{f_j} P(f_j) \times H(C|f_j), \qquad (11.6)$$

the conditional entropy in C given F, and

$$H(C|f_j) = \sum_{c_i} P(c_i|f_j) \times \log_2 \frac{1}{P(c_i|f_j)}, \qquad (11.7)$$

the entropy in C given a particular feature f_j.

11.1.3 *ReliefF*

ReliefF is an exponent of a multivariate correlation-based feature selection
method, repeatedly sampling instances, comparing feature values of the k
nearest instances for the same (hits) and the different classes (misses). The
selection of k hits and misses is the main difference to the original Relief
[Kira and Rendell (1992)] and ensures greater robustness of the algorithm
concerning noise (Robnik-Sikonja and Kononenko, 2003). For most purposes k can be safely set to 10 [Kononenko (1994)].

11.1.4 *Biomarker Identifier*

The biomarker identifier (BMI) was originally applied to metabolic data
to identify disease specific changes of concentrations of metabolites. This
approach combines various statistical measures (the product of sensitivity
and specificity, the effect size and variance) to calculate an evaluation score
for feature ranking. The BMI score for a feature f, a variant of the initial
method (Baumgartner and Baumgartner, 2006), is defined as:

$$BMI(f) = \lambda \times TP^2 \times \sqrt{|\Delta_{diff}| \times \frac{CV_{ref}}{CV}} \text{ with} \qquad (11.8)$$

$$\Delta_{diff} = \begin{cases} \Delta & \text{if } \Delta \geq 1 \\ -\frac{1}{\Delta} & \text{else} \end{cases} \text{ with } \Delta = \frac{\bar{x}}{\bar{x}_{ref}} \qquad (11.9)$$

where λ is a scaling factor and TP^2 is the product of the true positive
(TP) values determined for both classes using logistic regression analysis.

By default λ is set to 10 for ensuring that score values range between 1 and ~ 1000, which is of practical advantage. The parameter Δ_{diff} calculates relative changes in levels with respect to a reference group. $\Delta_{diff} \geq 1$ denotes a concentration enhancement, $\Delta_{diff} \leq 1$ a decrease of concentration. The ratio $\frac{CV_{ref}}{CV}$ considers changes in the variance of data across the two cohorts. $\overline{x}_{ref}$ and $\overline{x}$ is the mean value of levels in the reference and the comparison class.

In general, univariate feature ranking methods are very efficient and the provided output is intuitive and easy to understand. Univariate filter techniques, however, consider each feature separately, thereby ignoring feature dependencies, which may lead to worse classification performance (Saeys *et al.*, 2007). To overcome the problem of ignoring feature dependencies, a number of multivariate filter techniques such as ReliefF were introduced. Another disadvantage of filter methods is that they ignore the interaction with the classifier. In contrary, wrappers use a classifier to evaluate the discriminatory ability of feature subsets (Inza *et al.*, 2004). In general, heuristic approaches like forward selection or backward elimination are used to search through the space of possible feature subsets. Forward selection starts with an empty set of features and adds at each step the feature which optimizes a criterion such as discriminatory power, whereas backward selection starts with the full set and removes at each step one of the features to optimize the criterion. A combination of both approaches is also possible deciding in each step whether to remove or to add a feature. Examples for other heuristic search methods are random or genetic based algorithms. Genetic based search methods are based on the genetic algorithm described in Goldberg [Goldberg (1989)]. Feature subsets selected by wrappers are highly discriminatory, but at an extensive computational cost.

11.2 Evaluation of Feature Selection Approaches

Probably the most widely used method to evaluate the quality of a feature ranking is to determine the discriminatory power of a ranking. Therefore, the set of the k top ranked features is used for building the classifier and its classification accuracy is calculated. Measures that denote the classifier's accuracy are built from a confusion matrix that lists correctly and incorrectly classified samples for each class. Table 1 depicts such a confusion

Table 11.1: Confusion matrix for a binary classification problem.

Class/Recognized	as Positive	as Negative
Positive	TP	FN
Negative	FP	TN

matrix for a binary classification problem, where TP are true positive, FP false positive, FN false negative, and TN true negative counts. The most often used empirically measure to assess the quality of a classifier is the accuracy [Sokolova *et al.* (2006)]:

$$accuracy = \frac{(TP + TN)}{(TP + FP + FN + TN)} \qquad (11.10)$$

More informally, accuracy measures the percentage of correctly classified test points. To separately estimate a classifier's performance on different classes (i.e., healthy versus diseased) sensitivity and specificity which are the two main features of a diagnostic test can be used:

$$sensitivity = \frac{TP}{TP + FN} \qquad (11.11)$$

$$specificity = \frac{TN}{FP + TN} \qquad (11.12)$$

Since accuracy does not focus on a certain class (e.g., healthy or disease) it is the most general way to compare classification performance. However, especially if dealing with imbalanced data, accuracy was shown to be an inappropriate measure (He and Garcia, 2009). Let us, for example, consider a data set that includes 10 percent samples of the minority class and 90 percent of the majority class. In this case an uninformed classifier, assigning all samples of the dataset to be the majority class, would provide an accuracy of 90 percent. Another method to measure the discriminatory ability of a classifier is the area under the ROC curve (AUC). For the example given above the AUC is 0.5 corresponding to the real situation that the classes are assigned randomly. Let us consider a binary classification problem with m samples of class 0 and n samples of class 1. Let $x_1, \ldots, x_m$ be the output for class 0 and $y_1, \ldots, y_n$ be the output for class 1. 1_X denotes the Boolean indicator function of a set X. Then, the AUC, associated to a classifier is given by [Cortes and Mohri (2005)]:

$$AUC = \frac{\sum_{i=1}^{m} \sum_{j=1}^{n} 1_{x_i > y_i}}{mn} \qquad (11.13)$$

which is the value of the Wilcoxon-Mann-Whitney statistics (Hanley and McNeil, 1982). It is an estimate of the probability P_{xy} that the classifier ranks a randomly chosen sample of class 0 higher than a sample of class 1 [Cortes and Mohri (2005)]. A perfect classifier has an AUC = 1, indicating that there exists a threshold that separates both classes without error. The AUC is probably the most commonly used global index of diagnostic accuracy. The Youden index (Youden, 1950) is also frequently used in a diagnostic setting [Fluss *et al.* (2005)]. It is defined as the sum of sensitivity and specificity minus 1 and provides a useful criterion for choosing the optimal threshold value for which sensitivity and specificity are maximized.

11.2.1 *Popular Classifiers for Assessing Discriminatory Ability of Selected Features*

The general process in classification is to train a classifier on labeled training samples and to classify future unlabeled samples with the trained model [Cho and Won (2003)]. In contrast to regression, where the target variable is numerical, the target value in classification is categorical (e.g. diseased or healthy). Formally, a dataset can be described as a set of tuples (x,c), where x is a n-dimensional vector of features and c is a class label. A classifier is then a model f(x) learned of the conditional probability P(c|x). Two very popular classifiers are the support vector machine and the logistic regression. More specifically, support vector machines (SVM) produce a separating hyperplane in a transformed feature space which is usually of higher dimension than the original space. The transformation is done by using a kernel technique. This procedure enables classes to make them linearly separable and forms the basis for constructing class boundaries by maximizing the margin between the groups (maximum margin) [Varmuza and Filzmoser (2009)]. In contrast, logistic regression analysis uses linear functions to calculate posterior probabilities of the classes. A logit transformation ensures that the predicted values are constrained to lie between 0 and 1 [Hosmer and Lemeshow (2000)]. The class membership c of an object x is predicted by a probability measure

$$P(c|x) = \frac{1}{1 + e^{-z}} \text{ and } z = b_0 + \sum_{i=1}^{m} b_i x_i \qquad (11.14)$$

where b_i are the regression coefficients describing the size of the contribution of the risk factors. The sum of all posterior probabilities is 1. The estimation of parameters $b_0, b_1, \ldots, b_m$ is done by the maximum likelihood method. The parameter b_0 (intercept) describes the value of z when the value of all risk factors is zero (Tripepi *et al.*, 2008). The logistic regression analysis which is widely used in many biomedical applications is very similar to linear discriminant analysis, where the posterior probabilities are modeled by a linear function [Varmuza and Filzmoser (2009)].

11.2.2 *Classifier Validation*

Cross validation is a well-established method for estimating the error rate of a classifier on a particular dataset. In k-fold cross-validation the data set is split into k parts. The process is then repeated k times, using k-1 partitions for training and the remaining part for testing. Finally the k measures for quality obtained for the k folds are averaged. If the number of folds equals the number of samples, especially in the data set, the validation procedure is called leave-one-out cross-validation. Other methods for validation include bootstrapping or permutation analysis which are based on statistical procedures of sampling with or without replacement.

11.3 Ensemble Feature Selection

When evaluating the quality of single feature ranking methods especially for small size data errors in the model strongly influence the quality of the method. The bias-variance decomposition (Geman *et al.*, 1992) distinguishes between three types of errors: 1) The bias error is a systematic component of the error and results from differences between the learning method and the domain (Van Der Putten and Van Someren, 2004). It is the mean-squared error expected when averaging over models built from all possible training datasets [Witten and Frank (2005)]. 2) The variance error is associated with differences between models of different samples. The sum of bias and variance is called total expected error, whilst 3) the intrinsic error (noise) is due to the uncertainty in the domain [Witten and Frank (2005)]. One approach to reduce the total expected error is the combination of multiple learning methods. The bias component can be diminished by averaging over multiple models built from independent training sets. The variance component of the expected error can be reduced by combining multiple classifiers. Different methods to design ensemble-based learning models are: Resampling techniques such as bootstrapping or bagging build varying models on a defined number of training datasets randomly drawn with replacement from the initial dataset (Polikar, 2006). Stacking [Wolpert (1992)], an ensemble approach, combines different models in a multi-layer architecture, where the base level or level-0 incorporates different classifiers. The predictions of level-0 serve as input for a level-1 classifier that aggregates level-0 results to the final class prediction.

The idea of ensemble learning has recently also been described for feature selection purposes. The basic idea is to combine multiple learning methods in order to reduce bias and variance in a classification task. As an example for feature selection, linear aggregation [Saeys *et al.* (2008)] builds up a consensus ranking where features contribute in a linear way with respect to their rank. Let us consider an ensemble $E = F_1, F_2, \ldots, F_s$ consisting of s feature selection approaches, and assuming each F_i provides a feature ranking $f_i = (f_i^1, \ldots, f_i^N)$ then the linear aggregation is defined as [Saeys *et al.* (2008)]:

$$f^l = \sum_{i=i}^{s} f_i^l \qquad (11.15)$$

Another method to get a consensus ranking relies on the concept of stacking as described above. The adaption of this concept for feature selection was recently described by Netzer and authors (Netzer *et al.*, 2009), termed Stacked Feature Ranking (SFR). SFR utilizes a two level architecture with a suggestion (level-1) and a decision layer (level-0). The decision layer uses different feature selectors as input to determine a final consensus ranking.

11.3.1 *Stacked Feature Ranking*

Various feature ranking methods produce different rankings due to the diversity of the underlying models. SFR uses these different ratings as input for an induced meta-level layer that enables an optimized feature ranking. Starting with an empty set of ranked features, SFR looks at the d-highest ranked features ($1 < d \leq$ m; m ... number of all features) of all n feature ranking methods (level-0), referred to as prediction-input (Netzer *et al.*, 2009). The parameter d is referred to as depth. The prediction input is then used as input for the level-1 classifier that determines those features that increase the discriminatory ability of the already ranked feature set best (empty in the first step). This procedure is repeated until all features are ranked and thus the final consensus ranking is determined. The next section demonstrates the application of SFR for the search for breath gas markers in liver disease.

11.4 Biomedical Example

Fatty liver disease (FLD) represents a common clinical entity and can be divided into alcoholic fatty liver disease (AFLD) and nonalcoholic fatty liver disease (NAFLD) (Mills and Harrison, 2005). AFLD primary emerges from excess alcohol consumption whereas NAFLD is caused by metabolism-associated causes. Other reasons for NAFLD include parenteral nutrition, gastric bypass surgery, and certain disorders of the fatty acid metabolism (Reddy and Rao, 2006). It is generally difficult to distinguish AFLD from NAFLD due to remarkably similar pathological and histological features. Despite these similarities, however, AFLD and NAFLD follow different clinical courses and thus different treatment strategies (Mills and Harrison, 2005; Reddy and Rao, 2006). Diagnostic methods in clinical hepatology are still poor at specificity and little invasive methods are desired. Levels of transaminases determined by blood tests point out liver cell damage, but there is neither any correlation to the aetiology nor to the severity of the chronic liver disease. Liver biopsy can give insight into the aetiology of liver cell damage regarding viral and nonviral hepatic damage, but nevertheless it is not feasible in differentiating alcoholic from nonalcoholic fatty liver. The liver as the central organ in synthesis and detoxification has great influence on key pathways of metabolism (Tanimizu and Miyajima, 2007). Changes in functioning or in the texture of the liver leads to altered pathways and the accumulation of metabolites. Many of these accumulated molecules are exhaled and modern sensitive screening techniques like mass spectrometry (MS) are able to detect minimal alterations in breath that might occur in earlier stages of liver disease. Analysis of volatile compounds in the human breath using MS has been reported to provide useful information in lung cancer (Mazzone, 2008), diabetes mellitus (Buszewski et al., 2007) or in the estimation of oxidative stress (Risby and Sehnert, 1999). Thus, mass spectrometry analysis of the exhaled breath might be a potential tool for the search of breath gas markers to distinguish between NAFLD, AFLD and healthy individuals. For identifying, verifying and interpreting robust and generalizable key compounds or features, however, sophisticated data mining methods are required.

11.4.1   Data Collection

The breath gas data set comprises IMR-MS (Ion molecule reaction-Mass spectrometry) data of 92 individuals (57 patients and 35 healthy controls). The patient cohort was divided into two well-phenotyped subgroups according to a standardized clinical protocol including abdominal ultrasound examinations, laboratory tests and the interpretation of patient history data: the NAFLD cohort (n=34, mean age 50.9 years) and the AFLD cohort (n=20, mean age 49.5 years). The control cohort (n=35, mean age 37.4 years) yielded no history of liver disease, showed no serological markers of acute or chronic hepatitis and all blood tests including iron and glucose metabolism were within normal ranges. All samples were obtained from patient breath samples enrolled in the Department of Internal Medicine, Division of Gastroenterology and Hepatology, Medical University of Innsbruck, Austria. Clinical protocols were approved by the Innsbruck University Hospital Institutional Review Board, and all individuals gave written informed consent. We examined the three following dichotomous problems for the search for breath gas marker candidates, distinguishing between:

- AFLD vs. healthy,
- NAFLD vs. healthy,
- AFLD vs. NAFLD.

11.4.2   Sample Preparation and Mass Spectrometry Analysis

The study subjects had to fast the night before the measurement was performed, were not allowed to use toothpaste within the last hour and smoking was not allowed for the last 20 minutes before the samples were taken. Patients also had to be at rest for at least 15 minutes. For breath collection, subjects exhaled once through a standard drinking straw into a small glass vial of 20 ml volume which was then crimped airtight. The vials were transferred for the subsequent IMR-MS analysis (Airsense, V&F medical development GmbH, Absam, Austria), measuring concentrations of 114 volatile compounds in the exhalation breath. The ionization process for the detection of sample molecules is performed via ion beams that interact with the gas sample. This procedure is termed Ion Molecule Reaction (Hornuss *et al.*, 2007), which allows distinguishing between mass identical components, e.g., carbon dioxide and acetaldehyde by using different primary energy levels. Subsequently, the breath ions are separated in a quadrupol mass filter and amplified by a conversion dynode. The whole gas transfer from the autosampler to the analyzer lasted five minutes. The measured gas compounds are given as absolute concentrations in ppm or volume percent for CO_2 or O_2, respectively.

11.5   Computational Approach

Our feature selection modality SFR is embedded into a knowledge discovery workflow including data preprocessing and feature selection. Therefore, we used an in-house developed workflow design tool, termed KD3 (Knowledge Discovery in Database Designer) to carry out all experiments related to datamining [Pfeifer *et al.* (2008)]. After data import into KD3, a common statistical model for outlier detection was applied, since outliers can bias the findings and may lead to incorrect biological interpretations. Outliers were defined as values outside the range [Q1 - k IQR; Q3 + k IQR], where Q1 and Q3 are the first and third quartiles and IQR is the interquartile range. Parameter k was set to 3 for removing, by definition, "strong" outliers in the data. The preprocessed data set is then provided for the search for potential biomarker candidates using SFR.

11.5.1   *Experimental Setup*

In the given experimental setup level-0 comprises four popular feature selection methods that are the information gain (IG), reliefF (RF), the χ^2 statistics (CHI) and a statistical null-hypothesis test using the P-Value as measure for discrimination (see also Fig. 11.1). χ^2 evaluates the worth of a feature by discretizing its numeric values and computing the value of the χ^2 statistic with respect to the class. For hypothesis testing we applied a two tailed, two-sample test (Student's t-test or Welch as parametric tests, and the Mann-Whitney test as nonparametric test, respectively). As level-1 classifier we chose a logistic regression model (LOG). As an objective measure for estimating the discriminatory ability we determined the area under the ROC curve (AUC) of the selected feature sets (Lasko *et al.*, 2005).

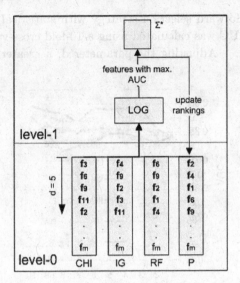

Fig. 11.1: The experimental design for the SFR using Information Gain (IG), ReliefF (RF), χ^2-Statistics (CHI), and null-hypothesis testing (P) serving as level-0 feature ranking methods and the logistic regression (LOG) employed as level-1 classifier.

11.6 Results

11.6.1 *Comparison of the Predictive Power of the Applied Feature Ranking Methods*

We evaluated the performance of the SFR by comparing SFR with each of the four single feature ranking methods IG, RF, CHI, statistical hypothesis testing (P-Value), and BMI as well as an ensemble-based feature selection modality that matches SFR best in structure and design. As ensemble feature selector we chose a paradigm described by Saeys and authors [Saeys *et al.* (2008)], performing a linear aggregation of features with respect to their ranks. We applied 10-fold cross-validation to validate the predicted feature rankings. It should be noted that the four single methods also serve as level-0 paradigms in SFR. Figure 11.2 shows that SFR outperforms each of the single methods as well as the linear aggregation of features with about 10% higher AUC when distinguishing between NAFLD and healthy controls using a depth d = 5. SFR also exceeds a wrapper based feature selection modality using logistic regression as classifier and using a greedy stepwise forward selection strategy with statistical significance (P < 0.001). The AUC was calculated using a 10-fold cross-validated logistic regression model.   Adjusting the parameter d, a greater depth (d > 5)

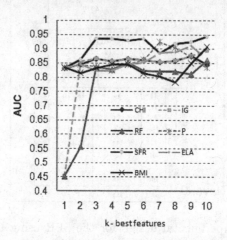

Fig. 11.2: AUC of the k top ranked features discriminating best between NAFLD and healthy controls, ranked by the single methods IG, RF, CHI, BMI, null-hypothesis testing (P-Value) and ensemble linear aggregation (ELA) vs. SFR.

further increases the predictive power of SFR (Fig. 11.3 a), but has the drawback of higher computational costs. Figure 11.3 b shows the linear correlation between depth and calculation time. A depth value of d > 6 does not lead to a further improvement of the discriminatory ability of the top five selected features.   Table 11.2 summarizes the mean AUC values for the 5, 10, 20 and 38 (= the first third of all features) top ranked features obtained for the three dichotomous problems AFLD vs. healthy, NAFLD vs. healthy and AFLD vs. NAFLD. It should be noted that logistic regression for classification was employed due to the model's simple applicability and interpretability, particularly in a clinical setting. Using a depth of d = 5, SFR achieved the highest AUC in 9 out of 12 (75%) subsets. It is important to note that in 11 of 15 (73%) comparisons SFR outperforms the other five methods with statistical significance for the top 33% selected features. Including BMI as additional level-0 feature ranking method the discriminatory power slightly increases in 3 of 12 (25%) subsets and remains constant in 6 of 12 (50%) subsets. The feature ranking methods signed by

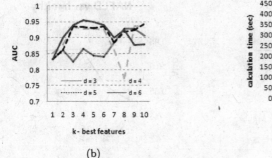

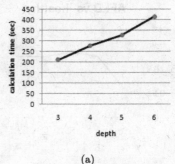

(b)

(a)

Fig. 11.3: (a) The AUC of the k ranked features discriminating best between
NAFLD and healthy controls for depth d = 3, 4, 5 and 6. (b)
The correlation between depth and calculation time for one fold.

"*" denote the different levels of significance for the AUC, i.e. * P < 0.05,
** P < 0.01, and *** P < 0.001 compared with SFR using the Wilcoxon
rank sum test.

11.6.2 *Identified Breath Gas Marker Candidates*

Figure 11.4 a) demonstrates the top five ranked breath gas marker candidates distinguishing between AFLD and healthy controls. The maximal
AUC of 0.93 for AFLD vs. controls refers to a subset of three compounds
which are M102, Isoprene and M60. Note that Mx indicates biochemically
unannotated compound masses. Figure 11.4 b) illustrates that the maximal AUC of 0.94 (NAFLD vs. healthy controls) is achieved with a set
of the three top ranked gas compounds namely CH_4, M39 and M20. The
set of the unannotated masses M75 and M102 discriminate best between
AFLD and NAFLD with an AUC of 0.96 as illustrated in Fig. 11.4 c).
Figure 11.5 illustrates the ROC curve, discriminating between AFLD and
NAFLD, and the corresponding Youden index (YI) = 0.86. The ROC curve
was calculated using logistic regression analysis.

11.7 Discussion

In this work we introduced SFR (Netzer *et al.*, 2009) as a powerful method
for the identification of potential breath gas markers in liver disease. Embedded into a stratified cross-validation strategy, SFR outperformed the

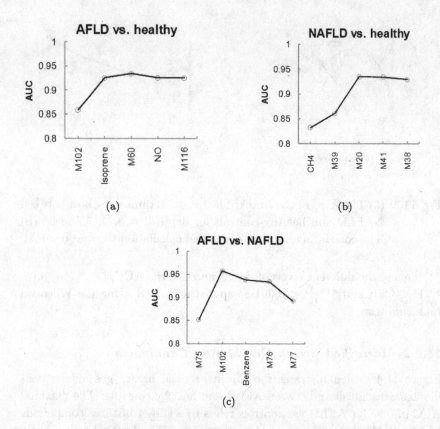

Fig. 11.4: Breath gas marker candidates for the investigated liver diseases (a
    - c) are depicted. The x-axis indicates the top 5 ranked gas com-
    pounds. The y-axis denotes the discriminatory ability (AUC) for
    the selected subsets 1...k obtained from the breath gas dataset
    (10-fold cross-validated).

other feature ranking methods significantly with the setting proposed in
this study. The experiments also showed that the performance parameter
d followed calculation time linearly. However, a depth of d = 5 appeared
to be a good tradeoff between discriminatory ability and calculation time.
One fold took roughly five minutes (less than one hour for 10-fold cross
validation) on an Intel Centrino 2x-1.83 GHz PC with 2048 MB RAM for
building up the entire feature ranking. A greater depth further increases
the predictive power of SFR, but has the drawback of higher computational
costs. Increasing the number of feature ranking methods using BMI did not

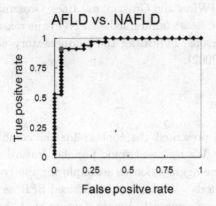

Fig. 11.5: The ROC curve for discriminating between AFLD and NAFLD. Dots in the curve are determined on the set of the two best ranked features (M75 and M102) with the maximum AUC of 0.96 using a logistic regression model. The grey dot in the left upper corner of the ROC curve indicates the Youden index (YI = 0.86, sensitivity = 0.91, specificity = 0.95).

significantly improve the predictive power of SFR. This might be explained due to correlation of BMI ranking with other level-0 feature ranking methods. With our proposed SFR setting we were able to discriminate between AFLD and NAFLD with an AUC of 0.96 with a set of two unannotated masses, namely M75 and M102. Interestingly, M75 showed a strong correlation with methylamine (r = 0.82, P < 0.01) that may play a significant role in the central nervous system disturbances observed during hepatic and renal disease (Mitchell *et al.*, 1999). Other top ranked compounds showing differences between the four groups comprised several still unidentified molecular masses. Mass 76 for example could be tentatively interpreted as carbon disulphide. Sehnert and authors (Sehnert *et al.*, 2002) described a triplet of carbon disulphide, carbonyl sulphide and isoprene greatly differentiating between healthy controls and patients with various liver diseases. Comparing alcoholic fatty liver disease with control we detected isoprene as putative marker candidate. Isoprene is linked to the cholesterol synthesis as a by-product derived from mevalonate (Stone *et al.*, 1993). Nitrogen monoxide (NO), which was the fourth top ranked compound when distinguishing between AFLD and healthy controls, was increased in portal hypertension, but still not enough to decrease sinusoidal pressure and allowed normal portal flow (Wiest and Groszmann, 1999; Groszmann, 1993). In patients suffering from heart failure, exhaled NO is increased compared with healthy control persons, indicating the compensatory circulatory mechanism (Hare *et al.*, 2002).

11.8   Conclusion

In this chapter we presented the context for the combination of feature selection methods. We reviewed some popular feature selection methods and described linear aggregation as example for the combination of feature selection methods. We further introduced SFR as a novel ensemble based feature ranking approach, demonstrating that this method greatly improved the predictive value of identified feature subsets compared with common feature selection methods. With the proposed setting SFR outperformed the other methods in 11 of 15 (73%) comparisons, identifying several expected and unexpected breath gas marker candidates, some of which could be verified from literature. We therefore propose SFR as a new representative of ensemble-based feature selection methods and as a powerful tool for the search for highly predictive biomarkers in complex biological and biochemical mixtures and settings using MS analysis.

Acknowledgment

The authors acknowledge the support from the Austrian Research Promotion Agency (KMT project 9a-b) and partly from the Austrian GEN-AU project "Bioinformatics Integration Network".

Table 11.2: Mean AUC values (10-fold cross validated) are denoted for the 5, 10, 20 and 38 (33%) top ranked features. Significance levels * P < 0.05, ** P < 0.01, *** P < 0.001 (Wilcoxon rank sum test) were calculated for the top 33% selected features. Bold numbers indicate maximal AUC values. CHI = χ^2 statistic, IG = information gain, RF = reliefF, P = statistical hypothesis testing (P-Value), ELA = ensemble linear aggregation, BMI = biomarker identifier, SFR = stacked feature ranking, SFR+BMI = SFR including BMI as additional level-0 feature ranking method.

AFLD vs. healthy	top 5	top 10	top 20	top 33%
CHI**	0.88	0.87	0.90	0.91
IG**	0.87	0.87	0.90	0.92
RF	0.87	0.91	0.93	0.94
ELA	0.88	0.90	0.92	0.93
P	0.89	0.89	0.92	0.94
BMI	0.88	0.88	0.91	0.94
SFR	0.91	0.88	0.91	0.93
SFR+BMI	0.92	0.88	0.91	0.93

NAFLD vs. healthy	top 5	top 10	top 20	top 33%
CHI***	0.85	0.86	0.86	0.91
IG**	0.78	0.82	0.85	0.91
RF***	0.70	0.77	0.78	0.86
ELA	0.83	0.86	0.89	0.93
P***	0.84	0.86	0.84	0.84
BMI	0.83	0.83	0.85	0.87
SFR	0.90	0.91	0.93	0.96
SFR+BMI	0.86	0.91	0.94	0.97

AFLD vs. NAFLD	top 5	top 10	top 20	top 33%
CHI***	0.86	0.86	0.89	0.92
IG***	0.87	0.88	0.90	0.93
RF**	0.87	0.84	0.90	0.94
ELA***	0.88	0.89	0.92	0.95
P***	0.90	0.89	0.91	0.94
BMI	0.89	0.85	0.91	0.94
SFR	0.91	0.91	0.95	0.97
SFR+BMI	0.91	0.89	0.94	0.97

Chapter 12

Analysis of Breast Cancer Genomic Data by Fuzzy Association Rule Mining

F. Javier Lopez[1], Marta Cuadros[1], Carlos Cano[1], Armando Blanco[1] and
Angel Concha[2]

University of Granada, Granada, Spain
[2]*Hospital Universitario Virgen de las Nieves, Granada, Spain*

Breast cancer is a great public health problem. It is the second most common cancer worldwide (one in eight women) and the fifth most common cause of cancer death. Its high incidence and mortality rate have made it to be the focus of a huge research effort. However, it is still unknown why some people (mainly women) get breast cancer. The exact causes of breast cancer remain unknown, although many epidemiological risk factors, such as hormone status, genetic factors, and environmental conditions, have been identified [Iselius *et al.* (1991)]. Indeed, modern technologies are allowing to better understand and identify prognostic factors in breast cancer. Moreover, there has never been more potentially available information to study this disease. However, it is a non-trivial task to transform the vast amount of biomedical data into useful knowledge.

In this context, computational techniques have been shown to be necessary to store, organize and analyze all this information. Hence, one of the main topics in bioinformatics research is to develop computational techniques that help to analyze such a huge amount of data [Kanehisa and Bork (2003)]. This chapter is thus focussed on one of the main techniques in knowledge discovery in databases: *association rule mining*. This methodology emerged recently as a powerful tool to analyze biological data, due to its ability to manage large datasets, its capacity to treat heterogeneous information and the intuitive interpretation of the results obtained with this technique. Thus, association rules have been widely used in bioinformatics, their applications spanning from pure data mining approaches to signaling pathways inference, protein-protein interaction prediction or regulatory modules discovery [Lopez *et al.* (2008); Carmona-Saez *et al.* (2006); Bebek and Yankg (2007); Morgan *et al.* (2007)].

In addition, genomic information and, in general any kind of biological information source, is likely to be imprecise and quite noisy. Advanced computational methodologies, such as fuzzy techniques, have been developed and have shown to be specially suitable to model this type of data [Zadeh (1965); Lopez *et al.* (2008)]. However, it is noteworthy the lack of works in the literature which make use of fuzzy techniques to analyze genomic data and, in general, any other type of biological information. Moreover, fuzzy concepts are easy to understand since they are very similar to the way a person might express knowledge. This makes them especially suitable for their application in this field in which experts must validate the results. Therefore, there is much room for improvement regarding the development and application of fuzzy techniques, and particularly, fuzzy association rule mining techniques for treating biological information.

In this work, we integrate information from the main prognostic factors in breast cancer with whole-genome microarray data to study the potential associations between these two types of data. The heterogeneity and noisy nature of the data along with its high dimensionality make necessary the use of data mining techniques to analyze the dataset. Thus, the attention of this chapter is focussed on the application of fuzzy association rule mining to analyze the above mentioned dataset. Many interesting associations have been obtained. Further studies and empirical evaluation of these associations are needed to obtain scientific evidence of such relations. Finally, a freely accessible web application has been developed which implements the fuzzy association rule mining algorithm used in this study (http://genome.ugr.es/biofar).

12.1   Introduction

This section reviews some concepts that may be useful in understanding the rest of the chapter. First, a brief introduction to the breast cancer disease is given along with a description of the main prognostic factors. Then, the basic notions of association rule mining and fuzzy association rule mining are presented.

12.1.1 Breast Cancer

Breast cancer is the most common cancer in the women of developed countries, accounting for 27% of cancers in European women. In general, breast cancer rates have risen about 30% in the past 25 years in western countries, due in part to increased screening which detects the cancer in earlier stages [Pollan *et al.* (2007)].

Breast cancer can be defined as the accelerated, disordered and uncontrolled proliferation of cells from different tissues of a mammary gland. It is a heterogeneous disease including a wide spectrum of clinical, histological and molecular subtypes. These differences may reflect genetic influences, differences in lifestyle or nutritional or environmental exposures [Slamon *et al.* (1989)]. Several molecular subtypes of breast tumors have been described by gene expression profiling. These molecular categories represent biologically distinct disease entities which correlate with biomarker phenotypes and show differences in clinical outcome [Perou *et al.* (2000); Rakha *et al.* (2006); Sorlie *et al.* (2001, 2003, 2006)]. For example, the basal like subtype, known as triple negative (TN), is related to aggressive histology, poor clinical outcome unresponsiveness to endocrine therapies [Lakhani *et al.* (2005); Mountain and Risch (2004)], and BRCA1-related breast tumors [Bauer *et al.* (2007); Guarneri *et al.* (2006)].

There are many prognostic factors associated with breast cancer. The most widely considered are primary tumor size, the lymph node[1] status, the tumor histological grade, and tumor receptor status (hormone receptors and human epidermal growth factor receptor 2, HER2) [Esteva *et al.* (2002)], p53 and ki67 status.

12.1.1.1 Tumor stage

In order to determine the most suitable treatment, it is important to precisely know the tumor stage. The most commonly used system to describe the stages of breast cancer is the so-called TNM. This staging system classifies cancers based on their tumor size (T), lymph nodes status (N), and metastasis[2](M) status. Taking into account these three features, breast cancer tumors are usually classified in one of the following stages:

- Stage 1. The tumor is no more than 2 cm across, there are no cancer

---

[1]Lymph node: small bean-shaped organ of the immune system, distributed widely throughout the body which acts as filters or traps for foreign particles.

[2]Metastasis is defined as the development of secondary malignant growths at a distance from a primary site of cancer.

cells in the lymph nodes in the armpit and the cancer has not spread anywhere else.

- Stage 2. Tumor size is between 2 and 5 cm, with or without cancer cells in the lymph nodes in the armpit and the cancer has not spread.
- Stage 3. The tumor may be bigger than 5 cm, it has spread to lymph nodes in the armpit and/or is fixed to the skin or chest wall.
- Stage 4. The tumor can be any size, the lymph nodes may or may not contain cancer cells and the cancer has spread (metastasised) to other parts of the body such as the lungs, liver or bones.

12.1.1.2 HER2/neu (Human Epidermal Growth Factor Receptor 2)

The HER2 oncogene[3] is a member of the human epidermal growth factor receptor family. It codifies a protein known to play an important role in the growth and development of epithelial-cells such as mammary glands cells. In each normal cell there are two copies of the HER2 gene (one for each chromosome-17), and about 50.000 copies of its corresponding protein in the cell surface. On the other hand, a tumor cell may present more than two copies of the gene and more than 1 million copies of the protein in the cell surface, thereby causing the cell to be extremely sensitive to growth factors [Slamon *et al.* (1987, 1989)].

Between 25% and 30% of breast cancer tumors present over-expression of the HER2 gene. In most of cases, this over-expression is also accompanied by HER2 amplification[4], though in the 3% − 7% of the cases the over-expression appears in absence of amplification, probably caused by chromosome-17 polisomy [Slamon *et al.* (2001); Vogel *et al.* (2002); Yaziji *et al.* (2004)]. The importance of determining the HER2 status relies on the fact that those patients with HER2 amplification present fast tumor growth, increased risk of recurrence after surgery, and poor clinical outcome [EBCTCG (2005); Vogel *et al.* (2002); Carey *et al.* (2006)].

A humanized monoclonal antibody[5] called *trastuzumab* (Herceptin ®) was developed some years ago. Trastuzumab is able of specifically blocking

---

[3] An oncogene is a mutated/desregulated gene that helps turn a normal cell into a tumor cell.

[4] Gene amplification is an increase in the number of copies of a gene.

[5] Antibodies are proteins found in blood or other bodily fluids of vertebrates, and are used by the immune system to identify and neutralize foreign objects, such as bacteria and viruses. Trastuzumab is specifically designed to identify and bind the extracellular portion of the HER2 receptor.

the action of the HER2 oncogene [Carter *et al.* (1992)]. It interrupts the signal transduction [6], inhibiting the proliferation of cells which over-express HER2. Therefore, HER2 positive tumors are expected to satisfactorily respond to the trastuzumab therapy. However, in practice only a 20% – 30% of these patients improve with this treatment [Ocana *et al.* (2006)]. This may be due to the appearance of resistance mechanisms, such as the loss of the HER2 protein in the cell surface, the activation of alternative signaling pathways or any other unknown molecular mechanisms [Ocana *et al.* (2006)]. Nevertheless, it has been shown that the trastuzumab therapy reduces the death risk by 30% [Slamon *et al.* (2006)].

All of this makes the HER2 status to be of great clinical value in breast tumors for the identification of those patients who are eligible for trastuzumab therapy [Yaziji *et al.* (2004)]. However, there is not a widespread consensus on the best technique to determine the HER2 status, being the immunohistochemistry (IHC) and fluorescence in situ hybridization (FISH) techniques the most widely used.

12.1.1.3   *HER2 Testing Methodologies*

Two diagnostic techniques are the tests of choice for most pathologists and are often used together on paraffin-embedded block tissue sections processed in routine practice, immunohistochemistry (IHC) and fluorescent in situ hybridization (FISH).

IHC techniques are used to determine the presence and level of specific cellular proteins. IHC measures protein expression using specially labeled antibodies that can bind to the proteins of interest. HER2 IHC is scored on a qualitative scale from 0 to 3, based on interpretation of staining intensity, with 0 and 1 classified as negative, 2 as equivocal, and 3 as positive (Table 12.1). Cytoplasmic staining is considered to be non-specific.

FISH is a cytogenetic technique used to detect and localize the presence or absence of specific DNA sequences on chromosomes. This technique is used to detect gene amplification. In this particular case, FISH testing results provide the average ratio of Her2/neu signals to CEP17 signals in non-overlapping interphase nuclei of the lesion. Tumors with a Her2/neu:CEP17 ratio $\geq 2 : 2$ are usually considered positive for HER2 gene amplification.

Comparative studies have shown high concordance rates between immunohistochemical analysis and FISH in tumors with immunohistochemical

---

[6]Signal transduction refers to any process by which a cell converts one kind of signal or stimulus into another.

Table 12.1: Interpretation of the IHC results

Value	Result	Visualization
0	Negative	Less than the 10% of the cells stained regardless of the staining intensity.
1	Negative	Incomplete membrane staining in more than the 10% of the cells
2	Equivocal	Incomplete membrane staining, weak or medium intensity in more than the 10% of the cells
3	Positive	Complete and intense membrane staining in more than the 10% of the cells

scores of 0 or 1 (negative) and 3 (strongly positive), and discordance rates among cases with undetermined immunohistochemical scores of 2. FISH is usually more reliable and reproducible than IHC, since it is less sensitive to the adverse effects of tissue handling and fixation. However, FISH is more complicated, time-consuming and it requires training, experience, and expensive equipment. Therefore, it is a common practice to firstly perform HER2 IHC in order to screen the HER2 status. Then, FISH is only carried out over IHC2 and IHC3 samples to confirm the HER2 status. Nevertheless, some studies stated that this strategy is not cost-effective, arguing that only FISH-positive cases benefit from trastuzumab therapy [Barlett *et al.* (2003); Bilous *et al.* (2003); Dressler *et al.* (2005)].

12.1.1.4 *Additional Biomarkers*

As commented above, some additional biomarkers are also considered in routine clinical management of breast cancer, such as hormone receptors (ER & PR), p53 and ki67. Hormone-receptor negative breast tumor patients present poor prognosis, since hormonal therapy cannot be used in their treatment [EBCTCG (2005)]. These patients are treated with traditional systemic chemotherapy [Guarneri *et al.* (2006)].

The presence of p53 gene mutations is also associated with worse prognosis. The p53 protein is a tumor suppressor encoded by a gene which disruption is associated with approximately 50 to 55 percent of human cancers. The p53 protein acts as a checkpoint in the cell cycle, either preventing or initiating programmed cell death.

The nuclear antigen ki67 is a proliferation marker expressed by cells in all phases of the active cell cycle [Gasparini *et al.* (1994)]. Ki67 antibodies are useful in establishing the cell growing fraction in neoplasms. Intuitively, proliferating tumors confer a poor prognosis, and the majority of studies confirm this association [Burcombe *et al.* (2006)].

The status of all of these biomarkers is usually determined by immuno-histochemical analysis. The expression of p53 and ki67 is assessed according to the estimated proportion of nuclear staining in tumor cells that are positively stained. The status of p53 is considered negative if this proportion is lower than the 5%. In the case of the ki67 marker the threshold value is usually set around the 10%.

The ER and PR expression is usually quantified by calculating the Allred scoring, which is a microscopic method conveying the estimated proportion and intensity of positive tumor cells (range from 0-8). Values of the Allred index over 3 are considered positive.

12.2   Microarrays

Microarray technology makes use of the sequence resources created by the genome projects and other sequencing efforts to monitor the expression of thousands of genes in particular cell samples, times and conditions. Thus, microarray data provide a global picture of the cell activities and open the way to a high-level understanding of its behavior.

The results of a set of microarray experiments are usually organized in the so-called *gene expression matrices*. Rows (columns) in these matrices represent genes, and columns (rows) the experimental conditions under study. Thus, each cell in the matrix contains the expression level of a gene under a certain experimental condition. The analysis of these matrices allows to get information about cellular operation in organisms. However, this analysis is very complex due to the large number of genes (even in the simplest organisms) and the noise that affects the whole process [Berrar *et al.* (2003)].

12.3   Association Rule Mining

Agrawal proposed in 1993 an algorithm for extracting association rules from large databases [Agrawal *et al.* (1993)]. The initial application of association analysis techniques was the study of the hidden relations in the commonly known as market basket databases. Typically, these databases contain information about the products bought by the customers in each

Table 12.2: Example of a market basket database.

Transaction	Items
1	Bread, Milk, Butter
2	Beer, Eggs, Milk, Butter, Fruit
3	Milk, Butter
...	...

purchase. Thus, a market basket database consists of a set of transactions each of them containing the items acquired in that transaction (Table 12.2). Hence, the main objective when an association analysis is carried out over this kind of databases is to obtain relations of the form:

$$Milk \rightarrow Butter$$

This is basically an *association rule*, and represents the expression: *Those who buy milk also buy butter*. This type of information may be of great interest for a supermarket administrator, since for example the sales might be increased by placing certain products together.

Association rules have also been successfully applied in many other different fields including web mining, advertising, bioinformatics, etc. Moreover, since they were first proposed in 1993 they have become one of the main techniques for Knowledge Discovery in Databases (KDD).

12.3.1   *Association Rules: Formal Definition*

Let $I = x_1, x_2, , x_n$ be a set of attribute-value pairs or *items*. Let D be a transactional database where each transaction is a set of items $T \subseteq I$. An association rule is an expression of the form:

$$X \rightarrow Y$$

where X and Y are sets of items (or *itemsets*) so that $X \cap Y = \emptyset$. The itemset X is called the antecedent of the rule while Y is called the consequent. An association rule like this indicates that if X occurs then Y is likely to occur. The probability that Y occurs, given that X has occurred is called the *confidence* of the rule. The probability that both X and Y occur is called the *support* of the rule. Thus, classical association rule mining algorithms aim to extract association rules with support and confidence greater than some user-specified threshold.

Table 12.3: Example of a data table.

Patient	ki67	IHC	FISH
1	POSITIVE	3	POSITIVE
2	NEGATIVE	3	NEGATIVE
3	NEGATIVE	1	POSITIVE
4	POSITIVE	0	NEGATIVE
5	NEGATIVE	0	NEGATIVE
6	POSITIVE	2	POSITIVE

Table 12.4: Table 12.3 transformed into a transactional data table.

Transaction	Items
1	{(ki67=POSITIVE),(IHC=3),(FISH=POSITIVE)}
2	{(ki67=NEGATIVE),(IHC=3),(FISH=NEGATIVE)}
3	{(ki67=NEGATIVE),(IHC=1),(FISH=POSITIVE)}
4	{(ki67=POSITIVE),(IHC=0),(FISH=NEGATIVE)}
5	{(ki67=NEGATIVE),(IHC=0),(FISH=NEGATIVE)}
6	{(ki67=POSITIVE),(IHC=2),(FISH=POSITIVE)}

A transaction T is said to support an itemset $X \subseteq I$, if $X \subseteq T$, i.e. T contains all the items in X. Thus, the support of an itemset X is the percentage of transactions in the database that supports X, i.e. the probability of finding the itemset X in the database. Therefore, the support of a rule $X \to Y$ can be calculated as:

$$Supp(X \to Y) = Supp(X \cup Y),$$

and the confidence of a rule $X \to Y$ can be defined as:

$$Conf(X \to Y) = \frac{Supp(X \to Y)}{Supp(X)}$$

Finally, an itemset X is said to be *frequent* if its support is greater than some user-specified threshold.

For example, consider the information in Table 12.3 which contains some structural data for a set of yeast genes. This table can be easily seen as a transactional database where each row represents a transaction and the attributes in each column form the items of the transaction (Table 12.4).

Consider now the itemset Z:

$$Z = \{(ki67 = POSITIVE), (IHC = 1), (FISH = POSITIVE)\}$$

This itemset is supported by transactions (patients) 7 & 9 and there are 13 transactions in total, therefore $Supp(Z) = 3/13 = 0.154$. Consider now the association rule:

$$R = \{(ki67 = POSITIVE), (IHC = 1)\} \rightarrow \{(FISH = POSITIVE)\},$$

The support of R is:

$$Supp(R) = Supp(Z) = 0.154$$

and the confidence of R can be calculated as:

$$Conf(R) = Supp(R)/Supp(\{(ki67 = POSITIVE), (IHC = 1)\})) =$$
$$= (2/13)/(3/13) = 0.67$$

The main drawback of association rule mining techniques is that the number of generated rules is often large, many of them providing redundant or non-relevant information. The support/confidence framework has been proven to be insufficient to deal with this problem. Therefore, additional strategies and interestingness measures have been proposed to enhance the interpretability of the resultant rule set. However, pattern interestingness is often confused with pattern accuracy. The majority of the literature focuses on maximizing the accuracy of the discovered patterns ignoring other important quality criteria. In fact, the correlation between accuracy and interestingness is not so clear. For example, the statement "men do not give birth" is highly accurate but not interesting at all [Freitas (2006)]. Hence, there is not a widespread agreement on a formal definition for the interestingness of a rule, some authors have even defined the interestingness of a pattern as a compendium of concepts such as conciseness, coverage, reliability, peculiarity, diversity, novelty, surprisingness, utility and actionability [Geng and Hamilton (2006)]. Thus, many rule interestingness measures and rule reduction strategies have been proposed (for a review see [Geng and Hamilton (2006); Ceglar and Roddick (2006)]).

Summarizing, the association rule mining process is generally divided in two steps:

- Finding the set of frequent itemsets. The majority of association mining research effort has been focused on this step, since it is the most computationally expensive phase.
- Deriving association rules with confidence greater than a user-specified threshold from the frequent itemsets.

A great number of algorithms have been proposed for association rule mining, the main ones being Apriori, Eclat, and Frequent-Pattern growth [Agrawal *et al.* (1993); Zaki *et al.* (1997); Han and Pei (2000); Pei *et al.* (2001)]. So far, there is no published implementation that outperforms every other implementation on every database with every support threshold [Goethals and Zaki (2003)]. The fundamentals of association mining are now well established and there appears little current research on the optimization of procedures for classical itemset identification. Hence, most of current works on association mining focus on the specialization of classic algorithms to address specific issues [Ceglar and Roddick (2006)]. A comprehensive listing and description of association rule mining algorithms can be found in [Ceglar and Roddick (2006); Tan *et al.* (2005)].

12.4 Fuzzy Association Rules

Classical crisp association rule mining algorithms partition continuous domains to deal with continuous attributes. For example, consider the data in Table 12.5. Attribute ki67 is continuous; therefore, it is infeasible to directly look for frequent itemsets that involve this attribute. A preprocessing step is needed to discretize the domain, or, in other words, to partition the continuous domain in intervals. After the partition is carried out, each continuous value is replaced by the interval to which it belongs. Several strategies have been proposed for discretizing the continuous domains [Srikant and Agrawal (1996); Miller and Yang (1997)].

Nevertheless, when dividing an attribute into intervals covering certain ranges of values, the *sharp boundary problem* arises. Elements near the boundaries of a crisp set (interval) will be either ignored or overemphasized. For example, rules like "If the ki67 is in the interval $[0, 10]$, then the IHC tends to be negative", and "Patients with low ki67 tend to be IHC negative" may all be meaningful depending on different situations. While the former is more specific and the latter is more general in semantic expressions, however, the former presents the previously called sharp

Table 12.5: Example of a data table with continuous variables.

Patient	ki67	IHC	FISH
1	50%	3	POSITIVE
2	5%	3	NEGATIVE
3	11%	1	POSITIVE
4	35%	0	NEGATIVE
5	3%	0	NEGATIVE
6	52%	2	POSITIVE

boundary problem, or, in other words, patients with $ki67 = 10.5\%$ may not be considered. In contrast, the latter is more flexible and can reflect these boundary cases [Chen *et al.* (2006)]. Moreover, fuzzy set theory has been proven to be a superior technology to enhance the interpretability of these intervals [Delgado *et al.* (2003a)]. Hence, in the fuzzy case, continuous domains are fuzzified by partitioning them into fuzzy sets (Figure 12.1). Therefore, fuzzy association rules are also expressions of the form: $X \rightarrow Y$, but in this case, X and Y are sets of fuzzy attribute-value pairs.

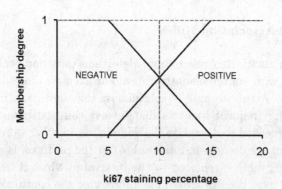

Fig. 12.1: An example of crisp and fuzzy partitions (discontinuous lines depict crisp borders).

When assessing a fuzzy association rule, the usual approach consists of using the fuzzy counterparts of the support and confidence measures. Several generalizations of these two measures have been proposed [Dubois *et al.* (2003)]. The standard approach is to replace the set-theoretic operations by their corresponding fuzzy set-theoretic operations. Thus, given a transactional database D, the membership degree of a transaction $t \in D$ to a fuzzy itemset X is calculated as $X(t) = \otimes_{X_i \in X} X_i(t)$, where $\otimes$ represents a *t-norm* [Dumitrescu *et al.* (2000)]. A so-called *t-norm* $\otimes$ is a generalized logical *conjunction*, or, in other words, a function $[0,1] \times [0,1] \to [0,1]$ which is associative, commutative, and monotone increasing, and which satisfies:

$$a \otimes 0 = 0,$$
$$a \otimes 1 = a, \ for \ all \ 0 \le a \le 1$$

Common examples of *t*-norms are:

$minimum(a,b) = min(a,b),$
$product(a,b) = a{\cdot}b,$
$Lukasiewiczt - norm(a,b) = max(a+b-1,0)$

Thus, *t-norms* are used for defining the *intersection* of fuzzy sets. Given two fuzzy sets defined over a domain Z and their corresponding membership degree functions $A : Z \to [0,1]$, $B : Z \to [0,1]$, the intersection of the two fuzzy sets, $A \cap B$, is defined as follows:

$$(A \cap B)(z) = A(z) \otimes B(z), \ for \ all \ z \in Z$$

Hence, considering all of this, the fuzzy support of an itemset X is usually defined as:

$$Supp(X) = \sum_{t \in D} [\otimes_{X_i \in X} X_i(t)]$$

that is, the sum of the membership degrees of the transactions in the database to the itemset X. Finally, the fuzzy support and confidence of a fuzzy association rule $X \to Y$ is given by:

$$Supp(X \to Y) = \sum_{t \in D} X(t) \otimes Y(t),$$

$$Conf(X \to Y) = \frac{\sum_{t \in D} X(t) \otimes Y(t)}{\sum_{t \in D} X(t)}$$

Even though the majority of fuzzy proposals are based on the fuzzy extensions described above, some alternative approaches have been reported [Delgado *et al.* (2003a); Dubois *et al.* (2006); Glass (2008)].

The development of efficient algorithms for fuzzy association rule mining has been paid little attention. This might be explained by the fact that, in general, standard crisp algorithms can be adapted for extracting fuzzy association rules in a straightforward way [Dubois *et al.* (2006); Delgado *et al.* (2003b)]. The first proposal for fuzzy association rule mining was reported in [Lee and Garrard (1991)]. The authors presented a straightforward approach in which a membership threshold is fixed for transforming fuzzy transactions into crisp ones before running an ordinary association rule mining algorithm. After this, some other authors presented algorithms for fuzzy association rule mining such as F-APACS and FARM [Au and Chan (1998, 1999)], extensions of the Equi-depth (EDP) algorithm [Zhang (1999)], and other Apriorilike methods [Gyenesey (2000); Hen *et al.* (1999)]. For a more extensive listing, please refer to [Delgado *et al.* (2003a)].

12.5 Dataset

Data used in this work were supplied by one of the Spanish National Centers for HER2 testing (Hospital Universitario Virgen de las Nieves). Gene expression data, tumor stage, histology and immunohistochemical markers were recorded for 58 tissue samples. In addition, clinical information was obtained from 2751 breast carcinoma patients which were diagnosed between September 2001 and December 2007. Two analysis were carried out separately: first, an exploratory analysis was performed over a data table comprising only the clinical data of these 2751 patients. Shedding light on the dependencies between prognostic factors values may help to better interpret the rule set obtained from the second analysis. Then, the main analysis was carried out, which comprehends the study of the relations between the gene expression data and the prognostic factors in the 58 tissues mentioned above.

12.5.1 *HER2 Testing Methodologies*

HER2 gene status of breast tumors was evaluated by both immunohistochemistry (IHC) and fluorescence in situ hybridization (FISH) analysis of paraffin-embedded tissue on conventional slide using FDA approval kits. HER2 test results were interpreted according to manufacturers' test protocols.

HER2 IHC was scored on a qualitative scale from 0 to 3 depending on the staining intensity: IHC0 and IHC1 were considered as HER2 IHC negative, IHC2 as equivocal, and IHC3 as HER2-positive. Cytoplasmic staining was considered to be non-specific. Heterogeneous HER2 staining pattern in different areas of the same tumor was also considered as an additional variable in the study.

FISH results were calculated as the average ratio of Her2/neu signals to CEP17[7] signals in non-overlapping interphase nuclei of the lesion. Tumors with a Her2/neu:CEP17 ratio $\geq$ 2 : 2 were considered positive for gene amplification. This test also allowed a simultaneous determination of the number of chromosome-17 copies. Polysomy was defined as the occurrence of three or more copies of chromosome-17.

12.5.2 *Immunohistochemical Data*

The estrogen-receptor (ER) and progesterone-receptor (PgR) expression was quantified in our laboratory using the Allred scoring (Section 12.1.1.4). Values of the Allred index values over 3 were considered as positive samples.

The expression of p53 and ki67 mitosis marker was assessed according to the estimated proportion of nuclear staining in tumor cells that were positively stained. For p53, values $\geq$ 5% were considered positive. For ki67 percentage values two fuzzy sets were defined as shown in Figure 12.1 according to expert knowledge, since percentages around 10% are in the border between positive and negative cases.

12.5.3 *Microarray Data*

Total RNAs were extracted from 46 frozen breast tumor tissues and 12 normal breast tissues using Trizol (Invitrogen,Carlsbad, CA). After quality control using a Bioanalyzer (Agilent 2100), RNAs were amplified, labeled, and hybridized onto whole genome microarrays U133 plus 2.0. according to Affymetrix protocol.

After all this process the raw gene expression values were obtained for each of the 58 samples. As commented above, microarray experiments inevitably introduce many sources of variation. A normalization step is essential to correct the effects of systematic sources of variation of non-biological origin. The well-known robust multiarray analysis method (RMA) [Irizarry *et al.* (2003)] was used to normalize the set of microarray experiments. Relative expression levels were then obtained by dividing each normalized value

---

[7]Chromosome-17 centromere Enumeration Probe

by a reference expression level and calculating its logarithm base-2 as shown in (12.1):

$$Expr'_{i,j} = \log_2(Expr_{i,j}/ref\_value_i), \qquad (12.1)$$

where:

- $Expr'_{i,j}$ represents the relative expression level of gene i for sample j,
- $Expr_{i,j}$ represents the normalized absolute expression level of gene i for sample j,
- ref_value_i represents the reference expression value for gene i. The twelve samples obtained from normal breast tissues were considered as the reference samples. Thus, for each gene i, a reference value was calculated as the median of the expression values of gene i for these samples.

We then removed those genes which did not change their expression level more than 0.5 fold in at least the 10% of the samples under study (*flat genes*). After filtering out these genes, we finally obtained a gene expression matrix of 46 rows (one for each tumor tissue), and 3708 columns (one for each remaining gene).

Finally, the fuzzy definitions of *over-expression* and *under-expression* were done as shown in Figure 12.2, taking into account that it is usually accepted that genes which change their expression level more than one fold with respect to the control sample are over/under-expressed.

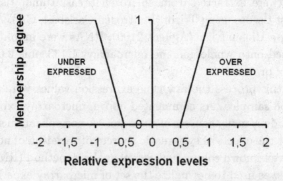

Fig. 12.2: Gene expression levels.

12.6 Extracting the Fuzzy Association Rules

At this point we had a gene expression matrix and a data table containing the information of the prognostic factors. Both tables were then combined thus forming a final data table of 46 rows and 3717 columns. This data table can be easily seen as a transactional database where each tumor tissue (i.e. row) represents a transaction and the values in each column form the items of the transaction (see Section 12.3.1). Table 12.6 shows a summary of the variables included in this dataset.

Table 12.6: Variables included in the study of 46 breast tissues

Variable	Possible values
IHC	0, 1, 2, 3
FISH	+, −
ER-Allred Index	+, −
PR-Allred Index	+, −
p53	+, −
ki67	[0, 100]
Polysomy 17	*yes, no*
Metastasis	*yes, no*
Stage	*I, II, III*
Gene expression values	] − ∞, +∞[

Table 12.7: Clinical data obtained from 2751 patients

Variable	Possible values
IHC	0, 1, 2, 3
FISH	+, −
ER-Allred Index	+, −
PR-Allred Index	+, −
p53	+, −
ki67	[0, 100]
Polysomy 17	*yes, no*
Heterogeneity	*yes, no*

In addition, another table was obtained containing clinical data of 2751 patients as commented at the beginning of section 12.5. In this case, each patient represents a transaction and the values of each clinical variable form the items of the transactions. Table 12.7 shows a summary of the variables included in this dataset.

Thus, the fuzzy association rule mining algorithm was run over both tables separately in order to obtain the set of potential relations between the corresponding variables.

12.6.1 *Fuzzy Top-Down Frequent-Pattern Growth Algorithm*

As previously commented, a fuzzy version of the Top-Down Frequent-Pattern Growth algorithm was used, since it previously showed a good performance over this type of datasets [Lopez *et al.* (2008)]. The main idea of the algorithm is to condense in a data structure (the Fuzzy Frequent-Pattern tree) all the information it needs from the transactions. This data structure is then efficiently traversed in order to get the list of frequent itemsets. Hence, the algorithm can be summarized in the following three steps:

(1) Scan the database to get the list of frequent items.
(2) Build the Fuzzy Frequent-Pattern tree (FFP-tree).
(3) Traverse the FFP-tree in order to get the list of frequent itemsets.

12.6.1.1   *Obtaining the List of Frequent Items*

As commented above, the algorithm starts by scanning the database in order to get a list of all the *frequent* items, i. e. items with support greater than a threshold. Then, the list is sorted by support in decreasing order. The position of the items in this list determines the order in which they are introduced into the Fuzzy Frequent-Pattern tree (FFP-tree). Even though there is not an optimal ordering of the frequent item list for every case, the decreasing order has been shown to generate efficient FFP-tree structures [Han and Pei (2000)]. Table 12.8 shows an example of a frequent item list. An index is associated to each item according to its position in the list. For example, item ki67=POSITIVE is associated with index 1 and item IHC=1 is associated with index 5.

Table 12.8: Sorted item list

Index	Item	Support
1	{ki67 = POSITIVE}	10.03
2	{FISH = POSITIVE}	7
3	{FISH = NEGATIVE}	6
4	{IHC = 3}	4
5	{IHC = 1}	4
6	{IHC = 0}	3
7	{ki67 = NEGATIVE}	2.92
8	{IHC = 2}	2

12.6.1.2 Building the Fuzzy Frequent-pattern Tree

A new scan of the database is carried out. Transactions are considered one by one. The items in each transaction that are present in the list of frequent items are inserted as nodes into the FP-tree according to their position in the frequent item list. Two transactions share the same upper-path if their first frequent items are the same. Each node contains two vectors indicating the membership degree of the transactions to the corresponding item. Thus, each time a node is visited its membership degree vectors are updated. Figure 12.3 shows how the three transactions of Table 12.9 are introduced into the FFP-tree.

Table 12.9: Three fuzzy transactions

Transaction ID	Items
1	$\{ki67=+:1, IHC=3:1, FISH=+:1\}$
1	$\{ki67=+:1, IHC=3:1, FISH=+:1\}$
3	$\{ki67=+:0.53, ki67=-:0.47, IHC=1:1, FISH=+:1\}$

Note the two lists of membership degrees in each node. Initially both lists contain the same values. In the figure each list is formed by pairs of values of the form *transaction : membreship degree*. These pairs indicate the membership degree of the corresponding item to the transactions that visit that node during the FFP-tree construction. For example, the pair 1 : 1 in the node of item 2 indicates that the membership degree of item 2 to transaction 1 is 1.

In addition, next step (frequent itemsets generation) requires the construction of a header table H that helps to locate the nodes of every item and to compute the fuzzy support of the itemsets. Each entry in H corresponds to an item I, and contains the membership degrees of the transactions to I and pointers to the nodes of this item. A final FFP-tree plus its header table H is shown in Figure 12.4. The Algorithm 3 describes the procedure for the FFP-tree construction.

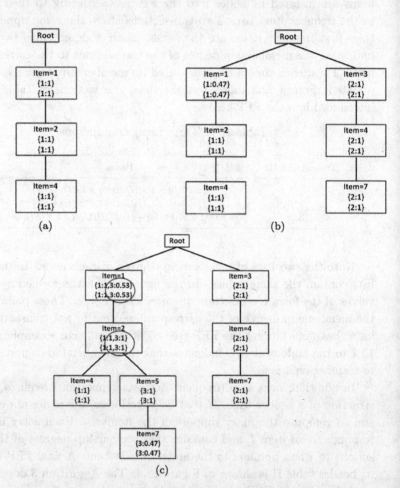

Fig. 12.3: The three transactions of Table 12.9 are introduced into a FFP-tree.

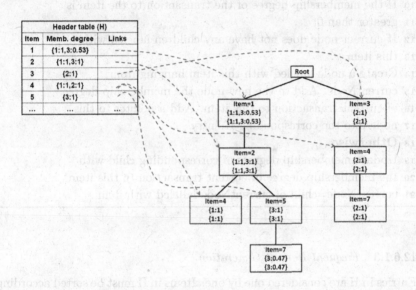

Fig. 12.4: Complete tree along with its header table.

```
 1 root=node()
 2 H=[] //Header table
 3 For each item in the ordered list:
 4 Initialize each entry in H with Links=[] and the corresponding
 5 membership
 6 degree for each transaction
 7 For each row (transaction) in the dataset:
 8 currentNode=root
 9 For each item from the ordered list:
10 If the membership degree of the transaction to the item is
11 greater than 0:
12 If current node does not have any children labeled with
13 this item:
14 Create a node labeled with this item hanging from
15 currentNode. Add to the new node the membership degree
16 of current transaction to this item. Add a pointer to this
17 node into the corresponding H entry.
18 Otherwise:
19 Update membership degrees of corresponding child with
20 the membership degree of current transaction to this item
21 currentNode=child of currentNode labeled with item
```

12.6.1.3 *Frequent Itemset Generation*

Entries in H are considered one by one. Items in H must be sorted according to their support. For each item I in the header table the tree is traversed in a down-top order starting from the nodes labeled with I. Nodes labeled with I can be reached following the side links of the corresponding H entry. Every frequent itemset whose last element is I is obtained during this walk up. Algorithm 4 describes this procedure. Note that one of the two membership degree lists in each node is considered as an auxiliary list, and will be modified during the process, while the other remains the same until the end of the procedure.

1 **Function frequent_itemsets(P, H):**
2 List=[] //Frequent itemsets will be stored here.
3 **For each** entry I in H:
4 **If** support(H(I).membership_degree)≥min_support:
5 Insert IP into List. Build sub-header table H_I by calling
6 create_subtable(I). Call frequent_itemsets(IP,H_I) and
7 concatenate the returned frequent itemset list with List.
8 **Return** List

---

1 **Procedure create_subtable(I):**
2 **For each** node n in I.Links:
3 **Walk up** the tree from n and each time a node c is visited do:
4 aux=min{n.aux_membership_degree,c.membership_degree}
5 **If** there is no entry in H_I for c.item:
6 Create a new entry in H_I for c.item. Initialize the
7 membership degree vector with aux. Append a link to c to
8 H_I[c.item].Links.
    c.aux_membership_degree=n.aux_membership_degree
9 **Otherwise:**
10 Update H_I[c.item].membership_degree with the values
11 in aux.
12 **If** c has not been visited yet in this call to
13 create_subtable:
14 c.aux_membership_degree = aux
15 Append a link to c to H_I[c.item].Links.
16 **Otherwise:**
17 Update c.aux_membership_degree with the values in aux.

Let us show the procedure functioning by carrying out some steps of the algorithm. Recall that the support threshold considered in this example is 0 for the sake of clarity. The algorithm starts by processing the first entry in H. Thus, the nodes corresponding to item 1 are considered. There is only one node for this item, the colored one in Figure 12.5. The algorithm proceeds to build sub-header table H_1 starting at this node. The root is reached in the first step, so no sub-header table needs finally to be built.

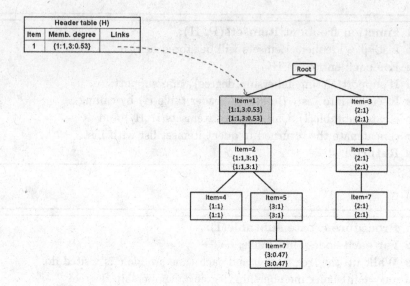

Fig. 12.5: Traversing the tree, first entry in H.

Next item in table H is item 2. This item is frequent and therefore table H_2 is created. There is one node labeled with item 2 in the tree (Figure 12.6). In the first step of the walk up a node labeled with item 1 is visited. A new entry for item 1 is added to sub-header table H_2 (Figure 12.7):

(1) The item associated with the new entry in H_2 corresponds to the item of the visited node, i.e. item 1.
(2) The membership degree list of the new entry is calculated as follows:

$$min(\{1:1,3:1\},\{1:1,3:0.53\}) = \{1:1,3:0.53\}$$

The auxiliary vector of the visited node is also assigned this minimum vector.
(3) A reference is added to the Links field in the new entry pointing to the visited node.

The algorithm then proceeds to process the sub-header table H_{21}. The itemset $\{1,2\}$ is inserted into the frequent itemsets list, since its support is greater than the support threshold. The first entry in this table corresponds to item 1. There is only one node for item 1 and the root is reached in the first step, therefore sub-header table H_{21} does not need to be built. Since there are not any more entries in table H_2, the algorithm continues

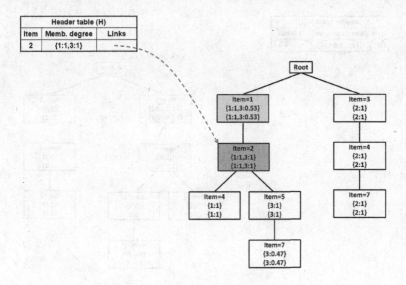

Fig. 12.6: Traversing the tree, second entry in H.

considering next entry in table H and so on. The procedure finishes when the header table and every sub-header table have been processed.

12.6.2 *Obtaining and Processing the Fuzzy Association Rules*

The last phase of the association rule mining process is the extraction of the rules from the frequent itemsets. This section describes the strategies and measures used to reduce the final rule set.

12.6.2.1 *Generating the Fuzzy Association Rules from the Frequent Itemsets*

Association rules are then derived from each frequent itemset. This phase is common to every association rule mining algorithm and therefore we will not go into deep details of the procedure. Given an itemset, the idea is to create a consequent with each possible subset of items in the itemset. The rest of the items in the itemset that are not in the consequent constitute the antecedent of the rule, and thus, in principle, a rule is generated from each subset. Furthermore, the efficiency of the process can be improved, since it is not necessary to consider every possible subset of items. A com-

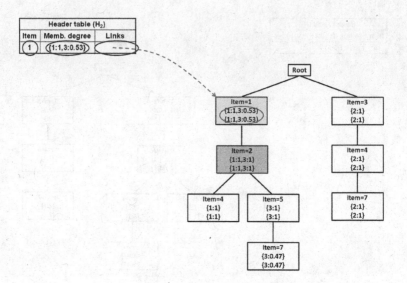

Fig. 12.7: Traversing the tree, building table H_2.

plete description of the procedure can be found in [Agrawal *et al.* (1993)].
Fuzzy support and confidence were calculated as described in [Delgado *et al.*
(2003b)].

12.6.2.2 *Deficiencies of the Confidence/Support Framework*

As it was previously commented in section 12.3.1 the support/confidence
framework has been proven to be insufficient to filter out uninteresting
patters. Thus, several authors proposed different properties which may
be desired for a rule interestingness measure [Geng and Hamilton (2006)].
In this particular study, the following properties were considered to be
interesting for a measure F and a rule $X \to Y$:

- $F = 0$ if X and Y are statistically independent, that is, $supp(XY) = supp(X)supp(Y)$.
- F monotonically increases with $supp(XY)$ when $supp(X)$ and $supp(Y)$ remain the same.
- F monotonically decreases with $supp(X)$ (or $supp(Y)$) when $supp(XY)$ and $supp(Y)$ (or $supp(X)$) remain the same.
- F is not be symmetric under variable permutation.
- F decreases if $supp(X \neg Y)$ increases.

Table 12.10: Contingency table for a rule $X \to Y$.

	Y	$\neg Y$	
X	$n(XY)$	$n(X\neg Y)$	$n(X)$
$\neg X$	$n(\neg XY)$	$n(\neg(XY))$	$n(\neg X)$
	$n(Y)$	$n(\neg Y)$	N

Table 12.11: Measures that fulfill the desired properties

Measure	Formula
Add value	$conf(X \to Y) - sop(Y)$
Klosgen	$\sqrt{supp(X \to Y)}(conf(X \to Y) - sop(Y))$
Certainty Factor	$\frac{conf(X \to Y) - supp(Y)}{1 - supp(Y)}$

- F is an increasing function of support if the margins in the contingency Table 12.10 are fixed.
- F has some relation with the count of records that do not contain X and Y.

Only three of the measures proposed so far fulfill all of these properties: the *added value* measure, the *Klosgen's* measure and the *Certainty Factors* (CF) [Delgado *et al.* (2003b); Geng and Hamilton (2006); Klosgen (1996)]. The definition of these three measures can be found in Table 12.11. As it can be seen from this Table, the Klosgen's measure includes the add value measure, since it is a combination of the latter with the support of the rule. However, it does not seem intuitive the fact that the measure takes values in $]-1, 1[$. In other words, it does not seem intuitive for example, the fact that given a "perfect" rule, there is not a maximum value of the measure defined for it (e.g. 1). Hence, certainty factors were finally used, which are also a combination of the add value measure.

In addition, we only allowed those *very strong rules* as defined by Berzal et al. [Berzal *et al.* (2004)]. That is, for each rule $X \to Y$, it was required that $\neg Y \to \neg X$ presents values of support, confidence and certainty factor greater than the user-specified thresholds.

Finally, in order to provide a global significance value of the obtained rule set, we estimated the number of rules that were obtained by chance. We generated 100 randomized independent datasets and extracted rules from each of them. The estimated number of false, rules was calculated as the mean of the number of rules obtained from each of these 100 randomized datasets. This way, we calculated a False Discovery Rate (FDR) which allowed us to check the quality of the rule sets [Zhang and Padmanabhan (2004)].

12.7   Results

First, the exploratory analysis of the clinical data from the 2751 patients is described. The previously described trends among the set of prognostic factors are captured as well as some other interesting associations. Then, the obtained relations between whole-genome expression data and prognostic factors variables are discussed. Again, the rules confirm previously published results and unveil potential novel biomarkers in breast cancer. In both cases CF, Confidence and Support thresholds were set according to expert knowledge and so that the FDR was low and that the number of obtained rules could be easily analyzed. A sample of the obtained rules is commented in the following two sections. The rules shown were selected according to expert knowledge and information extracted from the literature.

12.7.1   *Exploratory Analysis of 2751 Patients*

In order to get an overall impression of the data structure a descriptive study of the dataset was carried out. Frequencies of the items in the database are shown in Tables 12.12- 12.20 and Figure 12.8. The study was not without limitations, data were derived from many sources and lacked information about some of the variables, which is a common situation in biological data analysis. In addition, it can be seen that the minimum frequency value is 162, which corresponds to the item $\{Heterogeneity = yes\}$. This means that if the support threshold is set over 0.059, no rules will be obtained relating this item. In general, the support of the rest of the items is a bit high (usually over 0.10). This means that they very likely appear in the consequent of many rules, since they appear in many transactions of the data table [Delgado *et al.* (2003b)]. Therefore, low values for CF could be expected.

Table 12.12: Summary of the clinical data from the 2751 patients.

	IHC	FISH	Polysomy17	ER	PR	p53	Heterogeneity	Stage
Valid	2680	1960	1960	711	611	755	162	886
Missing	71	791	791	2040	2140	1996	2589	1865

Table 12.13: Frequencies of the IHC variable

Type	Value	Frequency	Percentage
Valid	0	696	25.3
	1	1012	36.8
	2	530	19.3
	3	442	16.1
	Total	2680	97.4
Missing		71	2.6
Total		2751	100.0

Table 12.14: Frequencies of the FISH variable

Type	Value	Frequency	Percentage
Valid	-	1498	54.5
	+	462	16.8
	Total	1960	71.2
Missing		791	28.8
Total		2751	100.0

Table 12.15: Frequencies of the polysomy-17 variable

Type	Value	Frequency	Percentage
Valid	no	1491	54.2
	yes	469	17.0
	Total	1960	71.2
Missing		791	28.8
Total		2751	100.0

Table 12.16: Frequencies of the ER variable

Type	Value	Frequency	Percentage
Valid	-	222	8.1
	+	489	17.8
	Total	711	25.8
Missing		2040	74.2
Total		2751	100.0

The fuzzy association analysis was then carried out. A value of 0.05 was finally selected for the support threshold and a value of 0.4 for the CF threshold. Thus, 69 rules were obtained. An FDR value of 0.00 was estimated, thereby indicating that every obtained rule very likely represents a real association. A sample of the obtained rules is shown in Table 12.21.

The first two rules in Table 12.21 support the previously described relation between the number of chromosome-17 copies and HER2 amplification [Chibon *et al.* (2009); Bempt *et al.* (2008)]. Likewise, the next four rules confirm the well known correlation between the ER and PgR sta-

Table 12.17: Frequencies of the PR variable

Type	Value	Frequency	Percentage
Valid	-	363	13.2
	+	392	14.2
	Total	755	27.4
Missing		1996	72.6
Total		2751	100.0

Table 12.18: Frequencies of the p53 variable

Type	Value	Frequency	Percentage
Valid	-	268	9.7
	+	343	12.5
	Total	611	22.2
Missing		2140	77.8
Total		2751	100.0

Table 12.19: Frequencies of the heterogeneity variable

Type	Value	Frequency	Percentage
Valid	yes	162	5.9
Missing		2589	94.1
Total		2751	100.0

Table 12.20: Frequencies of stage variable

Type	Value	Frequency	Percentage
Valid	I	177	6.4
	II	383	13.9
	III	326	11.9
	Total	886	32.2
Missing		1865	67.8
Total		2751	100.0

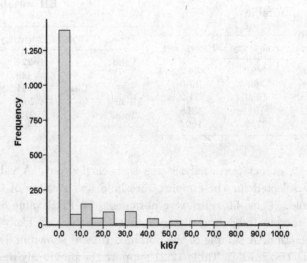

Fig. 12.8: Histogram showing the distribution of the ki67 values.

Table 12.21: Rules obtained from the 2751 patients dataset

Sup.	Conf.	CF	Association rule
0.44	0.81	0.58	$polysomy = no \rightarrow FISH = -$
0.44	0.80	0.57	$FISH = - \rightarrow polysomy = no$
0.13	0.91	0.89	$PR = + \rightarrow ER = +$
0.13	0.73	0.68	$ER = + \rightarrow PR = +$
0.07	0.83	0.81	$ER = - \rightarrow PR = -$
0.07	0.51	0.47	$PR = - \rightarrow ER = -$
0.09	0.58	0.50	$IHC = 3 \rightarrow FISH = +$
0.09	0.56	0.47	$FISH = + \rightarrow IHC = 3$
0.26	0.71	0.35	$IHC = 1 \rightarrow FISH = -$
0.06	0.77	0.50	$ki67 = Low \,\&\, IHC = 2 \rightarrow FISH = -$
0.09	0.75	0.45	$polysomy = no \,\&\, IHC = 2 \rightarrow FISH = -$

tus ($p < 0.0001$)[Burcombe *et al.* (2006)]. Another two rules show a good concordance between IHC3 and FISH-positive cases, which is also the conclusion of some previously published works [Cuadros *et al.* (2009)]. The no appearance of rules relating IHC0/1 and FISH-negative is justified by a certain bias present in the dataset. Recall that in most of cases FISH testing is only carried out if a previous immunohistochemical analysis yields an equivocal (IHC2) or a positive value (IHC3).

It would also be interesting to find some rules associating the itemset $\{IHC = 3, FISH = -\}$ with any other variable, since previous works described that only FISH-positive cases benefit from trastuzumab therapy [Barlett *et al.* (2003); Bilous *et al.* (2003); Dressler *et al.* (2005)]. However, no association was found involving this itemset. We checked the support of this itemset, which is 0.013. Then, an additional run of the algorithm was carried out setting the support threshold in 0.01. No relation was found anyway involving this itemset, showing that probably there is no dependency relation between this itemset and the rest of variables included in this study.

The last two rules are also specially interesting since they relate IHC-equivocal cases with FISH-negative samples. Let us first consider the one involving the ki67 marker. The rule $IHC = 2 \rightarrow FISH = -$ was not found in the resultant rule set, which means that the addition of the item $ki67 = Low$ to the antecedent increases the CF and Confidence values up to 0.5 and 0.77 respectively. This is, in our opinion, a significant difference. In other words, the 77% of IHC-equivocal cases with low proliferation rates ($ki67 = Low$) yield a FISH-negative result. A similar situation occurs with the last rule. This type of relations may be a good starting point to unveiling subtypes of tumors hidden in the IHC-equivocal samples.

Finally, it is noteworthy that no interesting associations were found relating the rest of variables (p53 & tumor stage). This is most probably due to the presence of missing values. Further studies are thus needed to clarify whether there exist additional relations between this variables and the rest of prognostic factors.

12.7.2 *Whole-genome Expression Data and Prognostic Factors*

The frequencies of the items in the data table used in this study are shown in Tables 12.22- 12.30 and Figure 12.9. In this case, the data set presents some important differences with the one analyzed in the previous section. Items present a very high support and are not well-balanced. For example, the support of the item $\{ER = +\}$ is 0.72, whereas the support of the item $\{ER = -\}$ is 0.28. This situation also appears in many of the genes. In addition, the number of items (7418) is much higher than the number of transactions (46). These features facilitate the appearance of fake rules. Therefore, in order to reduce the FDR an additional strategy is needed.

Table 12.22: Summary of the clinical data from the 46 tumor samples.

	IHC	FISH	Polysomy17	ER	PR	p53	Stage	Metastasis
Valid	45	42	46	46	46	46	39	31
Missing	1	4	0	46	46	0	7	15

Table 12.23: Frequencies of the IHC variable

Type	Value	Frequency	Percentage
Valid	0	3	6.5
	1	7	15.2
	2	22	47.8
	3	13	28.3
	Total	45	97.8
Missing		1	2.2
Total		46	100.0

Table 12.24: Frequencies of the FISH variable

Type	Value	Frequency	Percentage
Valid	-	22	47.8
	+	20	43.5
	Total	42	91.3
Missing		4	8.7
Total		46	100.0

Table 12.25: Frequencies of the polysomy-17 variable

Type	Value	Frequency	Percentage
Valid	no	32	69.6
	yes	14	30.4
	Total	46	100.0

Table 12.26: Frequencies of the ER variable

Type	Value	Frequency	Percentage
Valid	-	13	28.3
	+	33	71.7
Total	46	100.0	

Table 12.27: Frequencies of the PR variable

Type	Value	Frequency	Percentage
Valid	-	18	39.1
	+	28	60.9
	Total	46	100.0

Table 12.28: Frequencies of the p53 variable

Type	Value	Frequency	Percentage
Valid	-	30	65.2
	+	16	34.8
	Total	46	100.0

Table 12.29: Frequencies of the metastasis variable

Type	Value	Frequency	Percentage
Valid	yes	18	39.1
	no	13	28.3
	Total	31	67.4
Missing		15	32.6
Total		46	100.0

Table 12.30: Frequencies of the stage variables

Type	Value	Frequency	Percentage
Valid	I	3	6.5
	II	11	23.9
	III	25	54.3
	Total	39	84.8
Missing		7	15.2
Total		46	100.0

First, the set of "problematic" variables was identified. In order to do this, 100 randomized independent datasets were generated. The fuzzy association rule mining algorithm was run over each dataset, and the number of times each variable appears in a false rule was counted (Figure 12.10). Those variables which appeared in many false rules were considered to be undesirable. Therefore, the top-308 variables in this list were removed, which represented the 30% of the variables involved in any false rule. Some of the prognostic factors were included in this 30%: ki67, polysomy-17

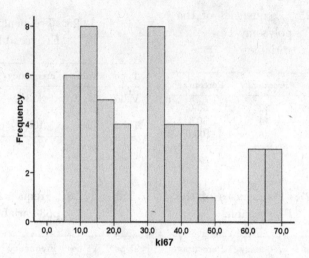

Fig. 12.9: Histogram showing the distribution of the ki67 values.

and ER. The ki67 variable was removed, since most of the samples were ki67-positive (Figure 12.9), therefore this variable could not provide much information. Observing the frequencies of the other two variables (Tables 12.25 & 12.26), we realized that the problem was caused by items $\{polysomy - 17 = no\}$ and $\{ER = +\}$, which actually do not represent interesting situations (Section 12.1.1). These two items were also removed from the data set. Thus, the final data table comprised 3205 variables and 46 samples.

A number of rules were obtained. CF, Confidence and Support thresholds were set so that the FDR was low and that the number of obtained rules could be easily analyzed by the expert. A value of 0.8 was finally selected for the CF threshold and a value of 0.1 was set for the support threshold. Thus, 1377 rules were retrieved and an FDR value of 0.06 was obtained, therefore very few rules were generated by chance and the majority of them may represent real biological associations. It is not the aim of this study to give a comprehensive list and biological interpretation of all of them, but to show that interesting associations can be obtained, which may allow to enunciate hypothesis for subsequent empirical evaluation.

Some of the rules linked prognostic factors and gene expression values. More concretely, 36 of the rules were of this type, a sample of them will be commented in this section (see Table 12.31). These rules were carefully selected according to expert knowledge and information extracted from the scientific literature. Association rules with more than one item in the antecedent/consecuent were also obtained and will be considered in future works. Complete rule sets are provided on request.

Table 12.31: Rules obtained from the 46 tumoral samples

Sup.	Conf.	CF	Association rule
0.11	0.95	0.90	$CDC6 = Over \rightarrow FISH = +$
0.11	0.98	0.97	$ESCO1 = Over \rightarrow FISH = +$
0.10	1.00	1.00	$BMPR1B = Over \rightarrow PR = +$
0.11	0.96	0.91	$THBS1 = Over \rightarrow PR = +$
0.18	0.88	0.80	$SOX11 = Over \rightarrow PR = -$
0.14	0.97	0.91	$SCUBE2 = Under \rightarrow PR = -$
0.26	0.93	0.81	$Metastasis = yes \rightarrow LPL = Under$
0.26	0.93	0.81	$Metastasis = yes \rightarrow EFEMP1 = Under$
0.12	1.00	1.00	$EREG = Over \rightarrow p53 = -$
0.12	1.00	1.00	$EREG = Over \rightarrow PR = +$
0.11	1.00	1.00	$PGR = Over \rightarrow PR = +$
0.10	0.96	0.93	$PAK6 = Over \rightarrow IHC = 2$
0.12	1.00	1.00	$CLDN11 = Sub \rightarrow Stage = III$

Some interesting rules related mRNA expression levels to HER2 amplification. For instance, HER2 FISH-positive breast tumors showed CDC6 over-expression. This gene is located on chromosome 17q21 near HER2, suggesting that both genes could be co-expressed. In addition, the ESCO1 over-expression also appears associated with HER2 FISH-positive cases. No direct mention to the association of the ESCO1 gene with HER2 FISH-positive cases was found in the literature. However, a deep study of this relation may be of interest since this gene has been repeatedly associated with a number of tumors [Stockert *et al.* (1998); Bownds *et al.* (2001)]. Actually, the ESCO1 gene has been described as an attractive candidate tumor antigen for the development of immunotherapy for a wide variety of cancers [Bownds *et al.* (2001)].

The next two rules in Table 12.31 involve high levels of BMPR1B and TSP1 (THBS1) mRNA, and PgR-positive breast tumors. BMPR1B over-expression was described in estrogen receptor-positive tumor [Esseghir *et al.* (2007); Helms *et al.* (2008)], suggesting a new breast cancer potential pathway target in the breast cancer treatment [Labhart *et al.* (2005)]. The levels of TSP1 mRNA were increased after incubation with progesterone [Iruela-Arispe *et al.* (1996)]. Invasive breast carcinomas showed higher contents of

TSP1 (an antiadhesive and antiangiogenic glycoprotein) than earlier lesions [Ito *et al.* (1997)].

Another interesting rule associates SOX11 with PgR-negative breast tumors. The SOX11 over-expression might contribute to a proliferative genotype which may be linked to poor prognosis in breast cancer patients [Brennan *et al.* (2009)]. On the other hand, another association linked PgR-negative stainning and SCUBE2 down-regulation. The expression levels of these genes could be an useful tool to predict benefit of hormonal therapy. Patients with negative SCUBE2 protein-expressing tumors, as well as those PgR-negative, present worse prognosis [Cheng *et al.* (2009)]. These findings could identify a breast cancer subgroup which might be associated with a poor clinical outcome.

Breast cancer is the most common cancer among women. Metastasis is the main cause of death of this disease. Two related related gene expression (EFEMP1 and LPL) to metastasis. EFEMP1 gene is an antagonist of angiogenesis that prevents angiogenesis and vessel infiltration [Albig *et al.* (2006)], while LPL plays an important role in lipid catabolism. EFEMP1 under-expression was associated with poor disease-free and overall survival [Sadr-Nabavi *et al.* (2009)]. LPL could be an candidate metastasis suppressor gene [Thomassen *et al.* (2009)].

Of special interest are also the relations between the epiregulin (EREG) over-expression, the p53-negative staining and the PgR-positive cases. Previous studies described that epiregulin is involved in certain physiological processes, such as maintenance or development of normal cell growth, and the progression of carcinomas [Toyoda *et al.* (1997)]. This makes sense, since the presence of the p53 is one of the mechanisms of the cell to avoid tumoral cells from reproducing (Section 12.1.1.4). Studies on a different type of tumor (bladder tumor) identified the members of the EGF family, especially EPI, as potential markers in this type of tumors [Thogersen *et al.* (2001)].

Finally, a rule relating the PgR mRNA overexpression and PgR positive staining is shown, which supports the central dogma of molecular biology. Two more associations are shown which link PAK6 & CLDN11 genes over-expression to $IHC = 2$ and $Stage = III$. The PAK6 was previously associated with breast cancer in the literature [Lee *et al.* (2002)]. However, no bibliographic evidence was found regarding its potential relation with IHC-equivocal cases. Likewise, no mention was found in the literature regarding a potential role of the CLDN11 gene in breast cancer. Further studies and empirical evaluations are thus necessary to confirm these rules, since these genes might be useful as novel prognostic markers in breast cancer.

12.8   Conclusion

An integrative and multi-disciplinary approach is presented in this work to study potential relations between prognostic factors and whole-genome expression data in breast cancer. The heterogeneity and imprecise nature of the data along with its high dimensionality make fuzzy association rules an appropriate tool for the analysis.

A number of interesting associations have been found. It was not the aim of this study to give a comprehensive list and biological interpretation of all of them, but to show that interesting associations can be obtained, which may serve to enunciate hypothesis for subsequent empirical evaluation. Therefore, a deep study and scientific evidences of the rules are needed to confirm such associations.

Finally, a web application was developed: BioFAR. This software aims to spread fuzzy techniques by providing a tool which helps to analyze heterogeneous and high dimensionality data. Results can be obtained in the form of a webpage. Few easy-understandable parameters (support, confidence and CF) describe the reliability of the associations, which are shown in an intuitive way by using linguistic labels. This web application has been shown to be very useful in the development of this work, future studies will include enhancements of this software.

Acknowledgements

This work has been carried out as part of projects P08-TIC-4299 of J. A., Sevilla, P06-CTS-02200 of J. A., Sevilla and TIN2009-13489 of DGICT, Madrid.

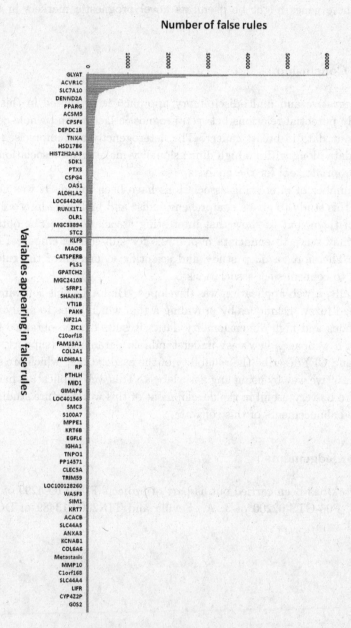

Fig. 12.10: Number of false rules generated by each variable. The red line approximately indicates the cut-point.

Chapter 13

Graph Mining on Brain Co-activation Networks

Bianca Wackersreuther[1], Annahita Oswald[1], Peter Wackersreuther[1],
Junming Shao[1] and Karsten M. Borgwardt[2]

[1] *University of Munich, Germany*
[2] *Max Planck Institute for Biological Cybernetics, Tübingen, Germany*

Graphs or networks are universal data structures[1]. In general, a graph models relationships between objects. This is interesting for two reasons: First, from a system-wide perspective, a graph represents a system and the interactions between its components. Second, from a component-centered point of view, a graph describes all relationships that link this object to the rest of the system. Furthermore, graphs are the most general data structures, as all common data types are simple instances of graphs. For example, a string can be considered as a graph in which each node represents one character, and consecutive characters are connected by an edge. In the following we demonstrate the advantages of graphs and networks in multiple application domains:

Medicine. The influence of chemical compounds on physiological processes, e.g. toxicity, or effectiveness as a drug and features of molecular structures are studied in the fields of chemoinformatics [Gasteiger and Engel (2003)] and bioinformatics. A large number of traditional benchmark datasets for graph mining algorithms originate from these domains, including MUTAG [Debnath *et al.* (1991)] and PTC [Toivonen *et al.* (2003)]. The MUTAG dataset consists of 230 mutagenic aromatic and heteroaromatic nitro compounds. Each of these molecules is known to possess a muta-

---

[1] We refer the interested reader to the awarded PhD thesis "Graph Kernels" [Borgwardt (2007)] for further details on graphs and networks.

genic effect in gram-negative bacterium *Salmonella typhimurium* or not. PTC (Predictive Toxicology Challenge) contains 417 chemical compounds which are tested for cancerogenicity in mice and rats. The classification task is to predict the cancerogenicity of compounds. As for MUTAG, each compound is represented as a graph, whose nodes or vertices are atoms and whose edges are bonds. Furthermore a high number of structured data comprises graph models of molecular structures, from RNA to proteins [Berman *et al.* (2000)], and of networks, which include protein-protein interaction networks [Xenarios *et al.* (2002a)], metabolic networks [Kanehisa *et al.* (2004)], regulatory networks [Davidson *et al.* (2002)], and phylogenetic networks [Huson and Bryant (2006)].

Social Network Analysis. Another important source of graph structured data is social network analysis [Wasserman and Faust (1994)]. In social networks, nodes represent individuals and edges represent interaction between them. The analysis of these networks is both of scientific and commercial interest. On the one hand, psychologists want to study the complex social dynamics between humans, and medical scientist want to uncover the spreading behaviour of a virus. On the other hand, industry wants to analyze these networks for marketing purposes. Detecting influential individuals in a group of people, often referred to as 'key-players' or 'trend-setters', is relevant for marketing, as companies could then focus their advertising efforts on persons known to influence the behavior of a larger group of people.

Internet, HTML, XML. A further application area for graph models is the internet which is a network and hence a graph itself. HTML documents are the nodes, and hyperlinks connect these nodes. In fact, Google exploits the Internet structure in its famous PageRank algorithm [Page *et al.* (1999)] for ranking websites. Furthermore, semi-structured data in form of XML documents is becoming very popular in the database community and in industry. The natural mathematical structure to describe semi-structured data is a graph. To quote the W3 Consortium:

> The main structure of an XML document is tree-like, and most of the lexical structure is devoted to defining that tree, but there is also a way to make connections between arbitrary nodes in a tree.[2]

---

[2]http://www.w3.org/XML/Datamodel.html

Consequently, XML documents should be regarded as graphs. Various tasks of data analysis can be performed on this graph representation, ranging from basic operations such as querying [Deutsch *et al.* (1999)] to advanced problems such as duplicate detection [Weis and Naumann (2005)].

13.1 Introduction

Understanding the mechanisms that govern neural processes in the is an important topic for medical studies. Recently the emergence of an increasing number of clinical diagnostics enable a global analysis of complex processes and therefore allow a better understanding of numerous diseases. We focus on the mechanisms in the brain that are associated with somatoform pain disorder. Somatization disorders constitute a large, clinically important health care problem that urgently needs deeper insight [Wessely *et al.* (1999)].

Earlier studies have revealed that different subunits within the human brain interact among each other, when particular stimuli are transmitted to the brain. Hence the different components form a network. From an algorithmic point of view, interacting subunits act as specific subgraphs within the network. From a medical perspective, it is interesting to ask to which degree interactions of subunits are correlated with medical disorders.

In this article, we study the question whether brain compartments of patients with somatoform pain disorder form motifs that differ from brain compartments of subjects that do not suffer from this disease. For this purpose, we analyze task-fMRI scans (a special form of neuroimaging) of the brain of 10 subjects, 6 patients with somatoform pain disorder and 4 healthy controls that attended the study of [Gündel *et al.* (2008)]. In this study both groups underwent alternate phases of non-pain and pain stimuli during the fMRI scanning. We construct a brain co-activation network for each subject where each node represents a voxel in the fMRI image. Voxels are grouped together in 90 so-called regions of interest (ROIs) using the template of [Tzourio-Mazoyer *et al.* (2002)]. We apply two approaches, the efficient heuristic approach GREW [Kuramochi and Karypis (2004b)] and the exhaustive sampling technique FANMOD by [Wernicke (2006)] to uncover frequent subgraphs in each of these networks. While an heuristic approach allows for finding motifs of arbitrary size, an exhaustive sampling algorithm can be applied to find *all* frequent subgraphs, but in this case we are limited in the size of the subgraphs. Both algorithms are designed to operate on one large graph and to find patterns corresponding to connected subgraphs that have a large number of vertex-disjoint embeddings. We demonstrate that patients with somatoform disorder show activation patterns in the brain that are different from those of healthy subjects.

The remainder of this article is organized as follows. Section 13.2 gives a brief survey of the previous work on frequent subgraph mining. Section 13.3 provides basic definitions from graph theory and subsequently describes our proposed framework. Experimental results of our method and an evaluation of the detected motifs are given in Section 13.4. Finally, Section 13.5 summarizes this work.

13.2 Related Work

Several algorithms have been defined for finding frequent subgraphs and their embeddings in one large graph or in a dataset of graphs. We distinguish algorithms for 'graph dataset mining' that work on a dataset of graphs, and algorithms for 'large graph mining' that discover frequent motifs in one large graph. While frequent subgraph algorithms that work on large graphs can directly be applied to datasets of graphs, the other direction is more complicated. However, by splitting a large graph into subgraphs, one can still use a graph dataset mining algorithm for frequent subgraph discovery on the large graph (albeit some subgraphs might be lost by the splitting).

13.2.1 *Graph Dataset Mining*

For the graph dataset mining task, approaches can be broadly divided into two classes, apriori-based approaches and pattern-growth based approaches. AGM (Apriori-based Graph Mining)[Inokuchi *et al.* (2003)] determines subgraphs G' in a dataset DS of graphs that occur in at least *minsup* percentage of all graphs in the dataset. AGM works on graphs with edge and node labels. In principle, AGM uses the famous apriori [Agrawal *et al.* (1993)] principle of iterated candidate generation and candidate evaluation. Candidate generation means that candidate subgraphs are created by joining subgraphs that have been shown to be frequent in earlier iterations. In the candidate evaluation phase, these candidates are tested, i.e. it is checked whether their frequency is greater than *minsup*, and then the whole process is iterated until all frequent patterns have been found. AGM uses a canonical form and a normal form to represent subgraphs to reduce runtime cost for subgraph isomorphism checking.

Similar to AGM, FSG (Frequent SubGraph Discovery) [Kuramochi and Karypis (2001)] uses a canonical labeling based on the adjacency matrix. Canonical labeling, candidate generation and evaluation are sped up in FSG by using graph invariants and the Transaction ID principle, which stores the ID of transactions a subgraph appeared in. This speed-up is paid for by reducing the class of subgraphs discovered to connected subgraphs, i.e. subgraphs where a path exists between all pairs of nodes.

The most well-known member of the class of pattern-growth algorithms, gSpan (graph-based Substructure pattern mining), discovers frequent substructures efficiently without candidate generation [Yan and Han (2002)]. Tree representations of graphs are encoded using a Depth First Search (DFS) code, amongst which a minimum DFS code is chosen according to some lexicographic order. Pre-order DFS-tree search is then conducted to find the complete set of frequent subgraphs in a set of graphs. gSpan is efficient, both with respect to runtime and memory requirements, making it one of the best state-of-the-art algorithms for graph dataset mining. CloseGraph [Yan and Han (2003)] extends gSpan by limiting the search to frequent complete graphs, i.e. subgraphs without supergraphs that have the same support, thereby increasing the efficiency of mining substantially.

13.2.2 *Large Graph Mining*

Unlike graph dataset mining, large graph mining intends to find subgraphs that have *minsup* embeddings in one large graph.

SUBDUE tries to minimize the minimum description length (MDL) of a graph by compressing frequent subgraphs. Frequent subgraphs are replaced by one single node and the MDL of the remaining graph is then determined. Those subgraphs whose compression minimizes the MDL are considered frequent patterns in the input graph. The candidate graphs are generated starting from single nodes to subgraphs with several nodes, using a computationally-constrained beam search.

GREW [Kuramochi and Karypis (2004b)] and SUBDUE [Cook and Holder (1994)] are greedy heuristic approaches to frequent graph mining that trade speed for completeness of the solution. GREW iteratively joins frequent pairs of nodes into one super-node and determines disjoint embeddings of connected subgraphs by a maximal independent set algorithm. Similarly, vSIGRAM and hSIGRAM [Kuramochi and Karypis (2004a)] find subgraphs that are frequently embedded within a large sparse graph, using "horizontal" (h) breadth-first search and "vertical" (v) depth-first search, respectively. They employ efficient algorithms for candidate generation and candidate evaluation that exploit the sparseness of the graph.

Several sampling methods for detecting motifs in a large protein network have been defined [Wernicke (2006); Kashtan *et al.* (2004)]. These algorithms sample subgraphs from a large network and estimate their frequency rather than resorting to heuristics. FANMOD, the algorithm by [Wernicke (2006)] uses a randomized enumeration strategy for sampling subgraphs. If one does not want to resort to any heuristics and miss out on any embeddings of a frequent subgraph, one may employ this enumeration strategy for exhaustively enumerating all subgraphs rather than randomly sampling from this enumeration.

13.3   Method

13.3.1   *Basics of Graph Theory*

We start with a brief summary of necessary definitions from the field of graph mining.

Definition 13.1 (Labeled graph / network). *A* **labeled graph** *is represented by a 4-tuple $G = (V, E, L, l)$, where V is a set of vertices (i.e. nodes), $E \subseteq V \times V$ is a set of edges, L is a set of labels, and $l : V \cup E \rightarrow L$ is a mapping that assigns labels to vertices V and edges E. If labels are not of decisive importance, we will use the* short *definition of a graph $G = (V, E)$. In the following we also use* **network** *as a synonym for graph.*

Definition 13.2 (Subgraph). *Let $G_1 = (V_1, E_1, L_1, l_1)$ and $G_2 = (V_2, E_2, L_2, l_2)$ be labeled graphs. G_1 is a* **subgraph** *of G_2 ($G_1 \sqsubseteq G_2$) if the following conditions hold: $V_1 \subseteq V_2$, $E_1 \subseteq E_2$, $L_1 \subseteq L_2$, $l_1 = l_2$. If G_1 is a subgraph of G_2, then G_2 contains G_1.*

Definition 13.3 (Isomorphism). *Two graphs are* **isomorphic** *if there exists a bijection f between the nodes of two graphs $G_1 = (V_1, E_1)$ and $G_2 = (V_2, E_2)$ such that $(v_{1a}, v_{1b}) \in E_1$ iff $(v_{2a}, v_{2b}) \in E_2$ where $v_{2a} = f(v_{1a})$ and $v_{2b} = f(v_{1b})$. If G_1 is isomorphic to G_2, we will refer to (v_{1a}, v_{1b}) and (v_{2a}, v_{2b}) as* **corresponding edges** *in the following.*

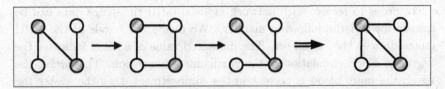

Fig. 13.1: Transformation from a time series of three labeled graphs into the corresponding union graph.

The problem to decide whether two graphs are isomorphic, i.e. the *graph isomorphism problem*, is not yet known to be NP-complete or in P. Given two graphs $G_1 = (V_1, E_1)$ and $G_2 = (V_2, E_2)$, the *subgraph isomorphism problem* consists in finding a subgraph of G_2 that is isomorphic to G_1. This problem is known to be NP-complete [Garey and Johnson (1979)].

Definition 13.4 (Embedding). *If graph G_1 is isomorphic to a subgraph S of graph G_2, then S is referred to as an* **embedding** *of G_1 in G_2.*

Definition 13.5 (Frequent subgraph / motif). *A graph G_1 is a* **frequent subgraph** *of graph G_2 if G_2 contains at least t embeddings of G_1, where t is a user-set frequency threshold parameter. Such a frequent subgraph is often called a* **motif.**

Definition 13.6 (Union graph). *Given a time series of graphs G_{ts} with n states. Then the* **union graph** *$DG(G_{ts})$ of G_{ts} is defined as $DG(G_{ts}) = (V_{DG}, E_{DG}, \ell)$, where $V_{DG} = V_i$ for all $1 \le i \le n$ and $E_{DG} = \cup_{1 \le i \le n} E_i$.*

An example for the transformation of a time series of graphs into a union graph is depicted in Figure 13.1. Note that the union of all edges of the time series is the set of edges of the union graph.

13.3.2 *Construction of Brain Co-activation Networks Out of fMRI Timeseries*

As we are interested in topological patterns that are characteristic for patients with somatoform pain disorder, we perform graph mining on brain co-activation networks. Each detected motif represents interacting regions of the brain.

In order to receive such network models, fMRI timeseries data can be transformed in the following manner. We define the voxels of the fMRI image data as the vertex set. The measured value of a voxel indicates the degree of blood circulation in the particular brain region. The *darker* the voxel, the *more* blood is present in the compartment, thus the *higher* the activation is. Edges between two vertices v_1 and v_2 stand for a similar level of activation of the two corresponding voxels. We distinguish two categories of activation levels for each voxel v at each time point i, denoted by v_i. $a(i)$ stands for its activation level at time point i. We determine an *activity–score* for each voxel v_i by comparing the median activation level of v across the time series with $a(i)$ in order to assign activation categories.

$$activity\text{-}score(v_i) = \frac{a(i) - median_{j \in \{1,..,n\}} a(j)}{median_{k \in \{1,..,n\}} \left| (a(k) - median_{j \in \{1,..,n\}} a(j)) \right|}$$

We use a median-based *activity–score* rather than a mean-based as we want to detect unusually high activation levels. In contrast to a mean-based *activity–score* a median-based *activity–score* is more robust with respect to these extremes and better suited for detecting them, as validated in initial experiments (not shown here).

- **High activation:** $a(i)$ is significantly higher than the median activation level of v.
  $(activity\text{-}score(v(i)) \geq 7.0)$
- **No significant activation:** $a(i)$ is not significantly higher than the median activation level of v.
  $(activation\text{-}score(v(i)) < 7.0)$.

Edges between vertices v_1 and v_2 are assigned if v_1 and v_2 both show high activation. Finally, we perform frequent subgraph mining on the resulting union graph.

13.3.3 Performing Frequent Subgraph Mining on Brain Co-activation Networks

In order to find frequent subgraphs in our network, we have to group our nodes and assign each group a labeling. A meaningful grouping of nodes when considering brain networks is a mapping of the nodes to their corresponding brain compartments. Hence motifs in those networks represent compartments of the brain that show a similar activation profile. We remove edges between nodes that share the same label, as a correlated degree of activation within one region is trivial, and we are interested in activity of different regions.

Then we apply two large graph mining algorithms for finding motifs in our labeled graphs. First, we employ the heuristic approach GREW [Kuramochi and Karypis (2004b)], as the runtime effort for exhaustive enumeration grows exponentially in the size of the subgraphs. This enables us to find frequent subgraphs in a large graph rather than to restrict ourselves to small frequent subgraphs. Nevertheless, as we want to in avoid missing out on embeddings of motifs that consist of a small number of vertices (up to 6), we also employ the exhaustive enumeration strategy FANMOD by [Wernicke (2006)].

13.3.4 *Evaluation of Detected Motifs*

To find motifs that are characteristic for a disease, we have to analyze the motifs separately. Therefore we want to detect motifs that occur in patients but not in the control group and vice versa. Another class of motifs that might be interesting are motifs that occur in all subjects that attend a certain study.

Another aspect that should be considered is the label distribution across motifs. A label that is used for a large number of vertices inside the network model of a particular subject s has a higher probability to appear in a motif than a label that covers a small number of nodes. Hence, we have to define the normalized frequency of a node label l, denoted by $freq_{norm}(l)$.

$$freq_{norm}(l) = \sum_{s \in S} \frac{freq_{m \in \{1,...,n\}}(l) \cdot \#Embeddings(m|s)}{freq_{Background}(l|s)}$$

$freq_{m \in \{1,...,n\}}$ stands for the number of occurences of label l in a motif m. This number has to be multiplied by the number of isomorphic subgraphs of m found in a subject s, its embeddings found in s. The $freq_{Background}(l|s)$ describes the number of occurences of label l with respect to all vertices of the network that refers to subject s. In our case this is equivalent to the *size* of a ROI. Finally, we sum up over all subjects given in the dataset.

13.4   Experiments

The experimental section is organized as follows. First, we summarize the construction of the network models, including a detailed description of the used dataset and the labeling scheme for the vertices of the networks. Then we perform motif discovery using the heuristic algorithm GREW to allow for finding motifs of arbitrary size. As an evaluation of these results indicates that a multitude of the motifs found by GREW consist of only a small number of vertices, we go a step further and additionally apply the exhaustive sampling technique FANMOD by [Wernicke (2006)] on the network models. Finally, we compare the results of both algorithms and give representative motifs for the group of subjects that suffer from the somatoform pain disorder and typical motifs for the group of healthy controls.

Construction of the Brain Network Models. We created networks for 10 subjects that attended the studies of [Gündel *et al.* (2008)]. The resulting networks comprise 66 to 440 nodes with 90 different classes of node labels and 358 to 13,548 edges. In addition, the network models indicate different number of edge types. These refer to the concatenation of the labels of the adjacent nodes. All edges are undirected because in the relationship 'both adjacent voxels show high activation' a direction makes no sense. The exact statistics of each subject are depicted in Table 13.4.

Subject	# Vertices	# Different Labels	# Edges	# Edge Types	# Different Motifs by GREW
Patient 1	102	31	453	91	38
Patient 2	185	32	1,961	84	706
Patient 3	241	35	3,506	90	505
Patient 4	263	46	5,152	293	752
Patient 5	313	46	10,977	372	4,154
Patient 6	440	58	13,548	475	4,256
Control 1	66	10	358	15	15
Control 2	99	33	407	111	32
Control 3	109	18	1,093	13	133
Control 4	202	35	2,045	133	236

Statistics of the network models for each subject.

Timeseries Datasets. We used fMRI timeseries data (1.5 T MR scanner) of 6 female somatoform patients and 4 healthy controls. Standard data preprocessing including realignment, correction for motion artifacts and normalization to standard space have been performed using SPM2 (available at http://www.fil.ion.ucl.ac.uk/spm/). In addition, to remove global effects the voxel time series have been corrected regressing out the global mean, as suggested in [Sarty (2007)].

Vertex Labels. We labeled all nodes in our network model by regional parcellation of the voxels into 90 brain regions using the template of Tzourio-Mazoyer *et al.* [Tzourio-Mazoyer *et al.* (2002)].

Finding Motifs With GREW. To allow for finding motifs of arbitrary size, we searched for topological motifs using GREW with a frequency threshold of $t = 5$. In these experiments, we searched for motifs with a minimum number of one edge. The total number of different motifs found in the 10 networks is depicted in the last column of Table 13.4.

Evaluation of the Motifs Detected by GREW. Altogether we found 10,530 different motifs in somatoform patients and healthy controls. 10,173 different motifs were detected among patients, 413 within the group of healthy subjects, where some of these motifs were also found among the patients and vice versa.

For validation we divided the subjects into three classes. Class (1) contains only the somatoform patients, class (2) consists of the controls exclusively and class (3) composes the union of class (1) and (2). Figure 13.2 shows typical representatives of each class. The two motifs on the left occur in 57% of the patients but in no healthy subject. The middle motif arises in 50% of the class (2)–subjects but in no patient. The upper motif on the right-hand side was found in 50% of the control group and in 14% of the patients, the lower motif in 25% of the control group and in 43% of the patient group. Most of the typical representatives of both groups comprise only a small number of vertices.

The largest motifs (highest number of vertices and edges) of class (1) were found in subject 'patient 5'. They consist of 28 vertices and 29 edges, five different brain compartments are involved in this motif. A total of 34 motifs of this kind were found in this subject. The largest motifs in class (2) were detected in subject 'control 3'. We found two motifs that comprise 12 nodes with two different labels and 17 edges. An example of the largest motifs found in class (1) and the two largest motifs of class (2) are shown

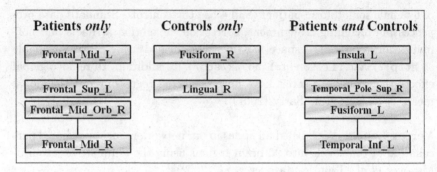

Patients *only*	Controls *only*	Patients *and* Controls
Frontal_Mid_L	Fusiform_R	Insula_L
Frontal_Sup_L	Lingual_R	Temporal_Pole_Sup_R
Frontal_Mid_Orb_R		Fusiform_L
Frontal_Mid_R		Temporal_Inf_L

Fig. 13.2: Typical representatives of motifs found in the groups of somatoform patients, healthy controls respectively and the group of all subjects.

in Figure 13.3. Note that no motif occurs in all subjects.

Evaluation of ROIs. We found motifs that can discriminate well between somatoform patients and controls. In the next step we determined the normalized frequencies of the ROIs in patients and controls, respectively. Figure 13.4(a) illustrates the results for the 15 most frequent ROIs with respect to the patient group, and Figure 13.4(b) for the group of healthy controls, respectively. Within the motifs found in the patient group, *Caudate_R* is the most frequent ROI ($freq_{norm} = 6.43\%$). The most frequent brain region with respect to the motifs of the control group is *Frontal_Mid_Orb_R* ($freq_{norm} = 22.04\%$). ROIs that show a small frequency are summarized by the label *Miscellaneous*. Our results are consistent with a previous study [Gündel *et al.* (2008)]. They report different activation pattern in the regions *Insula_L* (Patients: $freq_{norm} = 5.29\%$ Controls: $freq_{norm} = 1.95\%$) and *Frontal_Mid_Orb_R* (Patients: $freq_{norm} = 3.38\%$ Controls: $freq_{norm} = 22.04\%$), the key-player in the group of healthy controls. Our results of different activation of the parahippocampal cortex in patients and controls (not depicted in Figure 13.4) supports a recent study that suggests that patients with posttraumatic stress disorder showed also an altered activation pattern in the parahippocampal cortex in comparison to healthy controls when subjected to painful heat stimuli [Geuze *et al.* (2007)]. In addition, we found that patients show increased activation in *Rolandic_Oper_L*, *Caudate_R* and *Rectus_R* whereas the control group is activated in the regions *Temporal_Inf_L*, *Heschl_R* and *Lingual_R* to a higher degree. Also, the olfactory region shows alterations in the activation of pa-

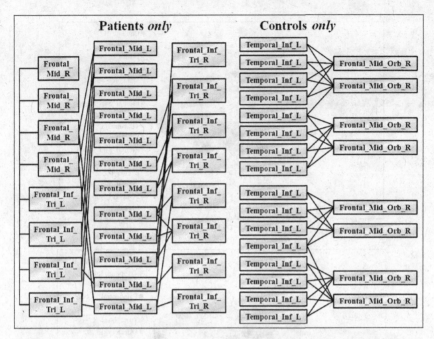

Fig. 13.3: Largest motifs found in the groups of somatoform patients and healthy controls.

tients and controls. Whereas *Olfactory_R* occurs to a much higher degree in motifs found in patients, motifs found in the networks of controls are labeled more often with *Olfactory_L*.

Finding Motifs With FANMOD. The public disposable implementation[3] of the exhaustive sampling algorithm by [Wernicke (2006)] is restricted to networks with a maximum number of 16 different vertex labels. Hence, we map the original network data to a modified version where only the 15 most frequent ROIs are kept. The remaining vertices are labeled by *Miscellaneous*. This labeling scheme refers to the ROI distribution among motifs detected by GREW as shown in Figure 13.4. As edges of the type *Miscellaneous–Miscellaneous* occur disproportional frequent within the network, and would therefore tamper with the real frequencies of the results, we deleted that kind of interaction.

We searched for motifs, consisting of up to 6 vertices and used a sample rate of 100,000 to estimate the number of subgraphs which is the default

---

[3]http://theinf1.informatik.uni-jena.de/motifs/

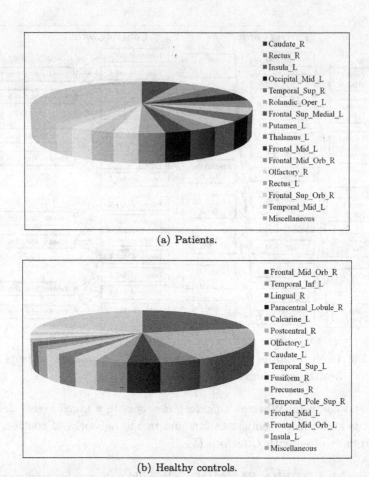

(a) Patients.

(b) Healthy controls.

Fig. 13.4: Frequencies of ROIs in motifs of patiens and controls, respec-
        tively.

parameterization, as recommended by the authors. Table 13.4 illustrates
the number of motifs that comprise $3 \leq k \leq 6$ vertices for each subject.
We compared these results by applying GREW ($t = 5$) to the same modified networks. The last column of Table 13.4 demonstrates that for small
subgraph sizes an exhaustive method provides significant more information
about the graph structure. Note that the total number of detected motifs
by FANMOD with a limited number of vertices exceeds the total number
of motifs found by GREW with arbitrary size in most cases. However, an

exhaustive method is only applicable for finding subgraphs that consist of a small number of vertices (cf. - in Table 13.4).

Subject	# Motifs $(k=3)$	# Motifs $(k=4)$	# Motifs $(k=5)$	# Motifs $(k=6)$	# Motifs $(3 \le k \le 6)$	# Motifs by GREW
Patient 1	9	13	28	42	92	4
Patient 2	42	121	288	-	451	406
Patient 3	5	6	7	8	26	4
Patient 4	22	91	374	-	487	56
Patient 5	139	509	-	-	648	988
Patient 6	431	3,292	-	-	3,723	1,861
Control 1	6	10	16	22	54	34
Control 2	18	32	51	78	179	56
Control 3	9	26	-	-	35	161
Control 4	137	565	2,399	-	3,101	472

Motifs detected by FANMOD for different number of vertices compared to the number of motifs found by GREW under the same conditions. For some motif sizes, FANMOD is not applicable as the runtime effort for exhaustive enumeration grows exponentially in the size of the subgraphs.

13.5 Conclusion

In this work, we have applied the heuristic algorithm GREW and FAN-MOD, an exhaustive sampling method for frequent subgraph discovery to time series data of 6 somatoform patients and 4 healthy controls. These motifs represent groups of brain compartments that covary in their activity during the process of pain stimulation. We evaluated the appearance of motifs for both groups. Our results let us suspect that somatoform brain disorder is caused by an additional pathogeneous activity, not by a missing physiological activity.

So far we care about the topology of the network, but ignore the temporal order of these interactions. When studying network topology, it is important to bear in mind that the network models currently available are simplified models of the systems that govern cellular processes. While these processes are dynamic, the models we consider so far are all static. In future research, we will look into the temporal order of the motifs, thus we want to determine dynamic motifs.

Chapter 14

Automatic Identification of Surgery Indicators

Marie Persson[1], Niklas Lavesson[1], Marteinn Magnusson[1] and
Johan Berglund[2]

[1] *Blekinge Hospital, Karlshamn, Sweden*
[2] *Blekinge Institute of Technology, Karlskrona, Sweden*

14.1 Introduction

Sweden is at present struggling with an increasing cost of its healthcare system as well as strong service demand from patients, similar to many other European countries. The old method of reducing the availability of service in favor of long waiting lists is no longer an option, especially in light of the fact that patients now have the right to seek treatment anywhere within the EU borders. There is therefore a strong enthusiasm in improving productivity and efficiency. One of the most expensive areas in healthcare is surgery, which necessitates many expensive resources in terms of staff, equipment, and medical resources. Generally, these resources have to be managed and divided between several departments, e.g., orthopaedics, gynecology or the general surgery, within the hospital in order to meet the total surgery demand (depicted in Fig. 14.1). The question is how and when in the planning process the surgery demand could be estimated.

Commonly, the patient queue, i.e., the waiting list for surgery, is viewed as the surgery demand. Let us review a quite common sequence of steps for processing a patient within the Swedish healthcare system: typically, the patient begins by contacting the general practitioner. If deemed necessary, the patient is then referred from the general practitioner to the hospital (specialist) care. The referral is assessed by an expert, e.g., a surgeon specialist. The patient is then, according to medical priority, put on wait for an appointment to meet a surgeon with the appropriate subspecialty. Next, the patient meets the appointed surgeon at the outpatient clinic, i.e., the hospital care, and together they decide upon treatment, e.g., surgery. If surgery is decided, the patient is added to the patient queue for surgery, again according to medical priority. At this point, when the patient has been added to the waiting list, the accumulated elective surgery demand in terms of number of patients can be estimated and hence provide information to facilitate and improve surgery management.

As stated above, the patient is usually referred from the general practitioner to hospital care. A patient referral contains information that indicates the need for hospital care and this information is differently structured depending on the medical needs. In practice, these needs can be viewed as the forthcoming patient demand at the hospital, analogous to a volume of orders. Today, the structure of referrals is very much up to the general practitioner who is referring the patient. This implies that the data provided to the hospital can vary extensively between cases. We suggest that, by enforcing a certain structure on the referral data, it may be possible to make early predictions about the patient demand. Such predictions could then be used as a basis for managing resources more efficiently, e.g., surgery management, to increase hospital productivity.

14.1.1   *Aims and Objectives*

We investigate whether it is possible to make predictions about the elective surgery demand by generating prediction models from surgery indicator variables that could be included in a structured referral. To find out which indicator variables are suitable we analyze data mining based models that are automatically generated from patient records in combination with surgery related statistics and the associated known outcomes. We argue that, if these predictions can be performed at the referral stage, the resource management and productivity related to surgery can be improved.

This work is an extension to a preliminary study [Persson and Lavesson (2009)], in which we first introduced the problem and our approach. We collaborate with domain experts from the Department of Orthopaedics at Blekinge hospital in Sweden and have gathered a small database of information extracted from patient records and the surgical suite. The idea is to provide a proof of concept and to perform initial validations of our the-

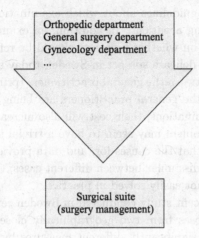

Fig. 14.1: The surgery demand. Several departments are managed by the surgical suite, which is responsible for operating room scheduling and resource allocation.

oretical models by using empirical data from the orthopaedic department.

14.1.2   *Outline*

The remainder of this chapter is organized as follows: first, we describe the problem more thoroughly from a healthcare point of view. We then review related work. In Sect. 14.3, our approach to address the problem is described and this is followed by a theoretical analysis. Finally, we perform an experiment in Sect. 14.4, discuss the results of the experiment in the subsequent section, and at the end present conclusions and some pointers to future work.

14.2   Background

In Sweden, there is an intense debate about, and work conducted on, the systematization and standardization of patient records, as well as of patient referral procedures from the general practitioner to hospital care. Consequently, the discussions about this referral standardization are of great interest for both the general practitioners and the hospital care.

The hospital care wants the referred patients to be more extensively and suitably examined on by the general practitioner. In turn, the general practitioners require guidelines about which examinations should be conducted before referring a patient. In addition, an examination could give valuable information on whether a patient should be referred or not. This is an interesting and delicate subject in Sweden today since the budgeted cost are separated between the general practitioners (primary care) and the hospital care and if the general practitioners are being forced to increase their number of examinations, their cost will also increase.

In theory, this problem may seem to have a trivial solution. However, considering the fact that the causes for, and data provided in, the patient referral can be quite dissimilar between different cases; this instead implies that the problem is not easily solved in practice.

Additionally, a recent study conducted in Sweden reveals that patients with identical diagnoses from two geographically close Swedish counties were managed using significantly different measures by the county hospitals [Ekblom *et al.* (2009)]. The study presents a variable, denoted surgery indication, which can be calculated given the appropriate information for different types of surgeries. However, they note that most referrals or patient records presently do not include the information necessary to calculate surgery indication.

14.2.1 *Referral Contents*

The main question is what kind of information should be included in the patient referral. This is indeed an interesting and difficult question. Despite the fact that a patient referral is strongly related to the symptoms and/or disorder/disease of the patient, the possibility of relying on diagnosis codes may be dismissed for two primary reasons: firstly, the patient might not have been given a diagnosis because the general practitioner has not been able to identify the disorder/disease with any degree of certainty. In many cases this is after all partly the motivation for having the patient referred to the hospital care. Secondly, the diagnosis of a patient may not in itself provide the necessary information on how to treat a patient. In other words, a diagnosis is a description of what is wrong rather than a description of how to treat a patient.

There are often several additional variables of interest that need to be known in order to provide effective treatment. Consequently, such variables would also be of interest when trying to predict future healthcare demand. The diagnosis, if available, is of course still an important variable. However, the question is which additional variables are important for different types of cases and how information about these variables may be extracted. Let us review an example case, where the described problem occurs. Consider a patient, referred from a general practitioner to an orthopaedic department at the hospital (as visualized in Fig. 14.2). One of the main interests of the

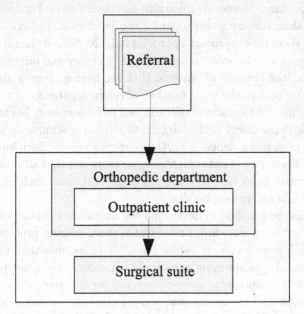

Fig. 14.2: A conceptual view of the studied healthcare process. The referrals from general practitioners are submitted to the hospital care.

orthopaedic department is that of knowing or being able to quickly find out what type of subspecialty is required, e.g., hip, knee, back, and so forth. Additionally, it is crucial to determine whether the patient needs surgery or not. In order to determine this, prerequisite medical examinations have to be conducted. Many of these medical examinations can be performed by the general practitioner. This may also be beneficial in terms of cost since hospital care is more expensive. Moreover, the patients will be prevented from burdening the surgery waiting list if the results of the medical examinations contraindicate surgery or if the prerequisite medical examination is incomplete and therefore has to be complemented at the hospital, which might lead to longer waiting times.

It also seems that the number of patients having orthopaedic surgery in comparison to the patients referred to the hospital care is lower than preferred. A small case study performed at the department of orthopaedic surgery at Blekinge hospital suggest that only 30–40% of the referred patients are having surgery. There will always be a certain amount of patients for which the decision about surgery cannot be determined accurately before specialist care. Moreover, some patients need a second opinion or other treatments than surgery at orthopaedic specialist care. Experience tells us that these two groups represent approximately 20–30% of the total number of referred patients. In order to achieve cost efficiency and minimize patient waiting time, the amount of patients that are having surgery should then be close to 70–80% of the total number of referred patients.

Which type of information is determined to be necessary in order for the Orthopaedic Department or the surgeon to be able to accurately predict the probability of surgery depends on the particular case. Each subspecialty requires a different set of data. However, we point out that all subspecialties have a collective need for several types of general data, such as: age, sex, and certain laboratory test results.

If it would be possible to determine the necessary information for a set of generic problems, e.g., hip, under which more specific problems can be sorted, e.g., hip arthrosis, it seems plausible to assume that the surgery prediction can be made more accurately. If sufficiently good predictions can be made, the upcoming surgery demand for different types of surgery can be estimated. This means that a more efficient resource planning can be performed.

If one type of surgery seems to increase in demand, certain actions can be taken to prevent waiting list congestions, e.g., operating room planning, scheduling of surgeons and/or more long-term actions like directions for education or employments to meet the approaching surgery demand. Instead of traditional waiting list management where the number of patients simply are counted to indicate future demand, we point out the advantages of considering the aggregated future patient demand in terms of surgery or no surgery, surgery duration, and surgery recovery when performing the resource planning.

This is also considered by Persson and Persson [Persson and Persson (2010)], where the problem of how to allocate the resources of surgeons between appointment and surgery in order to minimize total patient waiting time, is addressed. In their study, the first estimates of patient surgery demand are assumed to be made already at the referral level.

Accordingly, we want to find out which variables are of interest for an orthopaedic department in order to perform predictions about the future patient demand. We refer to these variables of interest as indicator variables. It should be observed that these predictions are by no means meant to serve as a substitution for the visit to the outpatient clinic. A physical visit at the outpatient clinic to meet the surgeon before surgery is in most cases a prerequisite for surgery (or other types of treatment). Indeed, the visit is also vital for patient trust. We have identified three target variables that are of great importance when making patient demand estimations:

- need for surgery (or probability of surgery),
- surgery duration, and
- surgery recovery or patient length of stay.

Consequently, we strive to identify which types of patient data have the potential to be good indicator variables for these three target variables. Obviously, if the probability of surgery is determined to be low, the two remaining variables are not of interest for the Orthopaedic Department. In the presented study, we focus on predicting the need for surgery.

14.2.2 *Related Work*

Throughout the last decades, quite a few studies have been conducted within the relatively new scientific field of healthcare management. Earlier, there has been a contrast between the rather haphazard approach of healthcare management and the more scientific approach related to the medical profession [Ozcan and Smith (1998)]. However, the field is now headed towards, what can be described as, evidence-based healthcare management.

The diversity of the healthcare management area is shown by the number of research directions and methods used as well as the broad field of application areas [Cardoen *et al.* (2009); Jun *et al.* (1999); Imhoff *et al.* (2001)]. Due to the many situations of uncertainty in healthcare (e.g., patient arrival, emergency cases and complications), different simulation techniques are widely used to study patient demand and waiting list management [Jun *et al.* (1999); Persson and Persson (2009)]. One application area of particular interest to the operations research field, besides healthcare management in general, is the management of operating room scheduling [Cardoen *et al.* (2009); Rauner and Vissers (2003)]. A number of different mathematical models are described in an attempt to analyze the complexity of operating room planning and scheduling. Another area of research relevant to healthcare management is healthcare informatics, which is about applying methods from, e.g., computer science, data mining, and statistics on different types of data to develop decision support systems that can improve healthcare management [Wan (2006)].

Data mining methods in general have been studied extensively in this respect [Obenshain (2004); Silver *et al.* (2001)]. However, studies about data mining-based approaches to waiting list management, and surgeon or operating room scheduling, are scarcer. One of the existing studies related to operating room scheduling compares the performance of four different machine learning techniques [Davies (2004)]. Many types of input data were collected for this study. However, potentially important variables such as age, sex, and morbidity, were left unused.

It is important to stress that most studies about operating room planning and scheduling are focusing on the patients that are already up for surgery. On the contrary, our chapter investigates the possibility to make predictions about the patient demand for surgery much earlier; namely at the referral stage. As the total amount of referrals constitute the out patient waiting list, this work also considers aspects of waiting list management, which is a well-studied phenomenon in healthcare management [Goddard and Tavakoli (1998); VanBerkel and Blake (2007)]. Vissers *et al.* [Vissers *et al.* (2001)] present a sound waiting list analysis based on four different levels of mechanisms that are described to underpin the problem of waiting list management. However, their study assumes that waiting lists represent the actual demand of service. Not only do we address the problem of assessing the actual demand of service given a certain waiting list, we also suggest the generation of prediction models that may assist the general practitioner in the referral process.

To our knowledge, the problem of predicting the probability or need for surgery based on referral data and patient records has not been studied previously.

14.3 Approach

We will now suggest an approach for solving some of the main problems discussed in the previous section. The motivation for this approach is primarily based on the fact that large amounts of potentially useful data about patients, procedures, and consumed resources are stored in the hospital databases. These data can quite possibly be associated with information about, e.g., the outcomes of treatments and decisions about whether to perform surgery or not. In the context of a major restructuring project related to surgery management at Blekinge hospital, this approach was introduced and received great interest.

Let us review the case under study: Blekinge hospital, which is a medium sized hospital in southeast Sweden, stores several types of structured data about the managed patients. At the surgical suite, additional, possibly important, stored data include: the type of surgery, as well as the duration of the surgery among several other data related to surgery, e.g., anesthesia methods and surgery preparation. Moreover, a number of variables are stored in the patient records, e.g., diagnoses, drug treatments, whether surgery was decided upon for a certain problem, length of stay, and so forth. However, the patient record data is presently unstructured, i.e., a patient record is stored as a digital text document.

We hypothesize that patterns may exist in the patient record data that can be used together with data from the surgical suite to predict the occurrence, type and, duration of surgery and recovery. Such predictions could then be used by the surgeon specialist (here, orthopaedic specialist) and surgery managers to schedule resources in terms of, e.g., staff, operating rooms, and beds more efficiently.

If the described patterns exist, it would be possible to generate surgery prediction models and surgery outcome prediction models. From these models, we may then extract indicator variables that could be included as required inputs for a structured referral. Of course, the generated models could then be used to predict the probability of surgery at the referral level since the variables needed for making the prediction have been included in the referral. In summary, we conclude that a machine learning-based data mining approach seems to be quite suitable for this purpose. In particular, there is one type of technique that could be useful to employ.

14.3.1 *Supervised Learning*

If our assumptions are correct, it would be possible to apply supervised learning algorithms for the task of generating classifiers, i.e., by generalizing from patient record data and the associated occurrence, type, duration of surgery and recovery for known cases. A classifier is a generated model that can categorize a certain type of data into a discrete number of classes. Many types of classifiers are also able to output probabilities for the complete set of classes [Lavesson and Davidsson (2007)]. These probabilities may be used by the domain experts, e.g., the surgeon specialists, to reason about which decision to make when presented with several possible options. For example, it would most certainly be beneficial for a surgeon specialist to know that the predicted probability of the need for surgery is 0.48 (i.e., a borderline case) as opposed to just knowing that the predicted action is to not perform surgery.

Generally, a supervised learning algorithm is given a data set that features inputs and the associated output. The objective is then to generalize from these known observations of input and output. The resulting generalization is represented either by a classifier, if the output is discrete, e.g., the need of surgery (true or false), or a regression function, if it is continuous, e.g., the duration of recovery.

The input variables, or attributes, of a data set can be represented using different data types out of which two of the most frequently employed are the nominal (discrete) and the numeric (continuous) type. More formally, we say that a data set is made up by a set of n instances, $X = \{x_1, \ldots, x_n\}$. In order to generalize from the results of the experiments, we theoretically assume that X represent a set of independent and identically distributed instances drawn from the same underlying distribution, which we may represent by the theoretical set, Z, consisting of all possible instances of the problem. Each instance, x_k, is labeled with a class, $y_k \in Y$ where $Y = \{y_1, \ldots, y_m\}$. In practice, the class labels for the instances are represented by a (nominal) target attribute.

A generated classifier, i.e., a model, $m : X \rightarrow Y$, may be used to predict the class, $\hat{y}_k \in Y$ of any provided instance, x_k. The objective is to find a model where $\hat{y}_k = y_k$ for all instances of Z. Since we will never get access to Z in practice, we instead seek a resonable estimation of the performance on Z. In order to evaluate this (generalization) performance it is crucial to divide the known data set, X, into subsets of data that can be used for training and testing the generated models, respectively. Naturally, these subsets should be disjoint. Otherwise, the performance estimate may be overly optimistic [Witten and Frank (2005)]. For example, X can be divided into two subsets, X_{test} and X_{train}, where $X_{\text{test}} \cap X_{\text{train}} = \emptyset$. We generate m from X_{train} and assume that $X \subset Z$ and that an evaluation result obtained on X_{test} is a resonable estimate of the performance on Z.

14.3.2   Theoretical Modeling

It would of course be interesting to generate a data set using existing referral data as the input and the occurrence of surgery as the output. We could then generate models that predict the occurrence or probability of surgery given the referral data. However, this only works in theory today since the currently used referrals are still represented by unstructured text, meaning that one would first need to extract pieces of information from these documents to transform them to structured representations, i.e., databases that could be mined. Of course, one could always employ text mining techniques on the unstructured data in order to extract useful information [Feldman and Sanger (2006)]. However, the lack of structure is not the only problem, as we have already discussed: the main problem associated with the referrals is that they do not necessarily include the type of information requested by the specialist.

Instead, we would like to approach this problem from another angle by trying to find out what kind of information is indeed required by the hospital care for different types of referrals. From a surgeon specialist, we may obtain a set of generic referral types, $R = \{r_1, \ldots, r_n\}$. For each type, we need to gather data from a large set of patients. Subsequently, for each patient, i, we need to obtain data about the target variable that is to be predicted at the referral stage. For example, we may obtain data from the hospital patient records about whether or not a surgery was carried out, s_i. Once we have gathered this data, it may even be possible to perform clustering to generate additional generic referral types; referral type definitions. A similar approach has been used to generate patient type definitions [Isken and Rajagopalan (2002)].

The difficulty lies in deciding on which input variables to include from the set of patient record variables, V, and this is indeed what we want to investigate, i.e., which variables, V_r, are good indicators of s for a certain referral type, r. Whether or not V represents the complete set of patient record variables or a subset, we would like use V as the set of input attributes, and s as the target attribute when applying the supervised learning algorithms. Our assumption is then that V_r can be extracted from the generated models on the condition that they are accurate in their prediction of s.

14.3.3 Models for Structured Referrals

If it is possible to generate accurate models for the prediction of s, the variables from V_r can be used as a basis for structuring the referral of type r. Consequently, the general practitioner would know which pieces of information need to be included in each specific type of referral. In fact, it would even be possible to design a software-based referral system, using domain expert knowledge. In this system, the general practitioner would specify the type of referral and in return the software application would describe what kind of information the general practitioner needs to provide and which tests and examinations to perform. Additionally, this type of interactive referral system may help the general practitioner in obtaining a better understanding of which possible actions e.g., surgery, that are needed to treat the patient and in taking decisions on whether it is useful or not to refer the patient. See Fig. 14.3 for an overview of the problem.

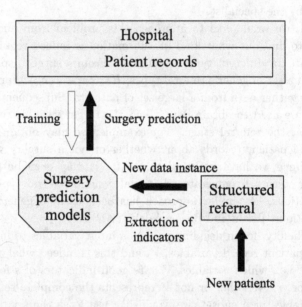

Fig. 14.3: Models for structured referrals.

14.3.4 *Prediction Models for the Surgical Suite*

Predicting whether surgery should be performed, or estimating the probability of surgery, at the referral stage would simplify resource allocation and staff management at the surgical suite and the orthopaedic department since it would allow the surgeon specialist to rule out patients with a low predicted probability of surgery in order to decrease the patient queue. However, the patients that are likely to need surgery would still pose a difficult problem of optimization and resource allocation.

14.3.5 *Algorithm Selection*

When presented with the task of constructing models for structured referrals, we first need to generate accurate surgery prediction models from data available in the various hospital databases. As suggested earlier, we may then extract suitable surgery indicators for each specific referral type from these prediction models. The set of identified indicators for each referral type (along with any known or uncovered relationships between them) would serve as a basis for constructing the structured referral models.

The first step in the data mining process would be to generate a data set that includes all possible variables that may be correlated with the target variable from the existing hospital databases. Feature selection can then be used in order to systematically reduce the effect of the curse of dimensionality and to generate robust prediction models.

With regard to the task of generating surgery prediction models, we have already indicated the possible benefit of using classifiers that are able to output probabilities in addition to the actual classification since this additional information may be used to make a more informed decision, e.g., about whether to perform surgery or not. Coincidentally, both of these tasks require the generation of surgery prediction models. However, the intended uses of the prediction models differ between the tasks.

For the second task, the goal is the prediction model itself. The intended use of this model is to serve as decision support for the surgeon specialist when allocating resources and scheduling personnel. Considering this intended use, we hypothesize that a human understandable (interpretable) model might be more valuable than one that is overly complex or opaque (assuming that both models are equally accurate in their predictions).

For example, neural network-based models or ensemble models, although accurate and robust for many domains, are generally considered as being opaque and incomprehensible. However, there are some possible approaches available to remedy this issue, e.g., by extracting transparent and comprehensive rule sets from the generated (opaque) models [Johansson (2007)]. A more common approach is to make use of learning algorithms that are able to generate interpretable models, e.g., decision tree inducers or rule-based learners, although it is important to recognize the fact that the models generated by these learning algorithms are not always interpretable. For example, we may generally regard tree-based models as an intuitive means for us to understand the decision process but if the tree structure is too complex (e.g., because of the high number of nodes, the existence of reoccurring sub trees, and so on) it might be time consuming or even impossible to understand the decision process.

For the first task, the model is merely used as a means to identify potential indicators that can be used as a basis for constructing a new referral system. Thus, we do not need to restrict ourselves to using learning algorithms that generate interpretable models. It is important, however, that we are able to understand (and perhaps rank) the importance of different input variables in predicting the target variable.

Up until now, we have presented the problem domain, our approach to solve two related problems in this domain, and we have also discussed some important aspects to consider when applying supervised learning in the domain. In order to further show the applicability of our approach, we will present a small experiment performed on real data from Blekinge hospital. This experiment is limited to the task of generating surgery prediction models from patient records.

14.4   Experiment

In this section, we first explain the process of data collection and preparation. We then motivate our selection of supervised learning algorithms and their configurations. Finally, we present the results of the experiments and finish off with some discussions.

14.4.1   *Data Collection*

We review the records of all new referrals seen at the outpatient clinic in the Department of Othropaedics at Blekinge Hospital during two subsequent months in 2008 with the ICD10 diagnosis M16 (Coxarthrosis, arthrosis of the hip). A total of 80 complete patient records were identified and their data included in the study.

14.4.2   *Data Preparation*

Information was gathered for both the surgery prediction case and the surgey outcome prediction case described earlier. The complete list of variables can be viewed in Tab. 14.1. Certain variables (*age*, *sex*) are of a general character and not specific for the type of patients included in this study while other variables are more specific for patients undergoing hip joint surgery.

Table 14.1: Data Set Statistics

Variable	Range/Values[a]	Mean/Ratio[b]	Missing
age[*]	43...92	70.7(10.6)	0%
asa	1,2,3	0.21,0.21,0.15	43%
b-hb	110...171	136.2(14.7)	45%
ecg	normal,borderline, pathologic	0.28,0.19, 0.09	45%
flexion[*]	no,yes	0.23,0.53	25%
had surgery[*]	no,yes	0.50,0.09	41%
home help	no,yes	0.43,0.03	55%
inrotation[*]	no,some,yes	0.50,0.13,0.16	21%
length of stay[c]	3...15	6.7(2.4)	41%
living alone	no,yes	0.43,0.26	31%
outrotation[*]	no,some,yes	0.36,0.18,0.28	19%
pain duration[*]	long,short	0.54,0.09	38%
residence	house,apartment	0.18,0.46	36%
s-krea	42...176	78.3(22.6)	45%
sex	male,female	0.43,0.56	0%
side	left,both,right	0.48,0.46	5%
walking aid[*]	0,1,2,3,4	0.49,0.08,0.10,0.05,0.06	23%
walking distance[*]	short,medium,long	0.18,0.16,0.19	48%
xray[*]	1,2,3,4	0.04,0.21,0.19,0.14	43%
surgery (target)[*]	no,yes	0.39,0.61	0%

[a]The minimum and maximum values for numeric variables or the categories of nominal variables.
[b]The mean and standard deviation for numeric variables or the ratio of instances belonging to each class for nominal variables.
[c]The length-of-stay variable could possibly be a suitable target attribute for the prediction of surgery outcome.
[*]The variables included in the experiment.

The *walking aid* variable indicates the level of aid needed for walking. A patient may be able to walk with; no aid (*0*), a cane (*1*), crutches (*2*), a walking frame (*3*), or he/she needs a wheel chair (*4*). Similarly, the *walking distance* variable indicates the distance a patient can walk. We discretisize this variable according to the interval: < 300 meter (*short*), < 1 kilometer (*medium*), ≥ 1 kilometer (*long*).

The b-hemoglobin (*b-hb*) and s-creatinine (*s-krea*) laboratory test variables give the level of hemoglobine and creatinine, respectively.

The *flexion, inrotation,* and *outrotation* variables represent different indicators of hip mobility. The patient records contained the degree of mobility for each of these variables. We discretisize the variables by the following intervals for *inrotation* and *outrotation*: 0 degrees (*no*), ≤ 10 degrees (*some*), > 10 degrees (*yes*), and the following interval for *flexion*: < 90 degrees (*no*), ≥ 90 degrees (*yes*).

The *side* variable indicates if it is the *right*, *left* or *both* hip joints that are affected. The *pain duration* variable gives the time the patient estimates he/she has been experiencing pain from the affected joint. The *had surgery* variable indicates whether the patient has previously had his contralateral hip joint replaced with a joint prosthesis. We discretisize *pain duration* according to the following interval: < 1 year (*short*), ≥ 1 year (*long*). The *had surgery* variable indicates whether the patient has previously had hip surgery (*yes* or *no*).

The type of residence (*residence*), whether the patient lives at home (*living home*), and whether the patient uses home help service (*home help*), are associated with the living conditions of the patient. *residence* may be either *apartment* or *house* while the two other variables can be either *yes* or *no*.

The x-ray variable (*xray*) indicates the grade of osteo-arthrosis as seen on an AP pelvic radiograph according to the Kellgren-Lawrence scale [Kellgren and Lawrence (1957)], which is a five-grade scale with the following possible grades: *0* (none), *1* (doubtful), *2* (minimal), *3* (moderate), and *4* (severe). The ECG variable (*ecg*) indicates the results of the electrocardiogram analysis, according to the following ordinal scale: *normal*, suspected pathologic (*borderline*), and *pathologic*.

The ASA variable (*asa*) is the patient's physical status classified according to the American Society of Anesthesiologists classification system. The ASA system is made up of six categories. Grade 1 is a normal, healthy patient. Grade 2 is a patient with a well-controlled disease of one body system but without functional limitations. Grade 3 is a patient with a controlled disease of more than one body system or one major system, with some functional limitations. Grade 4 is a patient with at least one severe disease that is poorly controlled or at end stage. Grade 5 is a patient in imminent risk of death. Grade 6 is a declared brain-dead patient whose organs are being removed for donor purposes.

The *surgery* and *length of stay* variables indicate whether surgery was carried out (*yes* or *no*) and the number of days of hospitalization, respectively.

Table 14.1 contains the 23 variables, of which 4 are numeric and 19 (including the target variable) are nominal. As we are limiting this article to just the surgery prediction case, then only 10 of these variables (indicated by an asterisk) are used for each instance.

14.4.3 *Algorithm Choice and Configuration*

The focus of this study is not to find the most appropriate algorithm(s) for solving the problem at hand but rather to study some possible algorithm candidates by investigating some of the previously highlighted aspects that need to be considered. Due to this fact, we choose to include a variety of algorithms from different learning paradigms, e.g.: decision trees, decision rules, function-based algorithms, Bayesian learners, and so on. The selected algorithms and their configurations are presented in Tab. 14.2.

We use algorithm implementations from the Weka machine learning workbench version 3.6.0 [Witten and Frank (2005)], which is an open source environment that includes a large set of algorithms as well as methods for evaluation and analysis. As can be seen in the table, we use the default Weka configurations for all algorithms, except IBk, for which we changed $k = 1$ to $k = 10$ since $k = 1$ is rather prone to overfitting and $k = 10$ is usually regarded as a resonable setting [Witten and Frank (2005)]. In addition, we opted to include the best performing algorithms from a preliminary experiment into the Stacking ensemble (see the table notes in Tab. 14.2) and we use IBk as a meta learner for the Stacking algorithm.

14.4.4 *Evaluation*

Before reviewing the evaluation metrics used in the experiment, we start by introducing some important concepts of classifier performance. A classification problem can involve learning how to distinguish between objects of any number of classes. However, a common case, which applies to our data set, is when the objects studied are of two classes. We refer to this particular case as the binary classification problem.

When studying this problem, we commonly select one of the classes and refer to it as the main class. The observations belonging to this class are called positives (P) and the remaining observations are negatives (N). Furthermore, we distinguish between the class labels assigned to the observations in the data set and the class labels assigned by a particular generated classifier. If the classifier assigns the correct label to an observation, we refer to the classification as being true (T). Likewise, if an incorrect classification is performed by the classifier, we label it as a false (F) classification. Using this terminology, we may now define a number of basic metrics, as

Table 14.2: Learning Algorithm Configurations

Weka Title	Algorithm	Configuration
AdaBoostM1	Ada Boost	default
BayesNet	Bayesian Belief Network	default
IBk	K-nearest Neighbor	$k = 10$
J48	C4.5 Tree Inducer	default
Logistic	Logistic Regression	default
MultilayerPerceptron	Back-propagated Neural Network	default
RandomForest	Random Forests	default
Ridor	Ripple Down Rule Learner	default
SMO	Support Vector Machines	default
Stacking	Stacking	classifiers[a]
ZeroR	Zero Rules (baseline)	default

Algorithm: Ada Boost [Freund and Schapire (1996)], Bayesian Belief Network [Kim and Pearl (1983)], K-nearest Neighbor [Aha and Kibler (1991)], C4.5 Tree Inducer [Quinlan (1993)], Logistic Regression [le Cessie and van Houwelingen (1992); Witten and Frank (2005)], Back-propagated Neural Network [Rumelhart *et al.* (1986)], Random Forests [Breiman (2001)], Ripple Down Rule Learner [Gaines and Compton (1995)], Support Vector Machines [Platt (1998)], Stacking [Wolpert (1992)], Zero Rules (baseline) [Witten and Frank (2005)]. [a]Meta classifier: IBk ($k = 10$), Ensemble classifiers: AdaBoostM1, BayesNet, RandomForest, Ridor, SMO

shown in Table 14.3. In this table, we also relate the outcomes of the target variable, surgery $\in \{\text{yes}, \text{no}\}$, to the basic metrics.

Table 14.3: Basic performance metrics

Abbreviation	Metric	Comment
TP	True positives	Correct predictions to not proceed with surgery
FP	False positives	Incorrect predictions to not proceed with surgery
TN	True negatives	Correct predictions to proceed with surgery
FN	False negatives	Incorrect predictions to proceed with surgery
TPR	True positive rate	$TP/(TP + FN)$
FPR	False positive rate	$FP/(FP + TN)$
ACC	Accuracy	$TP + TN/(TP + TN + FP + FN)$

Classification Accuracy (ACC) is still a commonly used evaluation metric in machine learning and data mining applications [Witten and Frank (2005)]. However, this metric assumes an equal class distribution and misclassification cost. These assumptions are rarely true for real-world applications [Provost *et al.* (1998)]. For example, the cost of classifying an ill patient as healthy may be more costly that the other way around. Regarding class distribution; when we study a database of patients in order to detect the presence of diabetes type II, the number of observations with this diagnosis may be far lower than the number of observations with diabetes type I or no diabetes at all.

Despite its apparent shortcomings, we still include ACC as a reference metric, since it is an intuitive and widely applied metric that can be useful if its issues are taken into consideration. However, more importantly, we also make use of some complementary metrics for evaluation. Firstly, we include the Area Under the ROC Curve (AUC) as our main metric [Fawcett (2003)]. AUC has been empirically shown to be more suitable than accuracy for many applications. It does not depend on an equal class distribution or an equal distribution of cost. AUC is a single-point measure derived from a Receiver Operating Characteristic (ROC) curve. ROC analysis was first introduced by Egan [Egan (1975)] to analyze the false alarm / hit rate in radar detection. It has since been introduced to the machine learning community [Provost and Fawcett (1997)] and it is now widely regarded as a suitable approach to analyze and evaluate classifier performance.

As mentioned in Sect. 14.3.1, the available data set should be divided into disjoint sets that are used for training and testing, respectively. This is to avoid a situation in which the results may be overly optimistic, which can occur if the models are evaluated on the same data that were used for generating the models. Since our available data set is rather small it makes sense to use a statistical resampling technique instead of dividing the data set into two disjoint sets. A resampling technique provides us with the possibility to systematically generate multiple disjoint training and testing sets. For our particular study, we use 10-fold cross-validation [Stone (1974)] for resampling.

14.4.5 *Results*

The experimental results are presented in Tab. 14.4. The network learners, MultilayerPerceptron (MLP) and BayesNet, outperformed the remaining algorithms in terms of AUC. The classifier generated by BayesNet also achieved the lowest amount of false positives. The two lowest performing algorithms, according to both the ACC and AUC metrics, were the rule learner (Ridor) and the decision tree inducer (J48). However, in both cases, the poor AUC performance is mostly attributed to a high amount of false negatives. The number of false positives achieved by Ridor and J48 is comparable to the other algorithms.

Next, AdaBoostM1 and IBk performed similarly, slightly outperforming each other on AUC and ACC, respectively. Stacking, SMO, and Logistic performed mediocre in terms of AUC while the first two (Stacking and SMO) were top scorers in terms of ACC. All algorithms outperformed ZeroR, which is the baseline classifier, in terms of both AUC and ACC. ZeroR generates a default rule that classifiers all instances as belonging to surgery = yes.

Table 14.4: Average Performance results for AUC and ACC (means and standard deviations) as well as the approximate number of TPs, FPs, TNs, and FNs from ten 10-fold cross-validation runs

Algorithm	AUC[a]	ACC[b]	TP[c]	FP[d]	TN[e]	FN[f]
AdaBoostM1	0.820(0.176)[*]	0.721(0.162)	19	10	39	13
BayesNet	0.834(0.168)[*]	0.755(0.168)	20	9	40	11
IBk	0.813(0.171)[*]	0.743(0.164)	22	12	37	9
J48	0.665(0.187)	0.651(0.132)	13	10	40	18
Logistic	0.806(0.185)[*]	0.755(0.150)[*]	24	12	37	7
MLP[g]	0.850(0.157)[*]	0.760(0.144)[*]	23	11	38	8
RandomForest	0.762(0.196)[*]	0.706(0.154)	18	10	39	13
Ridor	0.618(0.156)	0.653(0.146)	15	11	38	17
SMO	0.799(0.166)[*]	0.794(0.168)[*]	25	11	38	6
Stacking	0.806(0.170)[*]	0.770(0.165)[*]	24	11	38	7
ZeroR (baseline)	0.500(0.000)	0.613(0.377)	0	0	49	31

[a]Area Under the ROC Curve, [b]Accuracy, [c]True Positives, [d]False Positives, [e]True Negatives, [f]False Negatives, [g]MultilayerPerceptron, [*]$p < 0.01$, two-tailed corrected paired t-test

14.4.6 *Discussion*

We will now perform an analysis of the results presented in Sect. 14.4.5 and then we continue by discussing some of the implications of this analysis from the point of view of the domain experts.

14.4.6.1 *Analysis of Results*

It is evident that network learners generate the best classifiers, at least for this particular set of algorithms and data. Not only did BayesNet and MLP

Table 14.5: Ridor rule and exceptions to the rule, as generated from the complete data set

Surgery = yes
Except when (outrotation = yes) **and** (walking distance = long) **Except when** (walking aid = 0) **and** (age $\leq$ 66) **Except when** (xray = 2) **and** (age $\leq$ 68)

outperform the other algorithms in terms of AUC; BayesNet also yielded the lowest amount of false positives as well. In our case, this is particularly important since false positives represent patients for whom the incorrect prediction was to not proceed with surgery.

SMO performed poorly in terms of AUC but it generated the best performing classifiers according to ACC. The poor AUC performance of SMO, could perhaps be explained by the fact that SMO is not designed to predict probabilities [Caruana and Niculescu-Mizil (2006)]. MLP and Stacking did also manage to achieve good ACC scores, which is mostly attributed to the low number of false negatives.

All algorithms, except J48 and Ridor, significantly outperformed the baseline classifier ($p < 0.01$) in terms of AUC, according to a two-tailed corrected paired t-test. With regard to the area under the ROC curve, the baseline classifier can be regarded as a model of a random guesser. Thus, the statistical test lets us conclude that it is quite possible to find potential surgery indicators, i.e., correlations between the patient data and the target variable. However, because of the small amount of data, it is not possible to draw conclusions about whether these particular indicators would be suitable in the general case, i.e., that the discovered correlations are approximately identical to those that would be found on a larger sample from the same hospital or on samples from other hospitals.

Interestingly, J48 and Ridor performed poorly in the experiment. However, a J48 decision tree generated from the complete data set exhibits the use of indicators that are intuitively correct for a real-world situation (see Fig. 14.4). The performance on the training set is, not surprisingly, high but an additional test set from a larger sample would be needed to get a credible performance estimate. Similarly, the rules generated by Ridor for the training set seem to be intuitively realistic as well, as can be seen in Tab. 14.5. From a practical perspective, the false positives rate is too high. However, our general assumption is that this partly depends on the small amount of observations (and relatively large amount of input variables). An additional factor is no doubt the large number of missing values for each variable (ranging from 23–55 per cent). The negative impact of this factor could most likely be reduced by examining a larger set of patient records since one can adhere to a lower tolerance when omitting patient records on the basis of the amount of missing values.

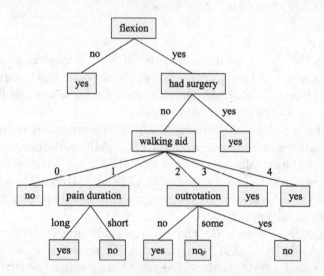

Fig. 14.4: J48 decision tree generated from the complete data set. The terminal nodes indicate whether surgery should be performed.

Moreover, in our study, it was necessary to minimize the number of categories for nominal variables since the inclusion of variables with a high number of categories could result in a loss of generality in the data, i.e., some combinations of a certain outcome of the target variable and a specific value of a specific input attribute would appear very infrequently. However, when decreasing the number of possible categories for a nominal variable, great care has to be taken both to ensure that the new categories are meaningful to the domain expert and that they do not result in a decrease in classification performance.

It should also be pointed out that false negatives (incorrect recommendations to perform surgery) can also be costly for the healthcare even though false positives arguably represent a higher cost (both financially and for the patient's well-being). We argue that the number of false negatives achieved by the included algorithms (ranging from 6 to 13 cases) is quite acceptable in relation to current practice. For example, the studied data set includes 80 referred patients and only 49 of these patients had surgery, indicating 31 false negatives.

14.4.6.2 *Implications*

The aim of this chapter is to present an approach to solve, at least partly, the problem of predicting patient demand. Our approach is to predict, at the referral stage, whether or not patients need surgery. The approach is based on the assumption that accurate predictions about whether to perform surgery would serve as valuable input when estimating the patient demand at the hospital. Since the surgery prediction can be conducted at the referral stage, the patient demand can be estimated very early compared to current practice.

Presently, the referrals are written as (unstructured) text documents. In fact, even the patient records are represented by unstructured text documents. Today, the referrals may be very brief and perhaps consist of a single statement or question addressed to the specialist. Obviously, it is difficult not to say impossible to accurately predict the need for surgery from this kind of information. One of the main difficulties in structuring different types of referrals (e.g. for various types of surgery or treatment) is that there is little or no consensus about which pieces of information should be included.

Conversely, in order to predict whether surgery should be performed or not, we need access to information that is currently only available in non-tabulated form in the patient records. To generate the prediction models we also need access to retrospective data about the real outcome (whether surgery was carried out or not) for a large group of patients as well as their patient records.

The idea is that, if our approach works well, it would be possible to extract surgery indicator variables from the generated prediction models. These surgery indicators could then be used as a basis for defining what information should be included in the referral. In the medical domain, work is already on-going to establish suitable indicators for different types of surgery or treatments. This work is mainly conducted on a national level but it is distributed across interest groups for different surgery types, e.g., cataract surgery [Lundström *et al.* (2006)]. We regard our approach, not as an alternative but, as a complement.

Our experiment, although conducted on a small sample of patients, has shown the applicability of our approach. Nevertheless, we need to gather a larger set of observations to further validate the approach. If we can increase the general performance and more specifically reduce the number of false positives, we hypothesize that this method could in fact be used in a real-world context. However, it is important to recognize that our approach should only be regarded as a decision support tool for domain experts. The generated prediction models do not represent a substitute for human knowledge of the problem domain. We do not suggest that this approach should replace the opinion of the domain expert in the decision about whether to perform surgery or not.

The objective of our approach is merely to help estimating the patient demand more accurately and at an earlier stage. This way, the problem of operation room planning and scheduling may be simplified and the results may be more accurate.

A secondary, but nevertheless important, aim of our approach is that it can be used by domain experts to periodically validate decisions, e.g. on whether surgery should be performed. For example, if a minority of the orthopaedic specialists at a particular hospital take decisions that are not correlated with the recommendations of the prediction models it might be possible to use the models to analyze the reasons behind wrongful decisions.

14.5   Conclusion

This chapter investigates issues related to the management of patient referrals from general practitioners to hospital care. In short, we begin by hypothesizing that hospital productivity could be increased if the surgical suite and the orthopaedic department would be able to predict the patient surgery demand at an earlier stage than what is possible today. We then suggest supervised learning as an approach to find patterns in patient and surgical suite records that could be used to predict whether a certain patient would need surgery and, if so, what would be the duration of the surgery and the subsequent recovery.

From the models generated by the supervised learning algorithms, we further assume that it is possible to extract information about which variables are good indicators for a particular type of referral. Our conclusion is that such a list of indicators, given for each referral type, would provide a good basis for developing a software-based patient referral system in which the general practitioner may specify the referral type and in return receive advice about which information to include in the referral.

We have obtained 80 patient records from the orthopaedic department at Blekinge hospital in Sweden. All records have been manually examined to extract a number of possible indicators, as well as additional variables of possible explanatory value. After careful review of each record, the extracted variables have been compiled into a data set in which each instance is described by 10 variables. We experimentally compare ten supervised learning algorithms on the problem of generating prediction models from this data set. Eight algorithms significantly outperformed the baseline. Thus, our conclusion is that our approach is viable. However, the number of false positives is too high for practical use. We assume that this is in large part due to the small number of instances and the large number of missing values. Nevertheless, there is a need to further study which variables should be included in the data set and how to discretisize these variables.

For future work, we intend to further establish our theoretical models of the studied problem and validate these models empirically by performing extensive experiments on a larger data set of hip arthrosis patients. We will also extend our investigation to include additional types of referrals. Moreover, the overall objective is to use surgery prediction models as a means for providing input to our simulation of operating room scheduling. We would also like to investigate whether it is possible to associate our data with information from the surgical suite in order to generate models that can predict the outcome of surgery, e.g., recovery time, length of stay, and so forth.

Finally, we intend to select a smaller number of suitable supervised learning algorithms to perform careful parameter tuning and analysis in order to gain more understanding of the problem, increase classification performance, and more specifically decrease the number of false positives.

Acknowledgments

We would like to thank Associate Professor Jan A. Persson at Blekinge Institute of Technology for his valuable comments and suggestions. Moreover, we acknowledge Leif Fransson at Blekinge Hospital for his comments and help in obtaining data. This work was supported in part by a grant from Blekinge County Council, Sweden.

Chapter 15

Incremental Learning of Medical Data for Multi-step Patient Health Classification

Philipp Kranen[1], Emmanuel Müller[1], Ira Assent[2], Ralph Krieger[1] and Thomas Seidl[1]

[1]*RWTH Aachen University, Germany*
[2]*Aalborg University, Denmark*

15.1 Introduction

Demographic change will pose a major challenge for our society as people get older due to enhanced living conditions. Especially the increasing amount of elderly people, which need medical assistance and supervision, has to be considered. In todays health environments medical supervision is an expensive task as it can only be achieved by health professionals in hospitals or other health facilities. A major contribution in this area is the development of remote monitoring systems that provide health assistance and supervision at home. Such a health monitoring provides not only economical savings as it can save expensive health professional costs, but it also increases the living quality of elderly people as they can stay in their familiar environment. One major task for such a remote health monitoring is to provide an emergency detection system. Based on a semi-automated classification of patient situation the system should automatically detect an emergency to pose an alert. This alert is then manually verified by a health professional. The applicability of this scenario to emergency detection has been shown as proof of concept in a framework for "Mobile Mining and Information Management in HealthNet Scenarios" [Kranen *et al.* (2008)].

However, such health monitoring tasks pose major challenges for data processing. In general, automated monitoring produces a huge amount of stream data that cannot be manually handled by humans. An automated analysis to assist the health professionals is essential for a scalable system monitoring hundreds of patients. Although automated analysis cannot take the final decision about an emergency, it can dramatically reduce the number of patients by highlighting the most urgent cases. The health professional can then focus on a more detailed analysis of these patients, which leads to an overall scalable semi-automated processing.

For the data analysis components in such an emergency detection system there are special requirements derived out of the health surveillance application. Due to the huge amount of streaming data one has to consider scalability issues for the automated analysis. While servers in a data farm might analyze terrabytes of data, computers in hospitals can only process gigabytes of data. Mobile clients, which collect the data from sensors, have even less resources and might process megabytes of data. Even the sensors in a body sensor network have capabilities of processing some kilobytes of data, however only with very restricted algorithms. A requirement in today's heterogeneous architectures is thus to design an adaptive analysis which scales with the available resources in a multi-step approach.

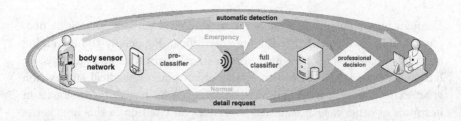

Fig. 15.1: Multi-step patient health classification from the body sensor network up to the health professional.

The general aim of such a multi-step classification is to provide an adaptive classifier applicable on various layers of the health surveillance process. Especially for mobile devices with limited resources an efficient pre-classifier is required. Based on the decision of the pre-classification the level of detail of the sensor measurements is decided. As shown in Figure 15.1 the full sensor information is sent only in emergency cases while only aggregated information is sent in normal situations. Adaptive aggregation thereby minimizes the communication cost and the energy consumption of the mobile devices. Every decision is refined on the next layer of the multi-step classification, since the pre-classification is optimized for limited resources and its lower classification accuracy may lead to false positives and false negative decisions..

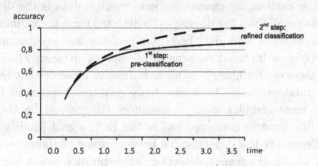

Fig. 15.2: Anytime classification accuracy.

Each of the classifiers on the different levels has to cope with streams of variable size and speed. This is on the mobile device due to the varying amount and frequency of data sent by the patients depending on their condition as preclassified locally on the sensor controller. The receiving server has to classify all incoming patient data as accurately as possible. With many patients potentially sending aggregated or detailed data, the amount of data and their arrival rate may vary widely. Additionally, the number of patient currently connected to the system may also vary. To treat each patient in a global emergency situation, e.g. an earthquake, classification for each individual observation must be performed quickly and be improved as long as time permits.

A solution to these requirements is offered by algorithms that are based on the so called anytime paradigm [Grass and Zilberstein (1996)]. Anytime algorithms improve the quality of their result with more time allowance, Figure 15.2 shows an ideal solution for a two-step anytime classification. Anytime algorithms are an active field of research and solutions have been proposed to many data mining problems such as clustering [Vlachos *et al.* (2003)], top k processing [Arai *et al.* (2007)] and anytime learning of classifiers [Street and Kim (2001); Wang *et al.* (2003)]. For classification under anytime constraints several well known classifiers have been adapted including support vector machines [DeCoste (2002)], decision trees [Esmeir and Markovitch (2006)], nearest neighbor classifiers [Keogh (1997)], Bayes classifiers [Seidl *et al.* (2009); Yang *et al.* (2007)], Bayesian networks [Liu and Wellman (1996); Hulten and Domingos (2002)] and boosting techniques [Myers *et al.* (2000)]. In this chapter we will present and extend the work described in [Seidl *et al.* (2009)], since it fulfills all requirements for medical applications as we will see in the following.

A further challenging characteristic of medical data is the diversity of the data. Depending on the disease to be detected there are various possible measurements to be sensored. ECG, temperature and accelerometer data has already been included in a proof of concept [Kranen *et al.* (2008)]. However, there are far more possible non-invasive measures like respiration quotient, pulse oximetry, humidity, body posture, respiration frequency and many more complex medical measures. There can be also derived measures like features extracted out of the ECG signal [Rodriguez *et al.* (2005)]. Especially the dependencies between some of these measures are important for an emergency detection, as respiration has a huge impact on ECG measurement artifacts, for example. The system has to fulfill this requirement of multivariate classification by handling many different measurements.

Finally, since new patient data is constantly coming in and parts of these data, e.g. from supervised hospital situations, can be used as additional training data, the classifier should be able to incrementally learn from new training data. Incremental learning is opposed to building a completely new classifier from scratch based on both old and new training data. The advantage of incremental learning is that it takes less time and that it can ideally be done online, i.e. new training data can be learned while the patient is supervised and in the next moment the status can be switched back to classification.

Summing up, the overall classification task has to fulfill three main requirements derived out of the health surveillance scenario:

- Anytime processing of varying stream rates
- Incremental learning based on multivariate data
- Multi-step processing for classification in a cascade of devices

In the following Sections we will give details about a classification technique called Bayes tree that fulfills all of the above requirements. The basic version of this technique was introduced in EDBT 2009 [Seidl *et al.* (2009)]. As an anytime classification approach it adapts to different classification times given for example by sensor measurement frequency. Furthermore, it can handle multivariate data provided by multiple different sensors. As the classifier includes an indexing structure for secondary storage it can handle huge amount of stream data collected at medical facilities. Parts of this index structure can be used in multi-step approaches in a cascade of classifiers with improving accuracy. Moreover, it also adapts to evolving data through an incremental learning of the underlying model. In addition to the basic technique we will present novel approaches that incorporate existing medical knowledge data bases and thereby improve the classification accuracy by up to 13%. Finally we will discuss an application of the presented approach in a patient health monitoring system that has been primary presented at MDM 2008 [Kranen *et al.* (2008)].

15.2   The Bayes Tree

We first briefly review Bayesian classification and density estimation in Section 15.2.1 and then describe the structure and working of the Bayes tree.

15.2.1   *Preliminaries*

Given a set C of classes, a classifier is a function G which maps an object x to a label $c_i \in C$. Here we focus on the Bayesian classifier which uses the statistical Bayesian decision theory for classifying objects. Based on a statistical model of the class labels, the Bayes classifier chooses the class with the highest posterior probability $P(c_i|x)$ for a given query object x according to the Bayes rule, i.e.

$$G_{Bayes}(x) = \underset{c_i \in C}{argmax}\{P(c_i|x)\} = \underset{c_i \in C}{argmax}\{P(c_i) \cdot p(x|c_i)\}$$

Note that $p(x)$ is left out in the last term, because it does not affect the $argmax$ evaluation. With $D_{c_i} = \{(x_j, y_j) \in D \,|\, c_i = y_j\}$ as the set of objects belonging to a specific class c_i, the a priori probability $P(c_i)$ can be easily estimated from the training data set D as the relative frequency of each class $P(c_i) = \frac{|D_{c_i}|}{|D|}$. Since x is typically multidimensional in medical applications (i.e. several different vital function are measured simultaneously), the task of estimating the class-conditional density $p(x|c_i)$ is not trivial.

A simple method is to assume a certain distribution of the data. Any model assumption (e.g. a single multivariate normal distribution) may not reflect the true distribution, as e.g. different diseases might be expressed in different areas of the data space. Mixture densities relax this assumption that the data follows exactly one unimodal model by assuming that the data follows a combination of probability density functions. The Bayes tree uses Gaussian mixture densities $p(\mathbf{x}|c_i) = \sum_{j=1}^{k} w_j \cdot g(\mathbf{x}, \mu_j, \sigma_j)$, where μ_j is the mean of the j-th Gaussian component, w_j its weight and σ_j its variance vector.

Another approach to density estimation are kernel densities, which do not make any assumption about the underlying data distribution (thus often termed "model-free" or "non-parameterized" density-estimation). Kernel estimators can be seen as influence functions centered at each data object. Thus, the class conditional probability density for any object $\mathbf{x}$ is the weighted sum of kernel influences of all objects $\mathbf{x_j}$ of the respective class. Gaussian kernel $\mathbf{K}_{Gauss}(\mathbf{x}) = \frac{1}{(2 \cdot \pi)^{d/2}} e^{-\frac{x^2}{2h_i}}$ are used along with Gaussian mixture models in a consistent model hierarchy to support mixing of models and kernels in the Bayes tree. In terms of classification accuracy, Bayes classifiers using kernel estimators have shown to perform well for traditional classification tasks. Especially for large training data sets (e.g. medical data bases) the estimation error using kernel densities is known to be very low and even asymptotically optimal. To set the bandwidth h_i for the d-dimensional kernel estimators a common data independent method according to [Silverman (1986)] is used in [Seidl *et al.* (2009)].

15.2.2 *Structure, Descent and Query Processing*

As stated above, the requirements described in the Section 15.1 are fulfilled by Bayes tree approach [Seidl *et al.* (2009); Kranen *et al.* (2010a,b)]. The achievement in [Seidl *et al.* (2009)] was to enable anytime kernel density estimation for efficient and interruptible classification. Incremental learning is inherently possible with the Bayes tree and we will discuss multi-step classification using the Bayes tree at the end of this section.

Indexing provides means for efficiency in similarity search and retrieval. By grouping similar data on hard disk and providing directory information on disk page entries, only the relevant parts of the data are accessed during query processing. In the Bayes tree, the data objects are stored at leaf level as in similarity search applications. As classification requires reading all kernel estimators of the entire model, accuracy would be lost if a subset of all kernel densities was ignored. Consequently, there is no irrelevant data, and hence the pruning as in similarity search is infeasible when dealing with density estimation. The Bayes tree solves this problem by storing aggregated statistical information in its inner nodes.

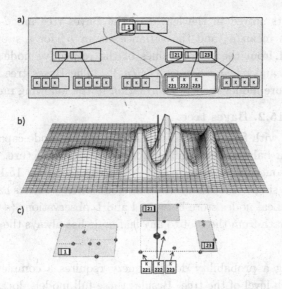

Fig. 15.3: a) Bayes tree and frontier. b) The resulting mixture model. c) The underlying R-tree structure.

The general idea of the Bayes tree is a hierarchy of mixture densities stored in a multidimensional index. Each level of the tree stores at a different granularity a complete model of the entire data. To this end, a balanced structure as in R-trees [Guttman (1984)] is used to store the kernels at leaf level. The directory on top is built in a bottom-up fashion, providing a hierarchy of node entries, each of which is a Gaussian that represents the entire subtree below it. To derive the mixture models the necessary information to compute parameters of the mixture densities, i.e. the mean and variance of the Gaussians, are stored in the entries.

Definition 15.1. Bayes tree node entry.

A subtree T_s of a d-dimensional Bayes tree is associated with the set of objects stored in the leaves of the subtree: $T_s = \{t_{(s,1)}, \ldots, t_{(s,n_s)}\}$. An entry e_s then stores the following information about the subtree T_s:

- The **minimum bounding rectangle** enclosing the objects stored in the subtree T_s as $MBR_s = ((l_1, u_1), \ldots, (l_d, u_d))$
- A **pointer** ptr_s to the subtree T_s
- The **cluster feature** CF $= (n_s, LS, SS)$ of the objects in T_s containing the number n_s of objects, their linear sum LS and their squared sum SS

All objects stored in the leaves of the Bayes tree are d-dimensional kernels. The mean μ_s and the variance vector σ_s^2 for a subtree $\mathbf{T_s}$ can be computed from the stored values of the respective node entry e_s as $\mu_s = LS/n_s$ and $\sigma_s^2 = SS/n_s - (LS/n_s)^2$. The Bayes tree extends the R*-tree to store model specific information in the following manner:

Definition 15.2. Bayes tree.

A Bayes tree with fanout parameters $\mathbf{m}, \mathbf{M}$ and leaf node capacity parameters $\mathbf{l}, \mathbf{L}$ is a balanced multidimensional indexing structure. Each inner node $node_s$ contains between $\mathbf{m}$ and $\mathbf{M}$ entries (see Def. 15.1). The root has at least a single entry and each inner node with ν_s entries has exactly ν_s child nodes. Leaf nodes store between $\mathbf{l}$ and $\mathbf{L}$ observations (d-dimensional kernels). A path from the root to any leaf node has always the same length (balanced).

Answering a probability density query requires a complete model as stored at each level of the tree. Besides these full models, local refinement of the model (to adapt flexibly to the query) provides models composed of coarser and finer representations. This is illustrated in Figure 15.3b. In any model, each component corresponds to an entry that represents its subtree. This entry may be replaced by the entries in its child node yielding a finer representation of its subtree. This idea leads to query-based refinement in the anytime algorithm. Each mixed granularity model corresponds to a frontier in the tree, i.e. a set of entries in the tree, such that each kernel estimator is represented exactly once. Figure 15.3 b) shows the resulting mixture density for the example frontier from part a). The leftmost Gaussian stems from the entry e_1 which is located at root level. The rightmost Gaussian and the one in the back correspond to entries e_{23} and e_{21} respectively, the remaining represent kernel densities at leaf level. Part c) of the image depicts the underlying R*-tree MBRs and the kernels as dots. The bigger blue dot and the vertical line represent the query object from which the above frontier originated.

Recall that an entry e_s represents all objects in its corresponding subtree by storing the necessary information to calculate its mean and variance. Hence, a set $E = \{e_i\}$ of entries defines a Gaussian mixture model, which can then be used to answer a probability density query.

Definition 15.3. Probability density query pdq.

Let $E = \{e_i\}$ be a set of entries, $\mathcal{M}_E$ the corresponding Gaussian mixture model and $\mathbf{n} = \sum_i n_{e_i}$ the total number of objects represented by E.

A probability density query pdq returns the density for an object $\mathbf{x}$ with respect to $\mathcal{M}_E$ by

$$pdq(\mathbf{x}, E) = \sum_{e_s \in E} \frac{n_{e_s}}{\mathbf{n}} \cdot g(\mathbf{x}, \mu_{e_s}, \sigma_{e_s})$$

where μ_{e_s} and σ_{e_s} are calculated as described above. For a leaf entry a kernel estimator as discussed in Section 15.2.1 is used and obviously μ_{e_s} is the object itself.

From time step t to $t + 1$, the set of entries in the frontier changes by adding all entries in the child node $node_s$ of one frontier entry $e_s \in E$. If $node_s$ has ν_s entries, then the frontier's entry set E_t changes to E_{t+1} by

$$E_{t+1} = (E_t \setminus \{e_s\}) \cup \{e_{so1}, \dots, e_{so\nu_s}\}$$

i.e. e_s is replaced by its children. The probability density for $\mathbf{x}$ in time step $t + 1$ is calculated taking the probability density for $\mathbf{x}$ in time step t, subtracting the contribution of the refined entry's Gaussian and adding the contributions of its children's Gaussians. Hence, the cost for calculating the new probability density for $\mathbf{x}$ after reading one additional node is very low due to the information stored for mean and variance.

For tree traversal three basic descent strategies were evaluated: breadth first (bft), depth first (dft) and global best descent (glo), which orders nodes globally with respect to a priority measure and refines nodes in this ordering. Two priority measure have been tested: a geometric measure, i.e. the distance from the query object to the MBR, and a probabilistic measure, i.e. the weighted probability density for the query object w.r.t. the Gaussian component of each entry.

One Bayes tree is built per class, therefore several improvement strategies have been proposed to decide which tree has the right to refine its model in the next time step. Extensive experiments showed that refining the k most probable classes (qbk) in turns yielded the best results throughout. $k = \min\{2, \lfloor \log(m) \rfloor\}$, where m is the number of classes, showed the best performance on all tested data sets. For more details please refer to [Seidl *et al.* (2009)].

To enable multi-step classification the Bayes tree offers a very simple yet very effective opportunity. To build a pre-classifier one can simply take the upper levels of the tree hierarchy and use these as a smaller model Hence, the pre-classifier is achieved easily without the need to train a second model. Moreover, the size of the pre-classifier (and with it the size of resources needed to store and use the classifier) can flexibly be adapted by taking

more or less levels of the full tree. We evaluate multi-step classification in
Section 15.3.3.

15.3 Experimental Evaluation

To test the Bayes tree approach for the requirements of the Health-
Net scenario we ran experiments on real world and synthetic data for
all requirements mentioned in Section 15.1, i.e. anytime classification,
incremental learning and multistep classification. The real world data
sets are taken from various repositories such as the UCI KDD archive
(http://kdd.ics.uci.edu) for two reasons: first, they contain labeled data
which is widely used as benchmark data sets for classification algorithms
and second, we do not yet have a representative amount of labeled medical
data to present reliable results. We discuss the collection of medical sensor
data and an application of the Bayes tree in Section 15.5. The synthetic
data sets are described in [Seidl *et al.* (2009)].

In all experiments we use a 4 fold cross validation. To evaluate anytime
accuracy we report the accuracy (averaged over the four folds) of the Bayes
tree classifiers after each node (corresponding to one page) that is read.
The first accuracy value corresponds to the classification accuracy of the
unimodal Bayes classifier that we use as an initialization. The roots of
the single trees are stored in a compressed way to use less storage pages
(cf. [Seidl *et al.* (2009)] for more details). Experiments were run using
2KB page sizes (except 4KB for Verbmobil and 8KB for the USPS data
set) on Pentium 4 machines with 2.4 Ghz and 1 GB main memory. To
set the bandwidth for the kernel estimators a common data independent
method according to [Silverman (1986)] is used as stated above. In the
following we first evaluate anytime classification performance of the Bayes
tree, results for the incremental learning are shown in Section 15.3.2 and
finally we discuss multi-step classification results in Section 15.3.3.

15.3.1 *Anytime Classification Performance*

For tree traversal depth first (*dft*), breadth first (*bft*) and global best first
(*glo*) strategies were evaluated as described above. Combined with both
the geometric (*geom*) and probabilistic (*prob*) priority measure compare
six approaches for model refinement in a Bayes tree have been compared.
Global best descent using the probabilistic priority measure was found to

deliver the best results in terms of anytime classification accuracy (cf. [Seidl *et al.* (2009)]). Here we restrict ourselves to the more interesting results regarding the improvement strategies.

The improvement strategy *unsorted* did not deliver competitive results throughout all experiments. For the *qb1* and *qbm* strategies no clear winner could be identified since on about half of the data sets the one outperformed the other and vice versa. Since none of the two was consistently better, we tested the *qbk* strategie for $k = \{1 \ldots m\}$ to see how the choice of k influences the anytime classification performance. Figure 15.4 shows the comparison of *qb1*, *qbm* and *qbk* for $k \in \{2, 4, 6, 8, 10\}$ on the Letter data set. On this data set, which contains 26 classes, *qb1* performs better than *qbm*.

The accuracy of the *qbm* strategy in Figure 15.4 initially increases steeply in the first three to four steps. It is clearly visible that the compressed root needs on average 19 pages for the 26 classes (recall the 4 fold cross validation). After the compressed root is read, the accuracy of the *qbm* strategy again steeply increases for the next four to five steps. A similar increase can be observed 26 steps later when all classes have been refined once more. Opposed to those three strong improvements are the rest of the steps, during which the accuracy hardly changes at all. For this data set we derive from Figure 15.4 that for an object that has to be classified there are on average five classes that are worth considering, the other 21 classes can be precluded.

The *qb10* strategy needs seven to eight pages to read the root information for the top ten classes from the compressed root. These steps show the same accuracy as the *qbm* approach, since the ordering according to the priority measure is equal. After that a similar pattern can be observed each ten steps, i.e. after reordering according to the novel density values. Continuing with the *qb8* variant, the "ramps" (steep improvements) move even closer together and begin earlier. Similar improvement gains are shown by *qb6* and *qb4*. An even smaller k ($k = 2$ in Figure 15.4) does no longer improve the overall anytime accuracy and *qb1* shows an even worse performance than *qb10*.

For an easier comparison of the *qbk* performance when varying k, we calculate the area under the anytime curve for each k and hence receive a single number for each value of k. The area fits the intuition of a best improvement, since *qbk* curves mostly ascend monotonically. Figure 15.4 (right) shows the area values corresponding to the anytime curves in the left part. As in the above analysis *qb4* turns out to perform best according

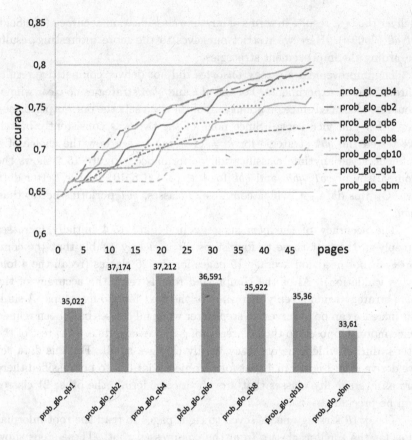

Fig. 15.4: Top: Anytime classification performance when varying k on
the Letter data set. Bottom: The corresponding area under the
anytime curves.

to this measure.

We evaluated qbk for $k \in \{1 \ldots m\}$ on all data sets and found the
same characteristic results. Figure 15.5 displays the results for Vowel and
Covtype. We found that the maximum value was always between $k = 2$
and $k = 4$ on the tested data sets. Moreover, with an increasing number
of classes, the k value for the best performance also increased, yet only
slightly. An exception is the Gender data set, where $k = m = 2$ showed the
best performance. This is due to the bad performance of $qb1$, therefore we
set k to be at least 2. To develop a heuristic for the value of k we evaluated
different data sets having different number of classes. It turned out that a

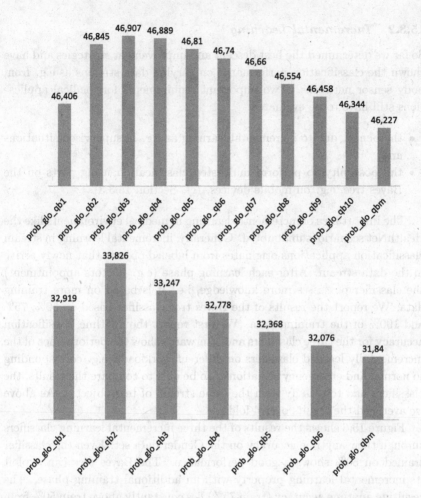

Fig. 15.5: Area values for $k \in \{1 \ldots m\}$ for Vowel (Top) and Covtype (Bottom).

good choice for k is logarithmic in the number of classes, i.e. $k = \lfloor \log_2(m) \rfloor$. Using this heuristic met the maximal performance for all our evaluations. Yet we set the minimum value for k to 2 as mentioned above. We use this improvement strategy along with the global best descent strategy in all further experiments.

15.3.2   *Incremental Learning*

So far we determined the best descent and improvement strategies and have shown the classification performance on varying data streams as e.g. from body sensor networks. Two important requirements for medical applications still have to be evaluated:

- the benefit due to incremental learning as e.g. in supervised situations and
- the possibilty to perform multi-step classification using parts on the Bayes tree, e.g. on mobile devices. (cf. Section 15.3.3).

The importance of incremental learning in medical environments like the HealthNet scenario is undoubted. Generally, incremental learning in stream classification applications originates from labeled objects that newly arrive in the data stream. After each learning phase (e.g. doctors appointment) the classifier possesses more knowledge, i.e. it is based on more training data. We report the results of the Bayes tree classifier based on 50%, 75% and 100% of the training data. We first report the anytime classification accuracy for the three classifiers and afterwards show the performance of the incrementally learned classifiers on different workloads, e.g. corresponding to normal and emergency situations. To be able to compare the results, the classifiers had to classify each the same stream of test objects . As above we averaged the results over 4 folds.

Figure 15.6 shows the results of the three incremental learning classifiers through their anytime accuracy on the Gender data set. Even the classifier trained on 50% shows a good performance. The Bayes tree can exploit its incremental learning property with an additional training phase. The resulting anytime accuracy (train 75%) lies constantly above train 50% from page three onwards. The Bayes tree that was trained on 100% performs consistently better then both the others, again highlighting the benefit of the incremental learning property and demonstrating the benefit for the HealthNet scenario.

To evaluate anytime classification under variable stream scenarios, we recapitulate a stochastic model that is widely used to model random arrivals [Duda *et al.* (2000)]. A Poisson process describes streams where the inter-arrival times are independently exponentially distributed. Poisson processes are parameterized by an arrival rate parameter λ. Exponential arrivals $F(t) = 1 - e^{-\lambda \cdot t}$ lead to an expected number of arrivals of $\lambda \cdot t$ in the time interval (0,t].

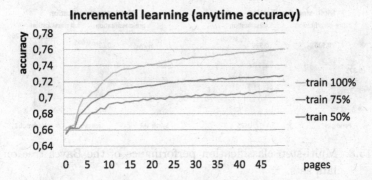

Fig. 15.6: Anytime classification performance after incremental learning on Gender.

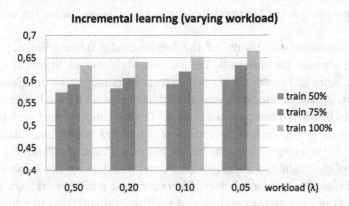

Fig. 15.7: Incremental learning performance for different workloads for Cover type.

Definition 15.4. Poisson stream.

A probability density function for the inter-arrival time of a Poisson process is exponentially distributed with parameter λ by $p(t) = \lambda \cdot e^{-\lambda t}$. The expected inter-arrival time of an exponentially distributed random variable with parameter λ is $E[t] = \frac{1}{\lambda}$.

We use a Poisson process to model random stream arrivals for each fold of the cross validation. We randomly generate exponentially distributed inter-arrival times for different values of λ. If a new object arrives (the time between two objects has passed) we interrupt the anytime classifier and measure its accuracy. We repeat this experiment using different expected

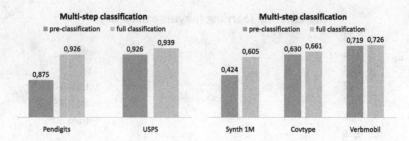

Fig. 15.8: Multi-step classification performance of the Bayes tree on five data sets.

inter-arrival times $\frac{1}{\lambda}$, where a unit corresponds to a page as in all previous experiments. We assume that any object arrives at the earliest after the initialization phase of the previous object, i.e. after evaluating the unimodal Bayes.

We evaluated the results of the incrementally trained Bayes trees on Poisson streams for various λ, i.e. various workloads as in hospital situations. Figure 15.7 shows the resulting stream accuracy values for Cover type data set. Again we used the same underlying stream models during classification to be able to compare the results. The anytime learning performance can be seen within each of the groups of three bars, where immediate comparison of the classifiers is possible through the Poisson stream evaluation. For all of the evaluated workloads (λ values) and data set the incrementally trained classifiers perform better. Moreover, with smaller workloads during classification, the stream accuracy of each individual Bayes tree improves. This property is especially advantageous in the medical context, since it is crucial to exploit the available time for classification improvement and yet to be able to treat each patient (i.e. data stream item) if time is bare.

15.3.3 *Evaluating Multi-step Classification*

Figure 15.8 shows the results for the classification accuracy of the Bayes tree in a multi-step approach on Pendigits, USPS, Covtype, Verbmobil and a large synthetic data set. The pre-classifier was created by taking only the three highest levels of the full tree for classification as described in Section 15.2.2. The pre-classifier is able to process all stream data items and often it already yields a decent classification accuracy despite its small model (i.e. small size of the tree). The difference in performance towards the full classifier varies among the different data sets. However, as expected, on all data sets the full classifier yields higher accuracy values than the restricted pre-classifier.

The simple way of applying the Bayes tree in multi-step setting, e.g. a cascade of devices as in [Kranen *et al.* (2008)] (cf. Section 15.5), constitutes a great advantage over other approaches. Together with the incremental learning property it enables fast and easy updating of the classification model on both the server and the mobile device.

Evaluation summary. The evaluation shows that the Bayes tree efficiently supports incremental learning as well as anytime classification. Moreover, the underlying index structure ensures the ability to handle very large data sets as in the case of streaming data. Hence, it meets all requirements for the HealthNet scenario and shows good performance on all tested data sets. In the next section we propose novel approaches that further improve the performance of the Bayes tree.

15.4 Incorporating Medical Knowledge Data Bases

In nowadays medical Institutions there is often a solid basis on medical patient data present, e.g. in form of a data base. Hence, the training of a classifier that uses this data does not necessarily have to be done using the incremental insertion proposed in [Seidl *et al.* (2009)] that we described above. To incorporate the existing knowledge of medical data bases and to improve the performance of the actual classifier, more sophisticated training methods can be beneficial. To this end we investigate bulk loading approaches for the Bayes tree. Bulk loading is opposed to incremental learning or incremental insertion in that it tries to optimize the resulting model by looking at the entire training data at the same time. Thereby it is independent of the order of training objects and can for example overcome largely overlapping mixture components or MBRs. We describe in the next Section and present preliminary results in Section 15.4.2.

15.4.1 *Approaches*

Since the Bayes tree is a statistical approach to classification we looked for statistical methods to create a smaller mixture model from a given mixture model. Starting bottom up with a mixture model that contains a kernel estimator for each training set item we create successively coarser models that represent good approximations. We adapted two approaches, a virtual sampling approach described in [Vasconcelos and Lippman (1998)] and a second approach described in [Goldberger and Roweis (2004)]. We will describe our approach based on [Goldberger and Roweis (2004)], called Goldberger in the following, since it outperformed the first approach.

The Goldberger approach assumes two initial mixture models f and g to be given, where f is the finer model with r components and g an approximation with s components, hence $r > s$. Each component is assigned a weight and is specified by its mean and covariance matrix. To measure the quality of the approximation [Goldberger and Roweis (2004)] defines the distance between two mixture densities as follows:

Definition 15.5. Let $f = \sum_{i=1}^{r} \alpha_i f_i$ and $g = \sum_{j=1}^{s} \beta_j g_j$ be two mixture densities containing r and s Gaussian components f_i and g_j with their respective weights α_i and β_j. The distance between f and g is then defined using the Kullback-Leibler divergence KL [Chen *et al.* (2008)] as follows

$$d(f,g) = \sum_{i=1}^{r} \alpha_i \cdot \min_{j=1}^{s} \{KL(f_i, g_j)\}$$

The optimal mixture model $\hat{g}$ reducing f to s components is $\hat{g} = \arg\min_g(d(f,g))$. Since there is no closed form to compute $\hat{g}$, a local optimum is computed iterating the following two steps until the distance $d(f,g)$ does no longer decrease. Therein $\pi(i) : \{1 \ldots r\} \to \{1 \ldots s\}$ is a mapping function that assigns each component in f to a component in g.

(1) **regroup** - update π: $\pi(i) = \arg\min_{j=1}^{s}\{KL(f_i, g_j)\}$
(2) **refit** - for each component g_j recompute weight β_j, mean μ_j and covariance matrix Σ_j as follows

- $\beta_j = \sum_{i,\pi(i)=j} \alpha_i$
- $\mu_j = \frac{1}{\beta_j} \sum_{i,\pi(i)=j} \alpha_i \mu_i$
- $\Sigma_j = \frac{1}{\beta_j} \sum_{i,\pi(i)=j} \alpha_i \left(\Sigma_j + (\mu_i - \mu_j)^2 \right)$

We devise a bulk loading technique based on [Goldberger and Roweis (2004)] as follows. To initialize the mixture g we compute a first mapping π_0 by assigning $0.75 \cdot M$ components from f to one component in g according to the z-curve order of their mean values. M is given through the fanout, which in turn is dictated by the page size.

The components g_j are converted to Bayes tree nodes containing the entries f_i with $\pi(i) = j$. Since the final π might map more than M components from f to a single component in g, we investigated several strategies to restrict the fanout to the given boundaries. First we reformulated the regroup step into an integer linear program with constraints regarding the resulting fanout. However, for realistic problem sizes, this approach took way too long to compute a complete bulk loading. Hence, we decided for a post processing after the mapping π was computed, which splits the nodes that contain too many entries. Therefore two representatives are computed by moving the mean along the dimension with the highest variance by an ϵ in both direction. A Gaussian is placed over the two representatives and the mapping of the entries to the representatives is computed as in the regroup step. If a node contains too few entries it is merged with the node closest to it in term of the Kullback-Leibler divergence.

Besides the above mentioned bottom up approaches we implemented a top down approach that recursively splits the training set into several clusters. In contrast to the previous approach, where Gaussian components were merged and mapped, we now operate solely on the data objects. More precisely, we start by applying the EM clustering algorithm [Dempster *et al.* (1977)] to the complete training set. (An introduction to clustering can e.g. be found in [Han and Kamber (2001)]). The desired number M of resulting clusters is always set to the fanout which is again given through the page size. If the EM returns less than m clusters, the biggest resulting cluster is split again such that the total number of resulting clusters is at most M. In the rare case that the EM returns a single cluster, this cluster is split by picking the two farthest elements and assigning the remaining elements to the closest of the two. Finally, if a resulting cluster contains more than L objects (the capacity of a leaf node), the cluster is recursively split using the procedure described above. Otherwise the items contained in that cluster are stored in a leaf node, its corresponding entry is calculated and returned to build the Bayes tree. The EM approach may result in an unbalanced tree, which differs from the primary Bayes tree idea. However, as we will see in the next section, the results show that this is not a drawback but even leads to better anytime classification performance.

Finally we employed traditional R-tree bulk loading algorithms, i.e. we implemented space filling curves like Hilbert curve or z-curve and other partitioning approaches, e.g. sort-tile-recursive [Leutenegger *et al.* (1997)]. We briefly describe the Hilbert curve approach since we will present its results in the next section. The bulk loading according to the Hilbert curve is a bottom up approach where in the first step the Hilbert value for each training set item is calculated. Next the items are ordered according to their Hilbert value and put into leaf nodes w.r.t. the page size. After that the corresponding entry for each resulting node is created, i.e. MBR, cluster features (CF) and the pointer. These steps are repeated using the mean vectors as representatives until all entries fit into one node, the root node. Theory on creating multidimensional Hilbert curves can be found in [Alber and Niedermeier (1998)], for implementation guide lines see [Lawder (2000)].

15.4.2   *Results*

We use the same setting as in Section 15.3 and compare the three proposed bulk loading techniques to the previous results from [Seidl *et al.* (2009)] (called *Iterativ* in the graphs). Figure 15.9 (left) shows the results for the pendigits data set. The Goldberger approach fails to improve the accuracy over the iterative insertion for the first 50 nodes. After that it performs slightly better, but cannot increase the accuracy more than 1%. The curve corresponding to the Hilbert bulkload shows a steep increase similar to the iterative insertion and shows better performance in most cases. The EMTopDown bulkload outperforms all other approaches and improves the accuracy over the iterative insertion constantly by 3% or more on this data set.

The performance of the Goldberger bulkload stayed below the iterative insertion in the majority of our experiments. Just on the Letter data set it improved the accuracy for larger time allowances. Figure 15.9 (right) shows the results on Letter. For the first 40 nodes Goldberger and Iterativ perform equally well, after that the accuracy of Iterativ stays behind that of Goldberger. While the Hilbert bulkload shows similar performance to Iterativ, the EMTopDown again constantly yields the best accuracy up to 13% better than the iterative insertion.

In general the EMTopDown shows the best results in terms of anytime classification accuracy on all tested data sets and continuously improves the accuracy over that of the previous results in [Seidl *et al.* (2009)] up to 13%. This proves the effectiveness of bulk loading for the Bayes tree and offers great potiential for medical applications by incorporating existing knowledge data bases in the training process.

15.5   Application of Anytime Classification

The achieved results on benchmark data show the applicability of anytime classification, incremental learning and multi-step classification in future

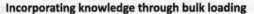

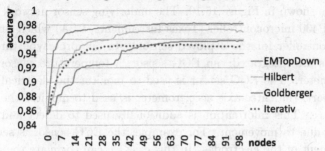

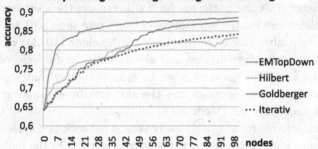

Fig. 15.9: Anytime classification accuracy on pendigits (top) and letter (bottom) using different bulk loading approaches.

body sensor network scenarios. For a remote health monitoring system, this ensures scalability as huge amounts of information from multiple hospitals can be collected, stored and processed in data farms. Moreover, incorporating existing medical data bases through the presented bulk loading approaches improves the resulting anytime classification performance.

With our anytime classification approach we focus on a multi-step patient health classification based on multivariate sensor data. As depicted in Figure 15.1 there are multiple steps from the body sensor network where we collect sensor measurements up to the health professional. Challenges for the overall system arise on multiple layers from the extraction of vital signals out of sensor measurements up to the health surveillance system for the health professional. Addressing all of these layers we have shown the applicability of this concept in a project for "Mobile Mining and Information Management in HealthNet Scenarios" presented for the first time at MDM 2008 [Kranen *et al.* (2008)].

The developed prototype provides an overall mobile system with textile sensors as shown in Figure 15.10. The underlying sensor network is based on a MSP430 microcontroller (Texas Instruments, USA) which serves as a master controller for the deployed sensors. In our prototype three types of sensors are integrated: an ECG sensor, a temperature sensor and an accelerometer. The ECG sensor is used to monitor the electrical activity of the heart, the three-axis accelerometer is used to monitor the activity of the user. This information is additionally used to detect and identify artefacts due to movement. For example, the ECG sensor is sensible to displacement of the electrodes. In this case we can correlate the acceleration data to distinguish movement artefacts from an irregular ECG due to disease related irregular patterns. As textile sensors the shirt has three integrated electrodes for the monitoring of heart rate signals. The electrodes are made from silver coated polyamide yarn (Shieldex 110/34) which yields both highly conductive surfaces and elastic behavior for ease of use and wearing comfort. The garment must be close-fitting so that a permanent contact between the electrodes and the skin can be guaranteed both for direct and capacitive use [Medrano *et al.* (2007)].

The master controller of this body sensor network is connected to the mobile device via a wireless communication channel. On the mobile device a J2ME application processes the sensor data stream and decides on the data to be forwarded to the back-end server. In depth analysis can then be done on the server and detailed data can be requested automatically or by interaction of a health professional. Thus, in addition to the pre-classification on the mobile device, we included further decision refinement about emergency situation on a central server with a more complex classifier. The integration of our multiple classification steps into this process ensures a scalable emergency detection system. First, on a mobile device carried by the patient, which includes data aggregation based on our novel pre-classification technique. Second, classification on a central server in a health facility which collects data of various patients and performs a more accurate classification to refine the classification results of the mobile devices. Overall the system is controlled by a health professional taking final decisions about the patients situation.

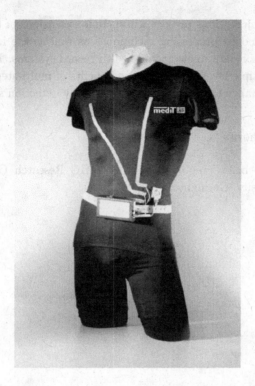

Fig. 15.10: Application of anytime classification in body sensor networks [Kranen *et al.* (2008); Medrano *et al.* (2007); Kim *et al.* (2009a,b)].

15.6 Conclusion

In this chapter we presented major challenges derived out of next generation mobile health surveillance. For the emergency detection task we highlighted semi-automated classification and showed how novel index-based classifiers build the core for multivariate multi-step classification in health surveillance. By supporting anytime learning and anytime classification the presented Bayes tree technique can handle huge amounts of data, which makes it a consistent solution for the described medical scenario. Moreover, as we laid out in this chapter, the Bayes tree fulfills all requirements which are crucial for classifying medical patient data in a scalable health surveillance.

Future challenges include extending the existing framework and evaluating the Bayes tree classifier based on sensor measurements in a broad health surveillance project. This project will include extensions of textile sensors, body sensors and preprocessing techniques as well as the integration and merging of sensor data in electronic health record systems. Emergency detection on multiple levels will show the benefits of multi-step classification and further enhance the scalability of emergency detection systems.

Acknowledgments

This work has been supported by the UMIC Research Centre, RWTH Aachen University, Germany.

Bibliography

Aamodt, A. and Plaza, E. (1994). Case-based reasoning: foundational issues, methodological variations and systems approaches, *AI Communications* **7**, pp. 39–59.

Aggarwal, C. C. (2005). On k-anonymity and the curse of dimensionality, in *Proc. of Int. Conf. on Very Large Databases (VLDB)*, pp. 901–909.

Aggarwal, C. C. and Yu, P. S. (2008). *Privacy-Preserving Data Mining: Models and Algorithms* (Springer).

Aggarwal, G., Feder, T., Kenthapadi, K., Khuller, S., Panigrahy, R., Thomas, D. and Zhu, A. (2006). Achieving anonymity via clustering, in *Symposium on Principles of Database Systems (PODS)*, pp. 153–162.

Agrawal, R., Imielinski, T. and Swami, A. (1993). Mining association rules between sets of items in large databases, in *Proc. of the ACM SIGMOD International Conference on Management of Data*, pp. 207–216.

Aha, D. and Kibler, D. (1991). Instance-based learning algorithms, *Machine Learning* **6**, pp. 37–66.

Alber, J. and Niedermeier, R. (1998). On multi-dimensional hilbert indexings, in *4th Annual International Conference on Computing and Combinatorics COCOON*.

Albig, A. R., Neil, J. R. and Schiemann, W. P. (2006). Fibulins 3 and 5 antagonize tumor angiogenesis in vivo, *Cancer research* **66(5)**, pp. 2621–2629.

Altman, D. G. (1991). *Practical Statistics for Medical Research* (Chapman & Hall).

Ammenwerth, E., Ehlers, F., Hirsch, B. and Gratl, G. (2007). His-monitor: an approach to assess the quality of information processing in hospitals, *Journal of medical informatics* **76**.

Anderson, I., Sorokin, A., l. V. Kapatra, Reznik, G., Bhattacharya, A., Mikhailova, N., Burd, H., Joukov, V., Kaznadzey, D., Walunas, T., d'Souza, M., Larsen, N., Pusch, G., Liolios, K., Grechkin, Y., Lapidus, A., Goltsman, E., Chu, L., Fonstein, M., Ehrlich, D., Overbeek, R., Kyrpides, N. and Ivanova, N. (2005). Comparative genome analysis of bacillus cereus group genomes with bacillus subtilis, *FEMS Microbiology Letters* **2**, pp. 175–184.

Anderson, N. R., Lee, E. S., Brockenbrough, J. S., Minie, M. E., Fuller, S.,

Brinkley, J. and Tarczy-Hornoch, P. (2007). Issues in Biomedical Research Data Management and Analysis: Needs and Barriers, *J Am Med Inform Assoc* 14, 4, pp. 478–488.

Andoni, A., Dater, M., Indyk, P., Immorlica, N. and Mirrokni, V. (2006). Locality-sensitive hashing using stable distributions, in T. Darrell, P. Indyk and G. Shakhnarovich (eds.), *Nearest Neighbor Methods in Learning and Vision: Theory and Practice* (MIT-Press).

Arai, B., Das, G., Gunopulos, D. and Koudas, N. (2007). Anytime measures for top-k algorithms, in *Proc. of Int. Conf. on Very Large Databases (VLDB)*.

Arens, Y., Hsu, C.-N. and Knoblock, C. A. (1996). Query Processing in the Sims Information Mediator, in *Advanced Planning Technology*, pp. 61–69.

Arzberger, P. and Finholt, T. A. (2002). Report on data and collaboratories in the biomedical community workshop, .

Assent, I., Wenning, A. and Seidl, T. (2006). Approximation Techniques for Indexing the Earth Mover's Distance in Multimedia Databases, in *Proc. of IEEE Int. Conf. on Data Engineering (ICDE)*.

Au, W. H. and Chan, K. C. C. (1998). An effective algorithm for discovering fuzzy rules in relational databases, in *Proceedings of the IEEE Int. Conf. on Fuzzy Systems*, pp. 1314–1319.

Au, W. H. and Chan, K. C. C. (1999). Farm: A data mining system for discovering fuzzy association rules, in *Proceedings of the IEEE Int. Conf. on Fuzzy Systems*, pp. 22–25.

Bader, D., Betel, D. and Hogue, C. W. V. (2003). Bind: the biomolecular interaction network database, *Nucleic Acids Research* 31, pp. 248–250.

Bader, D., Donaldson, I., Ouellette, F. and Pawson, T. (2001). Bind – the biomolecular interaction network database, *Nucleic Acids Research* 29, pp. 242–245.

Bader, G. D. and Hogue, C. W. V. (2000). Bind – a data specification for storing and describing biomolecular interactions, molecular complexes and pathways, *Bioinformatics* 16, pp. 465–477.

Bales, N., Brinkley, J., Lee, E. S., Mathur, S., Re, C. and Suciu, D. (2005). A framework for xml-based integration of data, visualization and analysis in a biomedical domain, in *Proc. Int. XML database Symposium (XSym)*, pp. 207–221.

Barken, D., Joanne, C., Kearns, J., Cheong, R., Hoffmann, A. and Levchenko, A. (2005). Oscillations in NF-kappaB signaling control the dynamics of gene expression, *Science* 306, pp. 704–708.

Barlett, J., Mallon, E. and Cooke, T. (2003). The clinical evaluation of her-2 status: which test to use? *J Pathol* 199(4), pp. 411–147.

Batini, C. and Scannapieco, M. (2006). *Data Quality: Concepts, Methodologies and Techniques*, Data-Centric Systems and Applications (Springer).

Baud, V. and Karin, M. (2001). Signal transduction by tumor necrosis factor and its relatives, *Trends in Cell Biology* 11, pp. 372–377.

Bauer, K. R., Brown, M., Cress, R. D., Parise, C. A. et al. (2007). Descriptive analysis of estrogen receptor (er)-negative, progesterone receptor (pr)-negative, and her2-negative invasive breast cancer, the so-called triple-negative phenotype: a population-based study rom the california cancer registri, *Nat Genet* **109(9)**, pp. 1721–1728.

Baumgartner, C. and Baumgartner, D. (2006). Biomarker discovery, disease classification, and similarity query processing on high-throughput ms/ms data of inborn errors of metabolism. *J Biomol Screen* **11**, pp. 90–99.

Baumgartner, C. and Graber, A. (2007). *Successes and new directions in data mining*, chap. 7, Data mining and knowledge discovery in metabolomics (Idea Group Inc.), pp. 141–166.

Bebek, G. and Yankg, J. (2007). Pathfinder: mining signal transduction pathway segments from protein-protein interaction networks. *BMC Bioinformatics* **8**, pp. 335–347.

Bellahsene, Z. and Ripoche, H. (2001). *Succeeding with Object Databases: A Practical Look at Today's Implementations with Java and XML*, chap. 16, An Object-Oriented Database for Managing Genetic Sequences (Wiley).

Bellatreche, L., Pierra, G., Xuan, D. N., DehainsalaHondjack and Ait-Ameur, Y. (2004). An a Priori Approach for Automatic Integration of Heterogeneous and Autonomous Databases, in *Proc. Database and Expert Systems Applications (DEXA)*, pp. 475–485.

Bellazzi, R., Larizza, C. and Riva, A. (1998). Temporal abstractions for interpreting diabetic patients monitoring data, *Intelligent Data Analysis* **2**, pp. 97–122.

Bempt, V. *et al.* (2008). Polysomy 17 in breast cancer: clinicopathologic significance and impact on HER-2 testing, *Journal of Clinical Oncology* **26(30)**, pp. 4869–4874.

Beneventano, D., Bergamaschi, S., Guerra, F. and Vincini, M. (2003). Synthesizing an integrated ontology, *IEEE Internet Computing* **7**, 5, pp. 42–51.

Benferhat, S., Dubois, D., Kaci, S. and Prade, H. (2006). Bipolar possibility theory in preference modeling: Representation, fusion and optimal solutions, *Information Fusion* **7**, 1, pp. 135–150.

Benitez, K. and Malin, B. (2010). Evaluating risk with respect to the *hipaa* privacy policies, *Journal of the American Medical Informatics Association* **17**, pp. 169–177.

Bergamaschi, S., Guerra, F., Orsini, M., Sartori, C. and Vincini, M. (2009). An etl tool based on semantic analysis of schemata and instances, in *Knowledge-Based and Intelligent Information and Engineering Systems, LNCS*, Vol. 5712/2009 (Springer), pp. 58–65.

Berman, H. M., Westbrook, J. D., Feng, Z., Gilliland, G., Bhat, T. N., Weissig, H., Shindyalov, I. N. and Bourne, P. E. (2000). The Protein Data Bank, *Nucleic Acids Research* **28**, 1, pp. 235–242.

Berrar, D. P., Dubitzky, W. and Granzow, M. (2003). *A practical approach to microarray data analysis* (Kluwer Academic Pub).

Berry, S. and Rumberg, B. (2001). Kinetic modeling of the photosynthetic electron transport chain, *Bioelectrochemistry* **53**, pp. 35–53.

Bertalanffy, L. (1973). *General Systems Theory* (Penguin).

Bertoni, M., Furlini, G., Gozzoli, G., Landini, M. P., Magnani, M., Messina, A. and Montesi, D. (2009). A case study on the analysis of the data quality of a large medical database, in *International Workshop on Database Technology for Data Management in Life Sciences and Medicine*.

Berzal, F., Blanco, I., Sanchez, D. and Vila, M. A. (2004). Measuring the accuracy and interest of association rules: A new framework, *Intelligent Data Analysis* 6, pp. 221–235.

Bestehorn, K., Hönig, R., Clemens, N. and Kirch, W. (2006). Register für klinische Studien - eine kritische Bestandsaufnahme, *Medizinische Klinik* 101, 2, pp. 120–126.

Bhalla, U. S. and Iyengar, R. (1999). Emergent properties of networks of biological signaling pathways, *Science* 283, pp. 381–387.

Bianciotto, V., Lumini, E., Bonfante, P. and Vandamme, P. (2003). Candidatus glomeribacter gigasporarum, an endosymbiont of arbuscular mycorrhizal fungi, *Int. J. Syst. Evol. Microbiol.* 53, pp. 121–124.

Bilous, M., Dowsett, M., Hanna, W., Isola, J. *et al.* (2003). Current perspectives on HER2 testing: a review of national testing guidelines, *Mod Pathol* 16(2), pp. 173–182.

Birney, E. and Clamp, M. E. (2004). Biological database design and implementation, *Briefings in Bioinformatics* 5, 1, pp. 31–38.

Böhm, C., Berchtold, S. and Keim, D. A. (2001). Searching in high-dimensional spaces—index structures for improving the performance of multimedia databases, *ACM Computing Surveys* 33, 3, pp. 322–373.

Bonfante, P. and Anca, I. (2009). Plants, mycorrhizal fungi, and bacteria: A network of interactions, *Annu. Rev. Microbiol.* 63, pp. 363–383.

Borgwardt, K. M. (2007). *Graph Kernels*, Ph.D. thesis, Ludwig-Maximilians-University Munich.

Borkar, V., Deshmukh, K. and Sarawagi, S. (2001). Automatic segmentation of text into structured records, in *Proc. of the ACM SIGMOD International Conference on Management of Data*, pp. 175–186.

Bower, J. M. and Bolouri, H. (eds.) (2001). *Computational Modeling of Genetic and Biochemical Networks* (MIT Press).

Bownds, S., Tong-On, P., Rosenberg, S. A. and Parkhurst, M. (2001). Induction of tumor-reactive cytotoxic T-lymphocytes using a peptide from NY-ESO-1 modified at the carboxy-terminus to enhance HLA-A2. 1 binding affinity and stability in solution, *Journal of Immunotherapy* 24(1), pp. 1–9.

Breiman, L. (2001). Random forests, *Machine Learning* 45, 1, pp. 5–32.

Brennan, D. J., Ek, S., Doyle, E., Drew, T. *et al.* (2009). The transcription factor Sox11 is a prognostic factor for improved recurrence-free survival in epithelial ovarian cancer, *European Journal of Cancer* 45(8), pp. 1510–1517.

Burcombe, R., Wilson, G. D., Dowsett, M., Khan, I. *et al.* (2006). Evaluation of Ki-67 proliferation and apoptotic index before, during and after neoadjuvant chemotherapy for primary breast cancer, *Breast Cancer Res* 8(3), pp. 31–33.

Burt, P. J. and Adelson, E. H. (1983). The laplacian pyramid as a compact image code, *IEEE Trans. Commin* COM-31, 4, pp. 532–540.

Buszewski, B., Kesy, M., Ligor, T. and Amann, A. (2007). Human exhaled air analytics: biomarkers of diseases. *Biomed Chromatogr* **21**, pp. 553–566.

Byun, J., Sohn, Y., Bertino, E. and Li, N. (2006). Secure anonymization for incremental datasets. in *Secure Data Management*, pp. 48–63.

Calvanese, D., Giacomo, G. D. and Lenzerini, M. (2002). Description logics for information integration, in A. Kakas and F. Sadri (eds.), *Computational Logic: Logic Programming and Beyond: Essays in Honour of Robert A. Kowalski*, no. 2408 in Lecture Notes in Computer Science (Springer-Verlag), pp. 41–60.

Cardoen, B., Demeulemeester, E. and Beliën, J. (2009). Operating room planning and scheduling: A literature review, *European Journal of Operational Research* .

Carey, L. A., Perou, C. M., Livasy, C. A., Dressler, L. G. *et al.* (2006). Race, breast cancer subtypes, and survival in the carolina breast cancer study, *Journal of the American Medical Assoc. (JAMA)* **295(21)**, pp. 2492–2502.

Carmona-Saez, P., Chagoyen, M., Rodriguez, A., Trelles, O. *et al.* (2006). Integrated analysis of gene expression by association rules discovery, *BMC Bioinformatics* **7**, pp. 54–69.

Carter, P., Presta, L., Gorman, C. M., Rdigway, J. B. *et al.* (1992). Humanization of an anti-p185her2 antibody for human cancer therapy, *Proc Natl Acad Sci* **89(10)**, pp. 4285–4289.

Caruana, R. and Niculescu-Mizil, A. (2006). An empirical comparison of supervised learning algorithms, in *23rd International Conference on Machine Learning*.

Catherine, M., Lloyd, M., Halstead, B. and Nielsen, P. (2004). Cellml: its future, present and past, *Progress in Biophysics and Molecular Biology* **85**, pp. 433–450.

Ceglar, A. and Roddick, J. F. (2006). Association mining, *ACM Computing Surveys* **38(2)**, pp. 1–42.

Chefd'hotel, C. and Bousquet, G. (2007). Intensity-Based Image Registration Using Earth Mover's Distance, in *Medical Imaging 2007: Image Processing*, pp. 65122B.1–65122B.8.

Chen, G., Wei, Q. and Kerre, E. E. (2006). *Fuzzy Logic in Discovering Association Rules: An Overview. Data Mining and Knowledge Discovery Approaches Based on Rule Induction Techniques* (Springer, New York, NY, USA).

Chen, J.-Y., Hershey, J., Olsen, P. and Yashchin, E. (2008). Accelerated monte carlo for kullback-leibler divergence between gaussian mixture models, in *Proc. of IEEE Int. Conf. on Acoustics, Speech and Signal Processing (ICASSP)*.

Chen, K. C., Calzone, L., Csikasz-Nagy, A., Cross, F. R., Novak, B. and Tyson, J. J. (2004). Integrative analysis of cell cycle control in budding yeast, *Molecular Biology of the Cell* **8**, pp. 3841–3862.

Cheng, C. J., Lin, Y. C., Tsai, M. T., Chen, C. S. *et al.* (2009). SCUBE2 suppresses breast tumor cell proliferation and confers a favorable prognosis in invasive breast cancer, *Cancer Research* **69(8)**, pp. 3634–3641.

Chibon, F., de Mascarel, I., Sierankowski, G., Brouste, V. *et al.* (2009). Prediction of HER2 gene status in Her2 2+ invasive breast cancer: a study of 108 cases comparing ASCO/CAP and FDA recommendations. *Modern pathology: an official journal of the United States and Canadian Academy of Pathology, Inc* **22(3)**, pp. 403–409.

Chin, G., Jr. and Lansing, C. S. (2004). Capturing and supporting contexts for scientific data sharing via the biological sciences collaboratory, in *Proc. of the ACM conf. on Computer supported cooperative work (CSCW)*.

Cho, K. H. and O.Wolkenhauer (2003). Analysis and modelling of signal transduction pathways in systems biology, *Biochemical Society Transactions* **31**, pp. 1503–1509.

Cho, K. H., Shin, S. Y., Kolch, W. and Wolkenhauer, O. (2003a). Experimental design in systems biology based on parameter sensitivity analysis with monte carlo simulation: A case study for the tnfalpha mediated nf-kappab-signal transduction pathway, *Simulation-transactions Of The Society For Modeling And Simulation International* **79**, pp. 726–739.

Cho, K. H., Shin, S. Y., Lee, H. W. and Wolkenhauer, O. (2003b). Investigations into the analysis and modeling of the tnfalpha-mediated NF-kappaB-signaling pathway, *Genome Research* **13**, pp. 2413–2422.

Cho, S.-B. and Won, H.-H. (2003). Machine learning in dna microarray analysis for cancer classification, in *APBC '03: Proceedings of the First Asia-Pacific bioinformatics conference on Bioinformatics 2003* (Australian Computer Society, Inc., Darlinghurst, Australia, Australia), pp. 189–198.

Chu, W., Cardenas, A. and Taira, R. (1994). Kmed: A knowledge-based multimedia distributed database system, *Information Systems* **19**, pp. 33–54.

Ciaccia, P. and Patella, M. (2002). Searching in metric spaces with user-defined and approximate distances, *ACM Transactions on Database Systems* **27**, 4.

Cimino, J. J. and Zhu, X. (2006). The practical impact of ontologies on biomedical informatics. *Methods Inf Med* **45 Suppl 1**, pp. 124–35.

Cohen, W. and Richman, J. (2002). Learning to match and cluster entity names, in *Proc. of ACM SIGKDD Int. Conf. on Knowledge Discovery and Data Mining (KDD)*, pp. 475–480.

Constrium, A. C. S. (2002). Overview of the alliance for cellular signaling, *Nature* **420**, pp. 703–706.

Cook, D. J. and Holder, L. B. (1994). Substructure Discovery Using Minimum Description Length and Background Knowledge. *J. Artif. Intell. Res. (JAIR)* **1**, pp. 231–255.

Cordero, F., Visconti, A. and Botta, M. (2009). A new protein motif extraction framework based on constrained co-clustering, in *Proceedings of the 24th Annual ACM Symposium on Applied Computing*, pp. 776–781.

Cortes, C. and Mohri, M. (2005). Confidence intervals for the area under the roc curve, in *Advances in Neural Information Processing Systems (NIPS)*, Vol. 17 (MIT Press).

Critchlow, T., Ganesh, M. and Musick, R. (1998). Automatic generation of warehouse mediators using an ontology engine, in *5th KRDB Workshop*, pp. 8.1–8.8.

Cruz, I. F. and Xiao, H. (2009). *Complex Systems in Knowledge-based Environments: Theory, Models and Applications*, chap. Ontology Driven Data Integration in Heterogeneous Networks, Studies in Computational Intelligence (Springer), pp. 75–98.

Cuadros, M., Villegas, R. *et al.* (2009). Systematic review of HER2 breast cancer testing, *Applied Immunohistochemistry & Molecular Morphology* **17(1)**, pp. 1–7.

Cullot, N., Ghawi, R. and Ytongnon, K. (2007). DB2OWL: A Tool for Automatic Database-to-Ontology Mapping, in M. Ceci, D. Malerba and L. Tanca (eds.), *Proceedings of the Fifteenth Italian Symposium on Advanced Database Systems*, pp. 491–494.

da Silva, V., Noya, R. and de Lucena, C. (2005). Using the uml 2.0 activity diagram to model agent plans and actions, in *Proceedings of the 4th International Conference on Autonomous Agents and Multiagent Systems, AAMAS*, pp. 594–600.

da Silva, V., Noya, R. and de Lucena, J. (2004). *Software engineering For multi-agent systems II : research issues and practical applications*, chap. Using the MAS-ML to model a multi-agent system (Springer), pp. 129–148.

Darwish, M. A., Veggerby, C., Robertson, D. H., Gaskell, S. J., Hubbard, S. J., Martinsen, L., Hurst, J. L. and Beynon, R. J. (2001). Effect of polymorphisms on ligand binding by mouse major urinary proteins, *Protein Science* **10**, pp. 411–417.

Davidson, E. H., Rast, J. P., Oliveri, P., Ransick, A., Calestani, C., Yuh, C.-H., Minokawa, T., Amore, G., Hinman, V., Arenas-Mena, C., Otim, O., Brown, C. T., Livi, C. B., Lee, P. Y., Revilla, R., Rust, A. G., Pan, Z., Schilstra, M. J., Clarke, P. J. C., Arnone, M. I., Rowen, L., Cameron, R. A., McClay, D. R., Hood, L. and Bolouri, H. (2002). A Genomic Regulatory Network for Development, *Science* **295**, 5560, pp. 1669–1678.

Davies, S. I. (2004). Machine learning at the operating room of the future: A comparison of machine learning techniques applied to operating room scheduling, Tech. rep., Master's Thesis, Massachusetts Institute of Technology, Cambridge.

de Maria, B., da Silva, V., Noya, R. and de Lucena, C. (2005). Visualagent: A software development environment for multi-agent systems, in *Proceedings of the 20th Brazilian Symposium on Databases and 19th Brazilian Symposium on Software Engineering, SBBD*.

Debnath, A., Lopez de Compadre, R., Debnath, G., Schusterman, A. and Hansch, C. (1991). Structure-Activity Relationship of Mutagenic Aromatic and Heteroaromatic Nitro Compounds. Correlation with Molecular Orbital Energies and Hydrophobicity, *J. Med. Chem.* **34**, 2, pp. 786–797.

DeCoste, D. (2002). Anytime interval-valued outputs for kernel machines: Fast support vector machine classification via distance geometry, in *Proc. of Int. Conf. on Machine Learning (ICML)*.

Delgado, M., Marin, N., Martin-Bautista, M. J., Sanchez, D. *et al.* (2003a). Mining fuzzy association rules: an overview, in *Proceedings of the BISC International Workshop on Soft Computing for Internet and Bioinformatics; Berkeley, CA, USA*.

Delgado, M., Marin, N., Sanchez, D. *et al.* (2003b). Fuzzy association rules: General model and applications, *IEEE Trans. Fuzzy Systems* **11**, pp. 214–225.

Demir, E., Babur, O., Dogrusoz, U., Gurosy, A., Nisanci, G., Atalay, R. C. and Oztruk, M. (2002). Patika: an integrated visual environment for collaborative construction and analysis of cellular pathways, *Bioinformatics* **18**, pp. 966–1003.

Dempere-Marco, L., Hu, X.-P., Ellis, S., Hansell, D. and Yang, G.-Z. (2006). Analysis of Visual Search Patterns with EMD Metric in Normalized Anatomical Space, *IEEE Transactions on Medical Imaging (TMI)* **25**, pp. 1011–1021.

Dempsey, W., Doyle, E., He, Q. and Cheng, G. (2003). The signaling adaptors and pathways activated by TNF superfamily, *Cytokine and Growth Factor Reviews* **14**, pp. 193–209.

Dempster, A. P., Laird, N. M. L. and Rubin, D. B. (1977). Maximum likelihood from incomplete data via the em algorithm, *Journal of the Royal Statistical Society, Series B* **39**, 1, pp. 1–38.

Deselaers, T., Keysers, D. and Ney, H. (2005). Discriminative Training for Object Recognition Using Image Patches, in *Proceedings of the IEEE Conference on Computer Vision and Pattern Recognition - Volume 2 (CVPR)*, pp. 157–162.

Deutsch, A., Fernández, M. F., Florescu, D., Levy, A. Y. and Suciu, D. (1999). A Query Language for XML, *Computer Networks* **31**, 11-16, pp. 1155–1169.

Deville, Y., Gilbert, D., van Helden, J. and Wodak, S. J. (2003). An overview of data models for the analysis of biochemical pathways, *Briefings in Bioinformatics* **4**, 3, pp. 246–259.

Dhillon, I., Mallela, S. and Modha, D. (2003). Information-theoretic co-clustering, in *Proc. of ACM SIGKDD Int. Conf. on Knowledge Discovery and Data Mining (KDD)*, pp. 89–98.

Dixit, V. and Mak, T. (2002). NF-kappaB signaling many roads lead to madrid, *Cell* **111**, pp. 615–619.

Donabedian, A. (1980). *The definition of quality and approaches to its assessment* (Health Administration Pr., Mich.).

Donnelly, P. (2008). Progress and challenges in genome-wide association studies in humans, *Nature* **456**, pp. 728–731.

Dressler, L. G., Berry, D. A., G, B., Cowan, D. *et al.* (2005). Comparison of her2 status by fluorescence in situ hybridization and immunohistochemistry to predict benefit from dose escalation of adjuvant doxorubicin-based therapy in node-positive breast cancer patients, *J Clin Oncol* **23(19)**, pp. 4287–4297.

Dubois, D., Prade, H. and Sudkamp, T. (2003). A discussion of indices for the evaluation of fuzzy associations in relational databases, in *Proceedings of the 10th Int. Fuzzy Systems Association World Congress (IFSA-03); Istambul, Turkey*, pp. 111–118.

Dubois, E., Hüllermeier, E. and Prade, H. (2006). A systematic approach to the assesssment of fuzzy association rules, *Data Mining and Knowledge Discovery* **2**, pp. 167–192.

Duda, R., Hart, P. and Stork, D. (2000). *Pattern Classification (2nd Edition)* (Wiley).

Dumitrescu, D., Lazzerini, B. and Jain, L. C. (2000). *Fuzzy Sets and Their Application to Clustering and Training* (CRC Press, Boca Raton, Florida, USA).

Dunckley, L. (2003). *Multimedia Databases, An Object-Rational Approach* (Addison Wesley).

EBCTCG (2005). Effects of chemotherapy and hormonal therapy for early breast cancer on recurrence and 15-year survival: an oveview of the randomised trials, *Lancet* **365(9472)**, pp. 1687–1717.

Edwards, J. S. and Palsson, B. O. (1997). How will bioinformatics influences metabolic engineering? *Biotechnology and Bioengineering* **58**, pp. 162–169.

Egan, J. (1975). *Signal detection theory and ROC analysis* (Academic Press, New York City, NY).

Eilbeck, K. and Lewis, S. (2004). Sequence ontology annotation guide, *Computational Functional Genomics* **5**, 8, pp. 642–647.

Ekblom, T., Bonnerstig, J., Vähärautio, S., Vikerfors, T. and Rytterberg, L. (2009). Olika indikation för knäplastik vid olika ortopedkliniker, *Läkartidningen* **106**, 13.

Esmeir, S. and Markovitch, S. (2006). Anytime induction of decision trees: An iterative improvement approach, in *AAAI Conf. on Artificial Intelligence*.

Esseghir, S., Todd, S. K., Hunt, T., Poulsom, R. *et al.* (2007). A role for glial cell derived neurotrophic factor induced expression by inflammatory cytokines and RET/GFR {alpha} 1 receptor up-regulation in breast cancer, *Cancer research* **67(4)**, pp. 11732–11741.

Ester, M., Kriegel, H.-P., Sander, J. and Xu, X. (1996). A density-based algorithm for discovering clusters in large spatial databases with noise. in *Proc. of ACM SIGKDD Int. Conf. on Knowledge Discovery and Data Mining (KDD)*, pp. 226–231.

Ester, M. and Sander, J. (2000). *Knowledge Discovery in Databases - Techniken und Anwendungen* (Springer).

Esteva, F. J., Sahin, A. A., Cristofanilli, M., Arun, B. *et al.* (2002). Molecular prognostic factors for breast cancer metastasis and survival, *Semin Radiat Oncol* **12(14)**, pp. 319–328.

Faloutsos, C. (1999). Multimedia ir: Indexing and searching, in R. Baeza-Yates and B. Ribeiro-Neto (eds.), *Modern Information Retrieval* (Addison-Wesley), pp. 345–365.

Faloutsos, C., Barber, R., Flickner, M., Hafner, J., Niblack, W., Petkovic, D. and Equitz, W. (1994). Efficient and effective querying by image content, *Journal of Intelligent Information Systems* **3**, 3/4, pp. 231–262.

Fawcett, T. (2003). ROC graphs – notes and practical considerations for data mining researchers, Tech. rep., No. HPL-2003-4. Palo Alto, CA, USA: Intelligent Enterprise Technologies Laboratories.

Fayyad, U. M., Piatetsky-Shapiro, G. and Smyth, P. (1996). Knowledge discovery and data mining: Towards a unifying framework. in *Proc. of ACM SIGKDD Int. Conf. on Knowledge Discovery and Data Mining (KDD)*, pp. 82–88.

Feldman, R. and Sanger, J. (2006). *The text mining handbook: Advanced Approaches in Analyzing Unstructured Data* (Cambridge University Press).

Fellegi, I. and Sunter, A. (1969). A theory for record linkage, *Journal of the*

American Statistical Association **64**, pp. 1183–1210.

Fischer, R., Chiarugi, F., Schmidt, J., Norgall, T. and Zywietz, C. (2003). Communication and Retrieval of ECG Data: How Many Standards Do We Need? *Computers in Cardiology* **30**, pp. 21–24.

Fluss, R., Faraggi, D. and Reiser, B. (2005). Estimation of the youden index and its associated cutoff point. *Biom J* **47**, 4, pp. 458–472.

Fonseca, J., Mora, A. and Marques, A. (2005). Mamis - a multi-agent medical information system, in *Proceedings of 3rd IASTED International Conference on Biomedical Engineering, BioMED*.

Fonseca, M. J. and Jorge, J. A. (2003). Indexing high-dimensional data for content-based retrieval in large databases, in *Proceedings of the 8th International Conference on Database Systems for Advanced Applications*, pp. 267–274.

Freitas, A. (2006). Are we really discovering "interesting" knowledge from data? *Expert Update (the BCS-SGAI magazine)* **9(1)**, pp. 41–47.

Freund, Y. and Schapire, R. E. (1996). Experiments with a new boosting algorithm, in *Thirteenth International Conference on Machine Learning* (Morgan Kaufmann, San Francisco), pp. 148–156.

Friedman, T., Beyer, M. A. and Bitterer, A. (2008). Magic quadrant for data integration tools, Tech. rep., Gartner.

Gagneur, J., Jackson, D. B. and Casari, G. (2003). Hierarchical analysis of dependency in metabolic networks, *Bioinformatics* **19**, pp. 1027–1034.

Gaines, B. R. and Compton, P. (1995). Induction of ripple-down rules applied to modeling large databases, *Intelligent Information Systems* **5**, 3, pp. 211–228.

Gardner, S. P. (2005). Ontologies and semantic data integration, *Drugs Discovery Today* **10**, 14, pp. 1001–1007.

Garey, M. R. and Johnson, D. S. (1979). *Computers and Intractability: A Guide to the Theory of NP-Completeness*, Series of Books in Mathematical Sciences (W. H. Freeman).

Gasparini, G., Boracchi, P., Verderio, P. and Bevilacqua, P. (1994). Cell kinetics in human breast cancer: comparison between the prognostic value of the cytofluorimetric S-phase fraction and that of the antibodies to Ki-67 and PCNA antigens detected by immunocytochemistry, *International Journal of Cancer* **57(6)**, pp. 822–829.

Gasteiger, J. and Engel, T. (2003). *Chemoinformatics: A Textbook* (Wiley-VCH).

Geisler, S., Brauers, A., Quix, C. and Schmeink:, A. (2007). An ontology-based system for clinical trial data management, in *Annual Symposium of the IEEE/EMBS Benelux Chapter 2007*, pp. 53–55.

Geman, S., Bienenstock, E. and Doursat, R. (1992). Neural networks and the bias/variance dilemma, *Neural Computation* **4**, pp. 1 – 58.

Geng, L. and Hamilton, H. J. (2006). Interestingness measures for data mining: A survey, *ACM Computing Surveys* **38(3) Article 9**, pp. 1–32.

Geuze, E., Westenberg, H., Jochims, A., de Kloet, C., Bohus, M., Vermetten, E. and Schmahl, C. (2007). Altered Pain Processing in Veterans with Posttraumatic Stress Disorder, *Arch. Gen. Psychiatry* **64**, pp. 76–85.

Glass, D. H. (2008). Fuzzy confirmation measures, *Fuzzy Sets and Systems* **159**, pp. 475–490.

Goddard, J. A. and Tavakoli, M. (1998). Referral rates and waiting lists: some empirical evidence, *Health Economics* **7**, 6, pp. 545–549.

Goethals, B. and Zaki, M. J. (2003). Advances in frequent itemset mining implementations: Report on fimi'03. *SIGKDD Explorations* **6(1)**, pp. 109–117.

Goldberg, D. E. (1989). *Genetic Algorithms in Search, Optimization, and Machine Learning* (Addison-Wesley).

Goldberger, J. and Roweis, S. T. (2004). Hierarchical clustering of a mixture model, in *Advances in Neural Information Processing Systems (NIPS)*.

Gomez-Perez, A. (2004). Ontology evaluation, in [Staab and Studer (2004)], pp. 250–273.

Gordis, L. (2008). *Epidemiology* (Elsevier Health Sciences).

Goryanin, I., Hodgman, T. C. and Selkov, E. (1999). Mathematical simulation and analysis of cellular metabolism and regulation, *Bioinformatics* **15**, pp. 749–758.

Grass, J. and Zilberstein, S. (1996). Anytime algorithm development tools, *SIGART Bulletin* **7**, 2, pp. 20–27.

Grauman, K. and Darrell, T. (2004). Fast Contour Matching Using Approximate Earth Mover's Distance, in *Proceedings of the IEEE Conference on Computer Vision and Pattern Recognition - Volume 1 (CVPR)*, pp. 220–227.

Groszmann, R. J. (1993). Hyperdynamic state in chronic liver diseases. *J Hepatol* **17 Suppl 2**, pp. S38–S40.

Gruber, T. (1993). A Translation Approach to Portable Ontology Specifications. *Knowledge Acquisition* **5**, pp. 199–220.

Guarneri, V., Broglio, K., Kau, S. W., Cristofanilli, M. *et al.* (2006). Assessing genetic contributions to phenotypic differences among racial and etnic groups, *Journal of Clinical Oncology* **24(7)**, pp. 1037–1044.

Gulcher, J., Kristjansson, K., Gudbjartsson, H. and Stefansson, K. (2000). Protection of privacy by third-party encryption in genetic research in iceland, *European Journal of Human Genetics* **8**, pp. 739–742.

Gündel, H., Valet, M., Sorg, C., Huber, D., Zimmer, C., Sprenger, T. and Tölle, T. R. (2008). Altered Cerebral Response to Noxious Heat Stimulation in Patients with Somatoform Pain Disorder, *Pain* **137**, 2, pp. 413–421.

Gurwitz, D., Lunshof, J. and Altman, R. (2006). A call for the creation of personalized medicine databases, *Nat Rev Drug Discov* **5**, pp. 23–26.

Guttman, A. (1984). R-trees: A dynamic index structure for spatial searching, in *Proc. of the ACM SIGMOD International Conference on Management of Data*, pp. 47–57.

Gyenesey, A. (2000). *A Fuzzy Approach for Mining Quantitative Association Rules. TUCS Technical Report 336.* (Department of Computer Science, University of Turku, Finland).

Hadzic, M. and Chang, E. (2005a). Medical ontologies to support human disease research and control, *International Journal of Web and Grid Service* **1**, pp. 139–150.

Hadzic, M. and Chang, E. (2005b). *Self-organization and Autonomic Informatics*, chap. Ontology-based multi-agent Systems Support Human Disease Study and Control (IOS Press), pp. 129–141.

Hahn, U. and Schulz, S. (2004). Building a very large ontology from medical thesauri, in [Staab and Studer (2004)], pp. 133–150.

Hammer, J., Garcia-Molina, H., Ireland, K., Papakonstantinou, Y., Ullman, J. D. and Widom, J. (1995). Information translation, mediation, and mosaic-based browsing in the TSIMMIS system, in *Proc. of the ACM SIGMOD International Conference on Management of Data*.

Han, J. and Kamber, M. (2001). *Data Mining: Concepts and Techniques* (Academic Press).

Han, J. and Pei, J. (2000). Mining frequent patterns by pattern growth: Methodology and implications, *SIGKDD Explorations* **2(2)**, pp. 14–20.

Hanley, J. A. and McNeil, B. J. (1982). The meaning and use of the area under a receiver operating characteristic (roc) curve. *Radiology* **143**, 1, pp. 29–36.

Hanover, J. and Julian, E. H. (2004). U.S. Clinical Trial Management Systems 2004 Vendor Analysis: Leadership Grid and Market Shares, *IDC* **1**, 32166.

Hao, N., Yildirim, N., Wang, Y., Elston, T. C. and Dohlman, H. G. (2003). Regulators of g protein signaling and transient activation of signaling: experimental and computational analysis reveals negative and positive feedback controls on g protein activity, *The Journal of Biological Chemistry* **278**, pp. 46506–46515.

Hare, J. M., Nguyen, G. C., Massaro, A. F., Drazen, J. M., Stevenson, L. W., Colucci, W. S., Fang, J. C., Johnson, W., Givertz, M. M. and Lucas, C. (2002). Exhaled nitric oxide: a marker of pulmonary hemodynamics in heart failure. *J Am Coll Cardiol* **40**, 6, pp. 1114–1119.

Hayward, S. W. (2002). Approaches to modeling stromal-epithelial interactions, *The Journal of Urology* **168**, pp. 1165–1172.

He, H. and Garcia, E. A. (2009). Learning from imbalanced data, *IEEE Transactions on Knowledge and Data Engineering* **21**, 9, pp. 1263–1284.

He, Y. and Naughton, J. F. (2009). Anonymization of set-valued data via top-down, local generalization, **2**, 1, pp. 934–945.

Helms, M. W., Kemming, D., Pospisil, H., Vogt, U. *et al.* (2008). Squalene epoxidase, located on chromosome 8q24. 1, is upregulated in 8q+ breast cancer and indicates poor clinical outcome in stage I and II disease, *British Journal of Cancer* **99(5)**, pp. 774–780.

Hen, T. P., Kuo, C. S. and Chi, S. C. (1999). A fuzzy data mining algorithm for quantitative values, in *Proceedings of the 3rd Int. Conf. on Knowledge-Based Intelligent Information Engineering Systems: 1999; Adelaide, Australia*, pp. 480–483.

Hermjakob, H., Montecchi, L., Bader, G., Wojcik, J., Salwinski, L., Ceol, A., Moore, S., Orchard, S., Sarkans, S., Mering, C., Roechert, B., Poux, S., Jung, E., Mersch, E., Kersey, P., Lappe, M., Lix, Y., Zeng, R., Rana, D., Nikolski, M., Husi, H., Brun, C., Shanker, K., Seth, G., Sander, C., Bork, P., Zhu, W., Pandey, A., Brazma, A., Jacq, B., Vidal, M., Sherman, D., Legrain, P., Cesareni, G., Xenarios, I., Eisenberg, D., Steipe, B., Hogue, C. and Apweiler, R. (2004). The HUPO PSI's molecular interaction format–

a community standard for the representation of protein interaction data, *Nature Biotechnology* **22**, pp. 177–183.

Hernandez, M. and Stolfo, S. (1995). The merge-purge problem for large databases, in *Proc. of the ACM SIGMOD International Conference on Management of Data*, pp. 127–138.

Hillier, F. and Lieberman, G. (1990). *Introduction to Linear Programming* (McGraw-Hill).

Hofestadt, R. and Thelen, S. (1998). Quantitative modeling of biochemical networks, *In Silico Biology* **1**, pp. 39–53.

Hoffmann, A., Levchenko, A., Scott, M. L. and Baltimore, D. (2002). The ikappab-nfkappab signaling module: Temporal control and selective gene activation, *Science* **298**, pp. 1241–1245.

Homer, N., Szelinger, S., Redman, M., Duggan, D., Tembe, W., Muehling, J., Pearson, J., Stephan, D., Nelson, S. and Craig, D. (2009). Resolving individuals contributing trace amounts of dna to highly complex mixtures using high-density snp genotyping microarrays, *PLoS Genetics* **4**, p. e1000167.

Horenko, I. (2003). Modellierung dynamischer prozesse in der zellbiologie, Seminar at FB Berlin.

Hornuss, C., Praun, S., Villinger, J., Dornauer, A., Moehnle, P., Dolch, M., Weninger, E., Chouker, A., Feil, C., Briegel, J., Thiel, M. and Schelling, G. (2007). Real-time monitoring of propofol in expired air in humans undergoing total intravenous anesthesia. *Anesthesiology* **106**, pp. 665–74.

Hosmer, D. W. and Lemeshow, S. (2000). *Applied logistic regression (Wiley Series in probability and statistics)* (Wiley-Interscience Publication), ISBN 0471356328.

Hu J, e. a. (2001). The arkdb: genome databases for farmed and other animals, *Nucleic Acids Res* **29**, pp. 106—110.

Huang, J., Jennings, N. and Fox, J. (1995). An agent-based approach to health care management, *International Journal of Applied Artificial Intelligence* **9**, pp. 401–420.

Hucka, M., Finney, A., Sauro, H. M., Bolouri, H., Doyle, J. and Kitano, H. (2002). The erato systems biology workbench: Enabling integration and exchanging between software tools for computational biology, in *Proceedings of the Pacific BioComputing Symposium*.

Hulo, N., Bairoch, A., Bulliard, V., Cerutti, L., Castro, E. D., Langendijk-genevaux, P., Pagni, M. and Sigrist, C. (2006). The prosite database, *Nucleic Acids Res* **34**, pp. 227–230.

Hulten, G. and Domingos, P. (2002). Mining complex models from arbitrarily large databases in constant time, in *Proc. of ACM SIGKDD Int. Conf. on Knowledge Discovery and Data Mining (KDD)*.

Huson, D. H. and Bryant, D. (2006). Application of Phylogenetic Networks in Evolutionary Studies, *Mol Biol Evol* **23**, 2, pp. 254–267.

Hyvärinen, A. and Oja, E. (2000). Independent component analysis: algorithms and applications. *Neural Networks* **13**, 4-5, pp. 411–430.

Ihekwaba, A., Broomhead, D., Grimely, R., Benson, N. and Kell, D. (2004). Sensitivity analysis of parameters controlling oscillatory signaling in the nf-kb pathway, *Systems Biology* **1**, pp. 93–102.

Imhoff, M., Webb, A. and Goldschmidt, A. (2001). Health informatics, *Intensive Care Medicine* .

Indyk, P. and Thaper, N. (2003). Fast Image Retrieval via Embeddings, in *Workshop on Statistical and Computational Theories of Vision (SCTV)*.

Inokuchi, A., Washio, T. and Motoda, H. (2003). Complete Mining of Frequent Patterns from Graphs: Mining Graph Data. *Machine Learning* **50**, 3, pp. 321–354.

Inza, I., Larrañaga, P., Blanco, R. and Cerrolaza, A. J. (2004). Filter versus wrapper gene selection approaches in dna microarray domains. *Artif Intell Med* **31**, pp. 91–103.

Ioannidis, Y. E., Livny, M., Ailamaki, A., Narayanan, A. and Therber, A. (1997). Zoo: a Desktop Experiment Management Environment, in *Proc. of the ACM SIGMOD International Conference on Management of Data*.

Irizarry, R. A., Bolstad, B. M., Collin, F., Cope, L. M. *et al.* (2003). Summaries of affymetrix genechip probe level data, *Nucleic Acids Research* **31(4)**.

Iruela-Arispe, M. L., Porter, P., Bornstein, P. and Sage, E. H. (1996). Thrombospondin-1, an inhibitor of angiogenesis, is regulated by progesterone in the human endometrium. *Journal of Clinical Investigation* **97(2)**, pp. 403–412.

Iselius, L., Slack, J., Littler, M. and Morton, N. E. (1991). Genetic epidemiology of breast cancer in Britain, *Ann Hum Genet* **55(Pt 2)**, pp. 151–159.

Isken, M. W. and Rajagopalan, B. (2002). Data mining to support simulation modeling of patient flow in hospitals, *Medical Systems* **26**, 2.

ISO (1998). ISO 9241-11:1998 Ergonomic requirements for office work with visual display terminals (VDTs) - Part 11: Guidance on usability, Tech. rep., International Organization for Standardization.

ISO05 (2005). Iso 9000:2005 quality management systems – fundamentals and vocabulary, .

ISO95 (1995). Iso 8402:1995 quality management systems – fundamentals and vocabulary, .

Ito, L. S., Iwata, H., Hamajima, N., Saito, T. *et al.* (1997). Expression of interleukin-1B in human breast carcinoma, *Cancer* **80**, pp. 421–433.

Jacobs, K. B., Yeager, M., Wacholder, S., Craig, D., Kraft, P., Hunter, D. J., Paschal, J., Manolio, T. A., Tucker, M., Hoover, R. N., Thomas, G. D., Chanock, S. J. and Chatterjee, N. (2009). A new statistic and its power to infer membership in a genome-wide association study using genotype frequencies, *Nature Genetics* **41**, pp. 1253–1257.

Jakobovits, R. M., Rosse, C. and Brinkley, J. F. (2002). WIRM: An Open Source Toolkit for Building Biomedical Web Applications, *JAMIA* **9**, 6, pp. 557–570.

Jedrzejek C., C. L. (1995). Fast closest codewordsearch algorithm for vector quantization, in *Proc. of the IEEE Information Theory Workshop ITW'95*.

Johansson, U. (2007). Obtaining accurate and comprehensible data mining models: An evolutionary approach, Tech. rep., Doctoral thesis, Linköping University, Sweden.

Jolliffe, I. (1986). *Principal Component Analysis* (Springer Verlag).

Joshi, G., Gillespie, M., Vastrik, I., D'Eustachio, P., Schmidt, E., de Bono, B., Jassal, B., Gopinath, G., Wu, R., Matthews, L., Lewis, S., Birney, E. and Stein, L. (2005). Reactome: a knowledgebase of biological pathways, *Nucleic Acids Research* **33**, pp. D428–D432.

Jun, J. B., Jacobson, S. H. and Swisher, J. R. (1999). Application of discrete-event simulation in health care clinics: A survey, *Journal of the Operational Research Society* .

Kaestle, G., Shek, E. C. and Dao, S. K. (1999). Sharing Experiences from Scientific Experiments, in *Proc. of Int. Conf. on Scientific and Statistical Database Management (SSDBM)*.

Kanehisa, M. (1997). A database for post-genome analysis, *Trends in Genetics* **13**, pp. 375–376.

Kanehisa, M. and Bork, P. (2003). Bioinformatics in the post-sequence era, *Nature Genet.* **33(Suppl)**, pp. 305–310.

Kanehisa, M., Goto, S., Kawashima, S., Okuno, Y. and Hattori, M. (2004). The KEGG Resource for Deciphering the Genome, *Nucleic Acids Res* **32**, pp. 277–280.

Karin, M. and Lin, A. (2002). NF-kappaB at the crossroads of life and death, *Nature Immunology* **3**, pp. 221–227.

Karp, P. D., Ouzounis, C. A., Moore-Kochlacs, C., Goldovsky, L., Kaipa, P., Ahren, D. and Tsoka, S. (2005). Expansion of the biocyc collection of pathway/genome databases to 160 genomes, *Nucleic Acids Research* **19**, pp. 6083–6089.

Kashtan, N., Itzkovitz, S., Milo, R. and Alon, U. (2004). Efficient Sampling Algorithm for Estimating Subgraph Concentrations and Detecting Network Motifs, *Bioinformatics* **20**, 11, pp. 1746–1758.

Katz, J. and Lindell, Y. (2007). *Introduction to modern cryptography: principles and protocols* (Chapman and Hall Crc).

Kavi, K., Kung, D., Bhambhani, H., Pancholi, G. and Kanikarla, M. (2003). Extending uml for modeling and design of multiagent systems, in *Proceedings of the 2nd International Workshop on Software Engineering for Large-Scale multi-agent Systems, SELMAS*.

Keller, T. and Jones, D. (1996). Metadata: The Foundation of Effective Experiment Management, in *First IEEE Metadata Conf.*

Kellgren, J. H. and Lawrence, J. S. (1957). Radiological assessment of osteoarthrosis, *Annals of the Rheumatic Diseases* **16**, 4, pp. 494–502.

Kensche, D., Quix, C., Chatti, M. A. and Jarke, M. (2007). GeRoMe: A generic role based metamodel for model management, *Journal on Data Semantics* **VIII**, pp. 82–117.

Keogh, E. (1997). Fast similarity search in the presence of longitudinal scaling in time series databases, in *Proc. Int. Conf. on Tools with Artificial Intelligence* (IEEE Computer Society Press, Washington, DC), pp. 578–584.

Kifer, D. and Gehrke, J. (2006). Injecting utility into anonymized datasets, in *Proc. of the ACM SIGMOD International Conference on Management of Data*, pp. 217–228.

Kim, J. and Pearl, J. (1983). A computational model for combined casual and diagnostic reasoning in inference systems, in *International Joint Conference on Artificial Intelligence*, pp. 190–193.

Kim, S., Beckmann, L., Pistor, M., Cousin, L., Walter, M. and Leonhardt, S. (2009a). A versatile body sensor network for health care applications, in *5th ISSNIP*.

Kim, S., Cousin, L., Beckmann, L., Walter, M. and Leonhardt, S. (2009b). A body sensor network base support system for automated bioimpedance spectroscopy measurements, in *World Congress on Medical Physics and Biomedical Engineering*.

Kimball, R. and Ross, M. (2002). *The Data Warehouse Toolkit: The Complete Guide to Dimensional Modeling (Second Edition)* (Wiley).

Kira, K. and Rendell, L. A. (1992). A practical approach to feature selection, in *ML92: Proceedings of the ninth international workshop on Machine learning* (Morgan Kaufmann Publishers Inc., San Francisco, CA, USA), ISBN 15586247X, pp. 249–256.

Kitano, H. (2002). Systems biology: A brief overview, *Science* **295**, pp. 1662–1664.

Klamt, S., Schuster, S. and Gilles, E. D. (2002). Calculability analysis in underdetermined metabolic networks illustrated by a model of the central metabolism in purple nonsulfur bacteria, *Biotechnology and Bioengineering* **77**, pp. 734–751.

Klamt, S. and Stelling, J. (2002). Combinatorial complexity of pathway analysis in metabolic networks, *Molecular Biology Reports* **29**, pp. 233–236.

Klein, O. and Veltkamp, R. C. (2005). Approximation Algorithms for the Earth Mover's Distance Under Transformations Using Reference Points, Tech. Rep. UU-CS-2005-003, Department of Information and Computing Sciences, Utrecht University.

Klosgen, W. (1996). *Explora: A multipattern and multistrategy discovery assistant. Advances in Knowledge Discovery and Data Mining.* (MIT Press, Menlo Park, CA, USA).

Kolpakov, F. A., Ananko, E. A., Kolesov, G. B. and Kolchanov, N. A. (1998). Genenet: a gene network database and its automated visualization, *Bioinformatics* **14**, pp. 529–537.

Kononenko, I. (1994). Estimating attributes: Analysis and extensions of relief, (Springer Verlag, Berlin/Heidelberg, Germany), pp. 171–182.

Korn, F., Sidiropoulos, N., Faloutsos, C., Siegel, E. and Protopapas, Z. (1996). Fast Nearest Neighbor Search in Medical Image Databases, in *Proc. of Int. Conf. on Very Large Databases (VLDB)*, pp. 215–226.

Kranen, P., Günnemann, S., Fries, S. and Seidl, T. (2010a). MC-tree: Improving bayesian anytime classification, in *Proc. of Int. Conf. on Scientific and Statistical Database Management (SSDBM)*.

Kranen, P., Kensche, D., Kim, S., Zimmermann, N., Müller, E., Quix, C., Li, X., Gries, T., Seidl, T., Jarke, M. and Leonhardt, S. (2008). Mobile mining and information management in healthnet scenarios, in *Int. Conf. on Mobile Data Management (MDM)*.

Kranen, P., Krieger, R., Denker, S. and Seidl, T. (2010b). Bulk loading hierarchical mixture models for efficient stream classification, in *Proc. of Pacific-Asia Conf. on Advances in Knowledge Discovery and Data Mining (PAKDD)*.

Kuffner, R., Zimmer, R. and Lengauer, T. (2000). Pathway analysis in metabolic databases via differential metabolic display (dmd), *Bioinformatics* **16**, pp. 825–836.

Kuramochi, M. and Karypis, G. (2001). Frequent Subgraph Discovery. in *Proc. of IEEE Int. Conf. on Data Mining (ICDM)*, pp. 313–320.

Kuramochi, M. and Karypis, G. (2004a). Finding Frequent Patterns in a Large Sparse Graph. in *SIAM Int. Conf. on Data Mining (SDM)*.

Kuramochi, M. and Karypis, G. (2004b). GREW-A Scalable Frequent Subgraph Discovery Algorithm. in *Proc. of IEEE Int. Conf. on Data Mining (ICDM)*, pp. 439–442.

Kuroda, S., Schweighofer, N. and Kawato, M. (2001). Exploration of signal transduction pathways in cerebellar long-term depression by kinetic simulation, *The Journal of Neuroscience* **21**, pp. 5693–5702.

Labhart, P., Karmakar, S., Salicru, E. M., Egan, B. S. *et al.* (2005). Identification of target genes in breast cancer cells directly regulated by the SRC-3/AIB1 coactivator, *Proceedings of the National Academy of Sciences* **102(5)**, pp. 1339–1344.

Lakhani, S. R., Reis-Filho, J. S., Fulford, L., Penault-Llorca, F. *et al.* (2005). Distinct molecular mechanisms underlyuing clinically relevant subtypes of breast cancer: gene expressio anaklyses across three different platforms, *Clin Cancer Res* **11(14)**, pp. 5175–5180.

Lang, S. (1970). *Linear Algebra* (Addison-Wesley).

Lasko, T. A., Bhagwat, J. G., Zou, K. H. and Ohno-Machado, L. (2005). The use of receiver operating characteristic curves in biomedical informatics, *J Biomed Inform* **38**, pp. 404–415.

Lavesson, N. and Davidsson, P. (2007). Evaluating learning algorithms and classifiers, *Intelligent Information & Database Systems* **1**, 1, pp. 37–52.

Lavin, Y., Batra, R. and Hesselink, L. (1998). Feature Comparisons of Vector Fields Using Earth Mover's Distance, in *Proceedings of the IEEE Conference on Visualization (Vis)*, pp. 103–109.

Lawder, J. (2000). Calculation of mappings between one and n-dimensional values using the hilbert space-filling curves, in *Technical Report JL1/00 Birkbeck College, University of London*.

Lazzarato, F., Franceschinis, G., Botta, M., Cordero, F. and Calogero, R. (2004). Rre: a tool for the extraction of non-coding regions surrounding annotated genes from genomic datasets. *Bioinformatics* **20**, pp. 2848—2850.

le Cessie, S. and van Houwelingen, J. (1992). Ridge estimators in logistic regression, *Applied Statistics* **41**, 1, pp. 191–201.

LeBeau, A. P., Goor, F. V., Stojilkovic, S. S. and Sherman, A. (2000). Modeling of membrane excitability in gonadotropin-releasing hormone-secreting hypothalamic neurons regulated by $Ca2+$-mobilizing and adenylyl cyclase-coupled receptors, *The Journal of Neuroscience* **20**, pp. 9290–9297.

Lee, M. S. and Garrard, W. T. (1991). Positive DNA supercoiling generates a chromatin conformation characteristic of highly active genes, in *Proceedings of the Natl Acad Sci: 1991; U. S. A.*, pp. 88:9675–9679.

Lee, S. R., Ramos, S. M., Ko, A., Masiello, D. *et al.* (2002). AR and ER interaction with a p21-activated kinase (PAK6), *Molecular Endocrinology* **16(1)**, pp. 85–99.

LeFevre, K., DeWitt, D. and Ramakrishnan, R. (2005). Incognito: efficient full-domain k-anonymity, in *Proc. of the ACM SIGMOD International Conference on Management of Data*, pp. 49–60.

Leff, D., Orihuela-Espina, F., Atallah, L., Darzi, A. and Yang, G. (2007). Functional Near Infrared Spectroscopy in Novice and Expert Surgeons – a Manifold Embedding Approach, *Medical Image Computing and Computer-Assisted Intervention – MICCAI 2007* , pp. 270–277.

Lehmann, T., Güld, M., Thies, C., Fischer, B., Spitzer, K., Keysers, D., Ney, H., Kohnen, M., Schubert, H. and Wein, B. (2004). Content-based image retrieval in medical applications, *Methods of information in medicine* **43**.

Leutenegger, S. T., Edgington, J. M. and Lopez, M. A. (1997). Str: A simple and efficient algorithm for r-tree packing, in *Proc. of IEEE Int. Conf. on Data Engineering (ICDE)*, pp. 497–506.

Li, H., Gennari, J. H. and Brinkley, J. F. (2006). Model Driven Laboratory Information Management Systems, in *AMIA 2006 Symposium Proceedings*, pp. 484–488.

Li, N., Li, T. and Venkatasubramanian, S. (2007). t-closeness: Privacy beyond k-anonymity and l-diversity, in *Proc. of IEEE Int. Conf. on Data Engineering (ICDE)*, pp. 106–115.

Lin, Z., Owen, A. B. and Altman, R. B. (2004). Genetics: genomic research and human subject privacy, *Science* **305**, pp. 183–183.

List, C. and Puppe, C. (2009). *Judgement aggregation: a survey* (Oxford University Press).

Liu, C.-L. and Wellman, M. P. (1996). On state-space abstraction for anytime evaluation of bayesian networks, *SIGART Bulletin* **7**, 2, pp. 50–57.

Ljoså, V., Bhattacharya, A. and Singh, A. K. (2006). Indexing Spatially Sensitive Distance Measures Using Multi-Resolution Lower Bounds, in *Proc. Int. Conf. on Extending Database Technology (EDBT)*, pp. 865–883.

Lodish, H., Berk, A., Matsudaira, P., Kaiser, C. A., Krieger, M., Scott, M. P., Zipursky, L. and Darnell, J. (2003). *Molecular Cell Biology*, 5th edn. (W. H. Freeman and Company, New York).

Lopez, F. J., Blanco, A., Garcia, F., Cano, C. *et al.* (2008). Fuzzy association rules for biological data analysis: a case study on yeast, *BMC Bioinformatics* **9**, pp. 107–115.

Loshin, D. (2001). *Enterprise knowledge management: the data quality approach.*

Loukides, G., Denny, J. C. and Malin, B. (2010). The disclosure of diagnosis codes can breach research participants privacy, *Journal of the American Medical Informatics Association.* In press.

Loukides, G., Gkoulalas-Divanis, A. and Malin, B. (2009). Coat: Constraint-based anonymization of transactions, Technical Report, arXiv:0912.2548v1 [cs.DB].

Loukides, G. and Shao, J. (2007). Capturing data usefulness and privacy protection in k-anonymisation, in *ACM Symposium on Applied Computing (SAC)*, pp. 370–374.

Loukides, G. and Shao, J. (2008). An empirical study of utility measures for k-anonymisation, in *British National Conference on Databases (BNCOD)*, pp. 15–27.

Lumini, E., Ghignone, S., Bianciotto, V. and Bonfante, P. (2006). Endobacteria or bacterial endosymbionts? to be or not to be, *New Phytol* **170**, pp. 205–208.

Lundström, M., Albrecht, S., Håkansson, I., Lorefors, R., Ohlsson, S., Polland, W., Schmid, A., Svensson, G. and Wendel, E. (2006). NIKE: a new clinical tool for establishing levels of indications for cataract surgery, *Acta ophthalmologica Scandinavica* **84**, pp. 495–501.

Lv, Q., Josephson, W., Wang, Z., Charikar, M. and Li, K. (2007). Multi-probe lsh: Efficient indexing for high-dimensional similarity search, in *Proceedings of the 33rd international conference on Very large data bases*, pp. 950–961.

Machanavajjhala, A., Gehrke, J., Kifer, D. and Venkitasubramaniam, M. (2006). l-diversity: Privacy beyond k-anonymity, in *Proc. of IEEE Int. Conf. on Data Engineering (ICDE)*, p. 24.

MacKay, V. L., Li, X., Flory, M. R., Turcott, E., Law, G. L., Serikawa, K. A., Xu, X. L. and Lee, H. (2004). Gene expression analyzed by high-resolution state array analysis and quantitative proteomics: response of yeast to mating pheromone, *Molecular and Cellular Proteomics* **3**, pp. 478–489.

Madnick, S. and Zhu, H. (2005). Improving data quality through effective use of data semantics, Tech. rep., Composite Information Systems Laboratory (CISL).

Mailman, M. D., Feolo, M. and et al., Y. J. (2007). The ncbi dbgap database of genotypes and phenotypes, *Nature Genetics* **39**, pp. 1181–6.

Malyankar, R. and Findler, N. (1998). A methodology for modeling coordination in intelligent agent societies, *Computational & Mathematical Organization Theory* **4**, pp. 317–345.

Mann, H. B. and Whitney, D. R. (1947). On a test of whether one of two random variables is stochastically larger than the other, *Annals of Mathematical Statistics* .

Marcus, D., Olsen, T. R., Ramaratnam1, M. and Buckner, R. L. (2007). The extensible neuroimaging archive toolkit: An informatics platform for managing, exploring, and sharing neuroimaging data, *Neuroinformatics* , pp. 11–33.

Markowitz, V. M., Chen, I. A., Kosky, A. S. and Szeto, E. (1997). Facilities for exploring molecular biology databases on the web: A comparative study, in *Proceedings of Pacific Symposium on Biocomputing*, pp. 256–267.

Matsuno, H., Tanaka, Y., Aoshima, H., Doi, A., Matsui, M. and Miyano, S. (2003). Biopathways representation and simulation on hybrid functional petri net, *In Silico Biology* **3**, pp. 389–404.

Mazzone, P. J. (2008). Analysis of volatile organic compounds in the exhaled breath for the diagnosis of lung cancer. *J Thorac Oncol* **3**, pp. 774–780.

McAdams, H. H. and Shapiro, L. (2003). A bacterial cell-cycle regulatory network operating in time and space, *Science* **301**, pp. 1874–1877.

McCallum, A., Nigam, K. and Unger, L. H. (2000). Efficient clustering of high-dimensional data sets with application to reference matching, in *Proc. of ACM SIGKDD Int. Conf. on Knowledge Discovery and Data Mining (KDD)*, pp. 169–178.

McIntyre, C. C., Richardson, A. G. and Grill, W. M. (2002). Modeling the excitability of mammalian nerve fibers: influence of afterpotentials on the recovery cycle, *Journal of Neurophysiology* **87**, pp. 995–1006.

Medes, P. (1997). Biochemistry by numbers: Simulation of biochemical pathways with gepasi 3, *Trends in Biochemical Sciences* **22**, pp. 361–363.

Medrano, G., Beckmann, L., Zimmermann, N., Grundmann, T., Gries, T. and Leonhardt, S. (2007). Bioimpedance spectroscopy with textile electrodes for a continous monitoring application, in *Int. Workshop on Wearable and Implantable Body Sensor Networks (BSN)*.

Mena, E., Illarramendi, A., Kahyap, V. and Sheth, A. P. (2000). Observer: An approach for query processing in global information systems based on inter-operation across pre-existing ontologies, *Distributed and Parallel Databases* **8**, pp. 223–271.

Mendes, P. and Kell, D. (1998). Non-linear optimization of biochemical pathways: applications to metabolic engineering and parameter estimation, *Bioinformatics* **14**, pp. 869–883.

Merelli, E., Culmone, R. and Mariani, L. (2002). Bioagent - a mobile agent system for bioscientists, in *Proceedings of the Network Tools and Applications in Biology Workshop Agents in Bioinformatics, NETTAB*.

Mesarovic, M. D. (1968). *System theory and biology view of a theoretician* (Springer), pp. 59–87.

Mewes, H. W., Frishman, D., Guuldener, D., Mannhaupt, G. and Mayer, K. (2002). Mips: a database for genomes and protein sequences, *Nucleic Acids Research* **30**, pp. 31–34.

Meyerson, A. and Williams, R. (2004). On the complexity of optimal k-anonymity. in *PODS '04*, pp. 223–228.

Micheau, O. and Tschopp, J. (2003). Induction of tnf receptor i-mediated apoptosis via two sequential signaling complexes, *Cell* **114**, pp. 181–190.

Miller, R. J. and Yang, Y. (1997). Association rules over interval data, in *Proc. of the ACM SIGMOD International Conference on Management of Data*, pp. 452–461.

Mills, S. J. and Harrison, S. A. (2005). Comparison of the natural history of alcoholic and nonalcoholic fatty liver disease. *Curr Gastroenterol Rep* **7**, 1, pp. 32–36.

Mitchell, S., Ayesh, R., Barrett, T. and Smith, R. (1999). Trimethylamine and foetor hepaticus, *Scand J Gastroenterol.* **34**, pp. 524–528.

Miyakis, S., Karamanof, G., Liontos, M. and Mountokalakis, T. D. (2006). Factors contributing to inappropriate ordering of tests in an academic medical department and the effect of an educational feedback strategy, *Postgrad. Med. J.* **82**.

Monk, B. C., Feng, W. C., Marshall, C. J., Seto-Young, D., Na, S., Haber, J. E.

and Perlin, D. S. (1994). Modeling a conformationally sensitive region of the membrane sector of the fungal plasma membrane proton pump, *Journal of Bioenergetics and Biomembranes* **26**, pp. 101–115.

Montani, S. (2008). Exploring new roles for case-based reasoning in heterogeneous ai systems for medical decision support, *Applied Intelligence* **28**, pp. 275–285.

Montani, S., Bottrighi, A., Leonardi, G., Portinale, L. and Terenziani, P. (2009). Multi-level abstractions and multi-dimensional retrieval of cases with time series features, in L. McGinty and D. Wilson (eds.), *Proc. International Conference on Case-Based Reasoning (ICCBR) 2009, Lecture Notes in Artificial Intelligence 5650* (Springer-Verlag, Berlin), pp. 225–239.

Moran, N., McCutcheon, A. and Nakabachi, P. (2008). Genomics and evolution of heritable bacterial symbionts, *Annu. Rev. Genet.* **42**, pp. 165–190.

Moreno, A. and Isern, D. (2002). A first step towards providing health-care agent-based services to mobile users, in *Proceedings of the 4th International Conference on Autonomous Agents and Multiagent Systems, AAMAS*, pp. 589–590.

Morgan, J. A. and Rhodes, D. (2002). Mathematical modeling of plant metabolic pathways, *Metabolic Engineering* **4**, pp. 80–89.

Morgan, X. C., Ni, S., Miranker, D. P. and Iyer, V. R. (2007). Predicting combinatorial binding of transcription factors to regulatory elements in the human genome by association rule mining, *BMC Bioinformatics* **8**, pp. 445–458.

Moss, S., Smith, J. and Nicholas, D. (1997). The quality of histopathology data in a computerised cancer registration system: implications for future audit of care, *Public Health* **111**, 2.

Mountain, J. L. and Risch, N. (2004). Assessing genetic contributions to phenotypic differences among racial and etnic groups, *Nat Genet* **36(11 Suppl)**, pp. S48–S53.

Muller, H., Rosset, A., Garcia, A., Vallee, J. and Geissbuhler, A. (2005). Benefits of content-based visual data access in radio graphics, *Informatics in radiology* **19**, pp. 33–54.

Murata, T. (1989). Petri nets: Properties, analysis and applications, in *Proceedings of the IEEE*.

Murtagh, F. (1983). A survey of recent advances in hierarchical clustering algorithms, *The Computer Journal* **26**, 4, pp. 354–359.

Myers, K., Kearns, M. J., Singh, S. P. and Walker, M. A. (2000). A boosting approach to topic spotting on subdialogues, in *Proc. of Int. Conf. on Machine Learning (ICML)*, pp. 655–662.

Nakayama, M., Kikuno, R. and Ohara, O. (2002). Protein-protein interactions between large proteins: Two-hybrid screening using a functionally classified library composed of long cDNAs, *Genome Research* **12**, pp. 1773–1784.

Nelson, J. D. (2005). Finding useful questions: on bayesian diagnosticity, probability, impact, and information gain. *Psychol Rev* **112**, 4, pp. 979–999.

Netzer, M., Millonig, G., Osl, M., Pfeifer, B., Praun, S., Villinger, J., Vogel, W. and Baumgartner, C. (2009). A new ensemble-based algorithm for identifying breath gas marker candidates in liver disease using ion molecule reaction mass spectrometry. *Bioinformatics* **25**, 7, pp. 941–947.

Newcombe, H. and Kennedy, J. (1962). Record linkage: Making maximum use of the discriminating power of identifying information, *Communications of the ACM* **5**, pp. 563–567.

Ng, R. T. and Han, J. (1994). Efficient and effective clustering methods for spatial data mining, in *Proc. of Int. Conf. on Very Large Databases (VLDB)*, pp. 144–155.

Novère, N. L., Bornstein, B., Broicher, A., Courtot, M., Donizelli, M., Dharuri, H., Li, L., Sauro, H., Schilstra, M., Shapiro, B., Snoep, J. L. and Hucka, M. (2006). Biomodels database: a free, centralized database of curated, published, quantitative kinetic models of biochemical and cellular systems, *Nucleic Acids Research* **34**, pp. 689–691.

Noy, N. F. and McGuinness, D. L. (2001). Ontology development 101: A guide to creating your first ontology, Tutorial, Stanford University.

Nwogu, I. and Corso, J. (2008). Exploratory Identification of Image-Based Biomarkers for Solid Mass Pulmonary Tumors, *Medical Image Computing and Computer-Assisted Intervention – MICCAI 2008* , pp. 612–619.

Obenshain, M. K. (2004). Application of data mining techniques to healthcare data, *Statistics for Hospital Epidemiology* **25**, 8.

Ocana, A., Cruz, J. J. and Pandiella, A. (2006). Trastuzumab and antiestrogen therapy: focus on mechanisms of action and resistance, *Am J Clin Oncol* **29(1)**, pp. 90–95.

Odell, J., Van Dyke, H. and Bauer, B. (2001). *Agent-Oriented Software Engineering* (Springer-Verlag).

Olafsson, A., Jonsson, B. and Amsaleg, L. (2008). Dynamic behavior of balanced nv-trees, in *International Workshop on Content-Based Multimedia Indexing Conference Proceedings, IEEE*, pp. 174–183.

Orphanoudakis, S., Chronaki, C. and Kostomanolakis, S. (1994). I2cnet: A system for the indexing, storage and retrieval of medical images by content, *Medical Informatics* **19**, pp. 109–122.

Osl, M., Dreiseitl, S., Cerqueira, F., Netzer, M., Pfeifer, B. and Baumgartner, C. (2009). Demoting redundant features to improve the discriminatory ability in cancer data. *J Biomed Inform* **42**, 4, pp. 721–725.

Osl, M., Dreiseitl, S., Pfeifer, B., Weinberger, K., Klocker, H., Bartsch, G., Schäfer, G., Tilg, B., Graber, A. and Baumgartner, C. (2008). A new rule-based algorithm for identifying metabolic markers in prostate cancer using tandem mass spectrometry. *Bioinformatics* .

Osprian, R. M., Breit, M., Visvanathan, V., Enzenberg, G. and Tilg, B. (2005). An integrative framework for modeling signaling pathways, in *1st FEBS Advanced Lecture Course: Systems Biology*.

Ozcan, Y. A. and Smith, P. (1998). Towards a science of the management of health care, *Health Care Management Science* **1**.

Page, L., Brin, S., Motwani, R. and Winograd, T. (1999). The PageRank Citation Ranking: Bringing Order to the Web. Tech. rep.

Pan, J.-Y. (2006). *Advanced Tools for Multimedia Data Mining*, Ph.D. thesis, Carnegie Mellon Univerity, Pittsburgh, PA.

Paolo Ciaccia, P. Z., Marco Patella (1997). M-tree: An efficient access method for similarity search in metric spaces, in *Proc. of Int. Conf. on Very Large Databases (VLDB)*, pp. 426–435.

Papadimitriou, S., Kitagawa, H., Gibbons, P. B. and Faloutsos, C. (2003). "LOCI: Fast Outlier Detection Using the Local Correlation Integral", in *Proc. of IEEE Int. Conf. on Data Engineering (ICDE)*, pp. 315–324.

Parka, S. and Sugumaran (2005). Designing multi-agent systems: a framework and application, *Expert Systems with Applications* **28**, pp. 259–271.

Pathak, J. S., Harold, R., Buntrock, J. D., Johnson, T. M. and Chute, C. G. (2009). Lexgrid: A framework for representing, storing, and querying biomedical terminologies from simple to sublime, *JAMIA* **16**, 3, pp. 305–315.

Paton, N. W. (2001). *Succeeding with Object Databases: A Practical Look at Today's Implementations with Java and XML*, chap. 15, Experience Using the ODMG Standard in Bioinformatics Applications (Wiley).

Peabody, J., Luck, J., Jain, S., Bertenthal, D. and Glassman, P. (2004). Assessing the accuracy of administrative data in health information systems, *Medical Care* **42**, 11.

Pei, J., Han, J. and Lakshamanan, L. V. S. (2001). Mining frequent itemsets with convertible cosntraints. in *Proc. of IEEE Int. Conf. on Data Engineering (ICDE)*, pp. 433–442.

Pensa, R., Boulicaut, J.-F., Cordero, F. and Atzori, M. (2010). Co-clustering numerical data under user-defined constraints. *Statistical Analysis and Data Mining* .

Perou, C. M., Sorlie, T., Eisen, M. B., van de Rijn, M. *et al.* (2000). Molecular portraits of human breast tumours, *Nature* **406(6797)**, pp. 747–752.

Persson, M. and Lavesson, N. (2009). Identification of surgery indicators by mining hospital data: A preliminary study, in *First International Workshop on Database Technology for Data Management in Life Sciences and Medicine*.

Persson, M. and Persson, J. (2009). Analysing management policies for operating room planning using simulation, *Health Care Management Science* .

Persson, M. and Persson, J. (2010). Waiting list management using early estimates of patient surgery demand, *Submitted for publication* .

Petricoin, E., Ardekani, A., Hitt, B., Levine, P., Fusaro, V., Steinberg, S., Mills, G., Simone, C., Fishman, D., Kohn, E. and Liotta, L. (2002a). "Use of proteomic patterns in serum to identify ovarian cancer", *Lancet* **359(9306)**, pp. 572–577.

Petricoin, E., Ornstein, D., Paweletz, C., Ardekani, A., Hackett, P., Hitt, B., Velassco, A., Trucco, C., Wiegand, L., Wood, K., Simone, C., Levine, P., Linehan, W., Emmert-Buck, M., Steinberg, S., Kohn, E. and Liotta, L. (2002b). "Serum proteomic patterns for detection of prostate cancer.", *J Natl Cancer Inst.* **94(20)**, pp. 1576–1578.

Pfeifer, B., Tejada, M., Kugler, K., Osl, M., Netzer, M., Seger, M., Modre-Osprian, R., Schreier, G. and Tilg, B. (2008). Biomedical knowledge discovery in databases design tool, in G. Schreier, D. Hayn and E. Ammenwerth (eds.), *eHealth2008 - Medical Informatics meets eHealth* (Österreichische

Computer Gesellschaft, Vienna), pp. 23–28.

Pfeiffer, T., Sanchez-Valdenebro, I., Nuno, J. C., Montero, F. and Schuster, S. (1999). Metatool: for studying metabolic networks, *Bioinformatics* **15**, pp. 251–257.

Phair, R. (1997). Development of kinetic models in the nonlinear world of molecular cell biology, *Metabolism* **12**, pp. 1489–1495.

Phair, R. D. and Misteli, T. (2001). Kinetic modeling approaches to in vivo imaging, *Nature Reviews: Molecular Cell Biology* **2**, pp. 898–907.

Pinto, H. S. and Martins, J. P. (2004). Ontologies: How can they be built? *Knowledge and Information Systems* **6**, 4, pp. 441–464.

Platt, J. (1998). Machines using sequential minimal optimization, in B. Schoelkopf, C. Burges and A. Smola (eds.), *Advances in Kernel Methods - Support Vector Learning* (MIT Press).

Polikar, R. (2006). Ensemble based systems in decision making, *IEEE Circuit and Syst. Mag.* **6**, pp. 21–45.

Pollan, M., Ramis, R., Aragones, N., Perez-Gomez, B. *et al.* (2007). Municipal distribution of breast cancer mortality among women in spain, *BMC Cancer* **7**, pp. 78–91.

Pomerantz, J. and Baltimore, D. (2002). Two pathways to NF-kappaB, *Molecular Cell* **4**, pp. 693–695.

Prokscha, S. and Anisfeld, M. H. (2006). *Practical Guide to Clinical Data Management*, 2nd edn. (CRC Press Inc).

Provost, F. and Fawcett, T. (1997). Analysis and visualization of classifier performance: Comparison under imprecise class and cost distributions, in *Proc. of Int. Conf. on Knowledge Discovery and Data Mining (KDD)*.

Provost, F., Fawcett, T. and Kohavi, R. (1998). The case against accuracy estimation for comparing induction algorithms, in *Proc. of Int. Conf. on Machine Learning (ICML)*, pp. 445–453.

Puzicha, J., Buhmann, J., Rubner, Y. and Tomasi, C. (1999). Empirical Evaluation of Dissimilarity Measures for Color and Texture, in *Proceedings of the IEEE International Conference on Computer Vision (ICCV)*, pp. 1165–1173.

Quinlan, R. (1993). *C4.5: Programs for Machine Learning* (Morgan Kaufmann Publishers, San Mateo, CA).

Quix, C., Kensche, D. and Li, X. (2007). Matching of ontologies with xml schemas using a generic metamodel, in *Proc. Intl. Conf. Ontologies, DataBases, and Applications of Semantics (ODBASE)*, pp. 1081–1098.

Rahm, E. and Bernstein, P. A. (2001). A survey of approaches to automatic schema matching, *VLDB Journal* **10**, 4, pp. 334–350.

Rakha, E. A., El-Rehim, D. A., Paish, C., Green, A. R. *et al.* (2006). Basal phenotype identifies a poor prognosis subgroup of breast cancer clinical importance, *European Journal of Cancer* **42(18)**, pp. 3149–3156.

Rao, A., Georgeff, M. and Kinny, D. (1996). *Agents Breaking Away*, chap. The methodology and modeling technique for systems of BDI agents (Springer Berlin / Heidelberg).

Rauner, M. S. and Vissers, J. M. H. (2003). OR applied to health services: Planning for the future with scarce resources, *European Journal of Operational Research* **150**, 1, pp. 1–2.

Ravikumar, P. and Cohen, W. (2004). A hierarchical graphical model for record linkage, in *Conference on Uncertainty in Artificial Intelligence*, pp. 454–461.

Reddy, J. K. and Rao, M. S. (2006). Lipid metabolism and liver inflammation. II. fatty liver disease and fatty acid oxidation. *Am J Physiol Gastrointest Liver Physiol* **290**, pp. G852–G858.

Redman, T. C. (1997). *Data Quality for the Information Age* (Artech House Publishers).

Ren, Z. and Anumba, C. (2004). Multi-agent systems in construction state of the art and prospects, *Automation in Construction* **13**, pp. 421–434.

Risby, T. H. and Sehnert, S. S. (1999). Clinical application of breath biomarkers of oxidative stress status. *Free Radic Biol Med* **27**, pp. 1182–1192.

Rivedal, E., Myhre, O. and Sanner, T. (2003). Supplemental role of the ames mutation assay and gap junction intercellular communication in studies of possible carcinogenic compounds from diesel exhaust particles, *Archives of Toxicology* **77**, pp. 533–542.

Rizzi, S., Abelló, A., Lechtenbörger, J. and Trujillo, J. (2006). Research in data warehouse modeling and design: dead or alive? in [Song and Vassiliadis (2006)], pp. 3–10.

Robnik-Sikonja, M. and Kononenko, I. (2003). Theoretical and empirical analysis of relieff and rrelieff, *Machine Learning* **53**, 1-2, pp. 23–69.

Rodriguez, J., Goni, A. and Illarramendi, A. (2005). Real-time classification of ecgs on a pda, *Trans. on Information Technology in Biomedicine* **9**, 1, pp. 23–34, doi:10.1109/TITB.2004.838369.

Rothstein, M. and Epps, P. (2001). Ethical and legal implications of pharmacogenomics, *Nature Rev. Genetics* **2**, pp. 228–231.

Rubin, D. L., Shah, N. H. and Noy, N. F. (2007). Biomedical ontologies: a functional perspective. *Brief Bioinform* .

Rubner, Y. and Tomasi, C. (2001). *Perceptual Metrics for Image Database Navigation* (Kluwer Academic Publishers).

Rubner, Y., Tomasi, C. and Guibas, L. J. (1998). A Metric for Distributions with Applications to Image Databases, in *Proceedings of the IEEE International Conference on Computer Vision (ICCV)*, pp. 59–66.

Rumbaugh, J., Jacobson, I. and Booch, G. (2004). *The Unified Modeling Language Reference Manual (2nd Edition)* (Addison Wesley).

Rumelhart, D. E., Hinton, G. E. and Williams, R. J. (1986). Learning representations by back-propagating errors, *Parallel Distributed Processing* **1**, pp. 318–362.

Saalbach, A., Twellmann, T., Nattkemper, T., Wismüller, A., Ontrup, J. and Ritter, H. (2005). A Hyperbolic Topographic Mapping for Proximity Data, in *Proceedings of the IASTED International Conference on Artificial Intelligence and Applications*, pp. 106–111.

Sabau, S., Hashimoto, S., Nemoto, Y. and Ihara, S. (2002). Cell simulation for circadian rhythm based on michaelis-menten model, *Journal of Biological Physics* **28**, pp. 465–469.

Sadr-Nabavi, A., Ramser, J., Volkmann, J., Naehrig, J. *et al.* (2009). Decreased expression of angiogenesis antagonist EFEMP1 in sporadic breast cancer is caused by aberrant promoter methylation and points to an impact of EFEMP1 as molecular biomarker, *International Journal of Cancer* **124(7)**, pp. 1727–1735.

Saeys, Y., Abeel, T. and Peer, Y. (2008). Robust feature selection using ensemble feature selection techniques, in *ECML PKDD '08: Proceedings of the European conference on Machine Learning and Knowledge Discovery in Databases - Part II* (Springer-Verlag, Berlin, Heidelberg), pp. 313–325.

Saeys, Y., Inza, I. and Larrañaga, P. (2007). A review of feature selection techniques in bioinformatics. *Bioinformatics* **23**, pp. 2507–2517.

Sakurai, Y., Yoshikawa, M., Uemura, S. and Kojima, H. (2002). Spatial indexing of high-dimensional data based on relative approximation, *VLDB Journal* **11**, 2, pp. 93–108.

Samarati, P. (2001). Protecting respondents identities in microdata release, *IEEE TKDE* **13**, 9, pp. 1010–1027.

Sankararaman, S., Obozinski, G., Jordan, M. I. and Halperin, E. (2009). *Nature Genetics* **41**, pp. 965–967.

Sarawagi, S. and Bhamidipaty, A. (2002). Interactive deduplication using active learning, in *Proc. of Int. Conf. on Very Large Databases (VLDB)*, pp. 269–278.

Sarty, G. E. (2007). *Computing Brain Activity Maps from fMRI Time-Series Images* (Cambridge University Press).

Sauro, H. M. (2000). Jarnac: A system for integrative metabolic analysis, in *Proceedings of the 9th International Meeting on BioThermoKinetics*.

Scannapieco, M., Figotin, I., Bertino, E. and Elmagarmid, A. (2007). Privacy preserving schema and data matching, in *Proc. of the ACM SIGMOD International Conference on Management of Data*, pp. 653–664.

Schacherer, F., Choi, C., Götze, U., Krull, M., Pistor, S. and Wingender, E. (2001). The transpath signal transduction database: a knowledgebase on signal transduction networks, *Bioinformatics* **17**, pp. 1053–1057.

Schaff, J., Slepchenko, B. and Loew, L. M. (2000). Physiological modeling with virtual cell framework, *Methods in Enzymology* **321**, pp. 1–23.

Schilling, C. H., Schuster, S., Palsson, B. O. and Heinrich, R. (1999). Metabolic pathway analysis: Basic concepts and scientific applications in the postgenomic era, *Biotechnology Progress* **15**, pp. 296–303.

Schoeberl, B., Eichler-Jonsson, C., Gilles, E. D. and Müller, G. (2002). Computational modeling of the dynamics of the map kinase cascade activated by surface and internalized egf receptors, *Nature Biotechnology* **20**, pp. 370–375.

Schoeberl, B., Gilles, E. D., Scheurich, C. and Pasadena, P. (2001). A mathematical vision of tnf receptor interaction, in *Proceedings of the International Congress of Systems Biology*, pp. 158–167.

Schuster, S., Dandekar, T. and Fell, D. A. (1999). Detection of elementary flux modes in biochemical networks: A promising tool for pathway analysis and metabolic engineering, *Trends in Biotechnology* **17**, pp. 53–60.

Sebat, J., Colwell, F. and Crawford, R. (2003). Metagenomic profiling: microarray analysis of an environmental genomic library. *Appl Environ Microbiol* **69**, pp. 4927—4934.

Sehnert, S. S., Jiang, L., Burdick, J. F. and Risby, T. H. (2002). Breath biomarkers for detection of human liver diseases: preliminary study. *Biomarkers* **7**, pp. 174–187.

Seidl, T., Assent, I., Kranen, P., Krieger, R. and Herrmann, J. (2009). Indexing density models for incremental learning and anytime classification on data streams, in *Proc. Int. Conf. on Extending Database Technology (EDBT)*.

Seidl, T. and Kriegel, H.-P. (1998). Optimal Multi-Step k-Nearest Neighbor Search, in *Proc. of the ACM SIGMOD International Conference on Management of Data*, pp. 154–165.

Shahar, Y. (1997). A framework for knowledge-based temporal abstractions, *Artificial Intelligence* **90**, pp. 79–133.

Shankaranarayanan, G., Wang, R. Y. and Ziad, M. (2000). Ip-map: Representing the manufacture of an information product, in *Fifth Conference on Information Quality* (MIT), pp. 1–16.

Silver, M., Su, H.-C. and Dolins, S. B. (2001). Case study: How to apply data mining techniques in a healthcare data warehouse, *Healthcare Information Management* **15**, 2.

Silverman, B. (1986). *Density Estimation for Statistics and Data Analysis* (Chapman & Hall/CRC).

Sivakumaran, S., Hariharaputran, S., Mishra, J. and Bhalla, U. S. (2003). The database of quantitative cellular signaling: management and analysis of chemical kinetic models of signaling networks, *Bioinformatics* **19**, pp. 408–415.

Skoutas, D. and Simitsis, A. (2006). Designing etl processes using semantic web technologies, in [Song and Vassiliadis (2006)], pp. 67–74.

Slamon, D. J., Clark, G. M., Wong, S. G., Levin, W. J. *et al.* (1987). Human breast cancer: correlation of relapse and survival with amplification of the HER-2/neu oncogene, *Science* **235(4785)**, pp. 177–182.

Slamon, D. J., Godolphin, W., Jones, L. A., Holt, J. A. *et al.* (1989). Studies of the HER-2/neu proto-oncogene in human breast and ovarian cancer, *Science* **244(4905)**, pp. 707–712.

Slamon, D. J., Leyland-Jones, B., Shak, S., Fuchs, H. *et al.* (2001). Use of chemotherapy plus a monoclonal antibody against HER2 for metastatic breast cancer that overexpresses HER2, *N Engl J Med* **344(11)**, pp. 783–792.

Slamon, D. J., Romond, E. H. and Perez, E. A. (2006). Advances in adjuvant therapy for breast cancer, *Clin Adv Hematol Oncol* **4(3)**, pp. suppl-9.

Snyder, A. and Weaver, A. (2003). The e-logistics of securing distributed medical data, in *Industrial Informatics '03*, pp. 207–216.

Sohma, Y., Gray, M. A., Imai, Y. and Argent, B. E. (2000). HCO3- transport in a mathematical model of the pancreatic ductal epithelium, *The Journal of Membrane Biology* **176**, pp. 77–100.

Sokolova, M., Japkowicz, N. and Szpakowicz, S. (2006). Beyond accuracy, f-score and roc: A family of discriminant measures for performance evaluation. in A. Sattar and B. H. Kang (eds.), *Australian Conference on Artificial Intelligence, Lecture Notes in Computer Science*, Vol. 4304 (Springer), pp. 1015–1021.

Song, I.-Y. and Vassiliadis, P. (2006) (ACM, Arlington, VA, USA).

Sorlie, T., Perou, C. M., Tibshirani, R., Aas, T. *et al.* (2001). Gene expression patterns of breast carcinomas distinguish tumor subclases with clinical implications, *Proc Natl Acad Sci* **98(19)**, pp. 10869–10874.

Sorlie, T., Tibshirani, R., Parker, J., Hastie, T. *et al.* (2003). Repeated observation of breast tumor subtypes in independent gene expression data sets, *Proc Natl Acad Sci* **100(14)**, pp. 8418–8423.

Sorlie, T., Wang, Y., Xiao, C., Johnsen, H. *et al.* (2006). Distinct molecular mechanisms underlying clinically relevant subtypes of breast cancer: gene expression analyses across three different platforms, *BMC Genomics* **26(7)**, pp. 127–141.

Sorribas, A., Curto, R. and Cascante, M. (1995). Comparative characterization of the fermentation pathway of saccharomyces cerevisiae using biochemical systems theory and metabolic control analysis: model validation and dynamic behavior, *Mathematical Biosciences* **130**, pp. 71–84.

Srikant, R. and Agrawal, R. (1996). Mining quantitative association rules in large relational databases, in *Proc. of the ACM SIGMOD International Conference on Management of Data*, pp. 1–12.

Srinivasan, P., Mitchell, J., Bodenreider, O., Pant, G. and Menczer, F. (2002). Web crawling agents for retrieving biomedical information, in *Proceedings of International Workshop on Agents in Bioinformatics, NETTAB-02*.

Staab, S. and Studer, R. (eds.) (2004). *Handbook on Ontologies*, International Handbooks on Information Systems (Springer).

Stallings, S., Huse, D., Finklestein, S., Crown, W., Witt, W., Maguire, J., Hill, A., Sinskey, A. and G.S.Ginsburg (2006). A framework to evaluate the economic impact of pharmacogenomics, *Pharmacogenomics* **7**, pp. 853–862.

Stockert, E., Jager, E., Chen, Y. T., Scanlan, M. J. *et al.* (1998). A survey of the humoral immune response of cancer patients to a panel of human tumor antigens, *Journal of Experimental Medicine* **187(8)**, pp. 1349–1354.

Stolte, E., v. Praun, C., Alonso, G. and Gross, T. (2003). Scientific Data Repositories: Designing for a Moving Target, in *Proc. of the ACM SIGMOD International Conference on Management of Data*.

Stone, B. G., Besse, T. J., Duane, W. C., Evans, C. D. and DeMaster, E. G. (1993). Effect of regulating cholesterol biosynthesis on breath isoprene excretion in men. *Lipids* **28**, 8, pp. 705–708.

Stone, M. (1974). Cross-validatory choice and assessment of statistical predictions, *Royal Statistical Society* **36**, 1, pp. 111–147.

Street, W. N. and Kim, Y. (2001). A streaming ensemble algorithm (sea) for large-scale classification, in *Proc. of ACM SIGKDD Int. Conf. on Knowledge Discovery and Data Mining (KDD)*, pp. 377–382.

Sun, X., Wang, H. and Li, J. (2009). Injecting purpose and trust into data anonymisation, in *Proc. ACM Conf. on Information and Knowledge Man-*

agement (CIKM), pp. 1541–1544.

Sweeney, L. (2002a). Achieving k-anonymity privacy protection using generalization and suppression, *Int. J. Uncertain. Fuzziness Knowl.-Based Syst.* **10**, 5, pp. 571–588.

Sweeney, L. (2002b). k-anonymity: A model for protecting privacy, *International Journal of Uncertainty, Fuzziness and Knowledge-Based Systems* **10**, 5, pp. 557–570.

Tan, P. N., Steinbach, M. and Kumar, V. (2005). *An Introduction to Data Mining* (Addison-Wesley Longman Publishing).

Tanimizu, N. and Miyajima, A. (2007). Molecular mechanism of liver development and regeneration. *Int Rev Cytol* **259**, pp. 1–48.

Tejada, S., Knoblock, C. and S. Minton, S. (2001). Learning object identification rules for information extraction, *Information Systems* **26**, 8, pp. 607–633.

Terrovitis, M., Mamoulis, N. and Kalnis, P. (2008). Privacy-preserving anonymization of set-valued data, *Proc. of Int. Conf. on Very Large Databases (VLDB)* **1**, 1, pp. 115–125.

Thogersen, V. B., Sorensen, B. S., Poulsen, S. S., Orntoft, T. F. *et al.* (2001). A subclass of HER1 ligands are prognostic markers for survival in bladder cancer patients. *Cancer Res* **61**, pp. 6227–6233.

Thomassen, M., Tan, Q. and Kruse, T. A. (2009). Gene expression meta-analysis identifies chromosomal regions and candidate genes involved in breast cancer metastasis, *Breast Cancer Research and Treatment* **113(2)**, pp. 239–249.

Toivonen, H., Srinivasan, A., King, R. D., Kramer, S. and Helma, C. (2003). Statistical Evaluation of the Predictive Toxicology Challenge 2000-2001, *Bioinformatics* **19**, 10, pp. 1183–1193.

Toyoda, H., Komurasaki, T., Uchida, D. and Morimoto, S. (1997). Distribution of mRNA for human epiregulin, a differentially expressed member of the epidermal growth factor family. *Biochemical Journal* **326(Pt 1)**, pp. 69–75.

Tripepi, G., Jager, K. J., Dekker, F. W. and Zoccali, C. (2008). Linear and logistic regression analysis. *Kidney Int* **73**, 7, pp. 806–810.

Tupek, A. R. (2006). *Definition of Data Quality* (Census Bureau Methodology & Standards Council, New York).

Tweedalea, J., Ichalkaranjeb, N., Sioutisb, C., Jarvisb, B., Consolib, A. and Phillips-Wren, G. (2007). Innovations in multi-agent systems, *Journal of Network and Computer Applications* **30**, pp. 1089–1115.

Typke, R., Giannopoulos, P., Veltkamp, R. C., Wiering, F. and van Oostrum, R. (2003). Using Transportation Distances for Measuring Melodic Similarity, in *Proceedings of the International Conference on Music Information Retrieval (ISMIR)*, pp. 107–114.

Tzourio-Mazoyer, N., Landeau, B., Papathanassiou, D., Crivello, F., Etard, O., Delcroix, N., Mazoyer, B. and Joliot, M. (2002). Automated Anatomical Labeling of Activations in SPM using a Macroscopic Anatomical Parcellation of the MNI MRI Single-subject Brain, *NeuroImage* **1**, 15, pp. 273–289.

Ulieru, M. (2003). *New Directions in Enhancing the Power of the Internet*, chap. Internet-enabled soft computing holarchies for e-Health Applications

(Springer), pp. 131–166.

Uzuner, O., Luo, Y. and Szolovits, P. (2007). Evaluating the state-of-the-art in automatic de-identification, *Journal of the American Medical Informatics Association* **14**, pp. 550–563.

Van Der Putten, P. and Van Someren, M. (2004). A bias-variance analysis of a real world learning problem: The coil challenge 2000, *Mach Learn* **57**, 1-2, pp. 177–195.

van Walraven, C. and Naylor, C. D. (1998). Do we know what inappropriate laboratory utilization is? *Journal of the American Medical Assoc. (JAMA)* **280**.

VanBerkel, P. T. and Blake, J. T. (2007). A comprehensive simulation for wait time reduction and capacity planning applied in general surgery, *Health Care Management Science* **10**, 4, pp. 373–385.

Varmuza, K. and Filzmoser, P. (2009). *Introduction to Multivariate Statistical Analysis in Chemometrics* (CRC).

Vasconcelos, N. and Lippman, A. (1998). Learning mixture hierarchies, in *Advances in Neural Information Processing Systems (NIPS)*, pp. 606–612.

Vassiliadis, P., Quix, C., Vassiliou, Y. and Jarke, M. (2001a). Data warehouse process management, *Information Systems* **26**, 3, pp. 205–236.

Vassiliadis, P., Simitsis, A., Georgantas, P., Terrovitis, M. and Skiadopoulos, S. (2005). A generic and customizable framework for the design of etl scenarios, *Information Systems* **30**, 7, pp. 492–525.

Vassiliadis, P., Vagena, Z., Skiadopoulos, S., Karayannidis, N. and Sellis, T. (2001b). ARKTOS: towards the modeling, design, control and execution of ETLprocesses, *Information Systems* **26**, pp. 537–561.

Verykios, V., Damiani, M. and Gkoulalas-Divanis, A. (2008). *Privacy and Security in Spatio-Temporal Data and Trajectories*, chap. 8, GeoPKDD Book: Geography, mobility, and privacy: a knowledge discovery vision (Springer), pp. 213–240.

Verykios, V. S., Karakasidis, A. and Mitrogiannis, V. K. (2009). Privacy preserving record linkage approaches, *International Journal of Data Mining, Modelling and Management* **1**, pp. 206–221.

Vissers, J. M. H., Bij, J. D. H. V. D. and Kusters, R. J. (2001). Towards decision support for waiting lists: An operations management view, *Health Care Management Science* **4**, 2, pp. 133–142.

Visvanathan, M., Breit, M., Enzenberg, G., Modre, R. and Tilg, B. (2005a). Mmd – a mathematical modeling database for cell signaling pathways, in *Proceeding of Workshop on Database Issues in Biological Databases (DBiBD-05)*.

Visvanathan, M., Breit, M., Enzenberg, G., Modre-Osprian, R. and Tilg, B. (2004). Integrative framework for signaling pathways, in *Proceedings of the 5th International Conference on Systems Biology*.

Visvanathan, M., Breit, M., Pfeifer, B., Osprian, R. M., Baumgartner, C., and Tilg, B. (2007). Systematic analysis of signaling pathways using an integrative environment, *Methods of Information in Medicine* **46**, pp. 386–391.

Visvanathan, M., Breit, M., Pfeifer, B., Osprian, R. M. and Tilg, B. (2005b). Dmsp – database for modeling signaling pathways, in *Proceeding as Inter-*

national Conference on Intelligent Systems for Molecular Biology (ISMB 2005).

Visvanathan, M., Enzenberg, G., Breit, M., Modre-Osprian, R. and Tilg, B. (2005c). A knowledge-base for modeling signaling pathways, in *Proceedings Keystone Symposia on Systems and Biology.*

Vlachos, M., Lin, J., Keogh, E. J. and Gunopulos, D. (2003). A wavelet-based anytime algorithm for k-means clustering of time series, in *ICDM Workshop on Clustering High Dimensionality Data and Its Applications.*

Vogel, C. L., Cobleigh, M. A., Tripathy, D., Gutheil, J. C. *et al.* (2002). Efficacy and safety of trastuzumab as a single agent in first-line treatment of HER2-overexpressing metastatic breast cancer, *J Clin Oncol* **20(3)**, pp. 719–726.

Vysniauskas, E. and Nemuraite, L. (2006). Transforming Ontology Representation from OWL to Relational Database, *Information Technology and Control* **35**, 3A, pp. 333–343.

Wache, H., Vgele, T., Visser, U., Stuckenschmidt, H., Schuster, G., Neumann, H. and Hbner, S. (2001). Ontology-Based Integration of Information - A Survey of Existing Approaches, in *Proceedings of Intrenational Workshop on Ontologies and Information Sharing*, pp. 108–117.

Wan, T. T. H. (2006). Healthcare informatics research: From data to evidence-based management, *Medical Systems* **30**, 1.

Wand, Y. and Wang, R. Y. (1996). Anchoring data quality dimensions in ontological foundations, *Commun. ACM* **39**, 11, pp. 86–95.

Wang, H., Fan, W., Yu, P. S. and Han, J. (2003). Mining concept-drifting data streams using ensemble classifiers, in *Proc. of ACM SIGKDD Int. Conf. on Knowledge Discovery and Data Mining (KDD).*

Wang, J., Du, Z., Payattakool, R., Yu, P. and Chen, C. (2007). A new method to measure the semantic similarity of go terms, *Bioinformatics* **23**, 10, pp. 1274–1281.

Wang, K., Fung, B. and Benjamin, C. (2006). Anonymizing sequential releases, in *Proc. of ACM SIGKDD Int. Conf. on Knowledge Discovery and Data Mining (KDD)*, pp. 414–423.

Wang, R., Li, Y. F., Wang, X., Tang, H. and Zhou, X. (2009). Learning your identity and disease from research papers: information leaks in genome wide association study, in *Proc. of ACM conference on Computer and communications security (CCS)*, pp. 534–544.

Wang, R. Y. and Strong, D. M. (1996). Beyond accuracy: what data quality means to data consumers, *J. Manage. Inf. Syst.* **12**, 4, pp. 5–33.

Wang, S. J., Wong, S. K. and Prusinkiewicz, P. (1988). An algorithm for multidimensional data clustering, *ACM Trans. on Mathematical Software* **14**, 2, pp. 153–162.

Wasserman, S. and Faust, K. (1994). *Social Network Analysis. Methods and Applications* (Cambridge University Press).

Watson, I. (1997). *Applying Case-Based Reasoning: techniques for enterprise systems* (Morgan-Kaufmann).

Wei, J. (2004). Markov edit distance, *IEEE Trans. on Pattern Analysis and Machine Intelligence* **26**, pp. 311–321.

Weis, M. and Naumann, F. (2005). Dogmatix tracks down duplicates in xml, in *Proc. of the ACM SIGMOD International Conference on Management of Data*, pp. 431–442.

Welch, B. L. (1947). The generalization of 'student's' problem when several different population variances are involved, *Biometrika* **34**, 1/2, pp. 28–35.

Wernicke, S. (2006). Efficient Detection of Network Motifs. *IEEE/ACM Trans. Comput. Biology Bioinform.* **3**, 4, pp. 347–359.

Wessely, S., Nimnuan, C. and Sharpe, M. (1999). Functional Somatic Syndromes: One or Many? *Lancet* **354**, pp. 936–939.

Westerhoff, H. V. and Palsson, B. O. (2004). The evolution of molecular biology into systems biology, *Nature Biotechnology* **22**, pp. 1249–1252.

Wichert, A. (2008). Content-based image retrieval by hierarchical linear subspace method, *Journal of Intelligent Information Systems* **31**, 1, pp. 85–107.

Wichert, A., Teixeira, P., Santos, P. and Galhardas, H. (2009). Subspace tree: High dimensional multimedia indexing with logarithmic temporal complexity, *Journal of Intelligent Information Systems* **doi:10.1007/s10844-009-0104-9**.

Wichterich, M., Assent, I., Kranen, P. and Seidl, T. (2008). Efficient EMD-Based Similarity Search in Multimedia Databases via Flexible Dimensionality Reduction, in *Proc. of the ACM SIGMOD International Conference on Management of Data*, pp. 199–212.

Wiechert, W. (2001). 13c metabolic flux analysis, *Metabolic Engineering* **3**, pp. 195–206.

Wiechert, W. (2002). Modeling and simulation: Tools for metabolic engineering, *Journal of Biotechnology* **94**, pp. 37–63.

Wiest, R. and Groszmann, R. J. (1999). Nitric oxide and portal hypertension: its role in the regulation of intrahepatic and splanchnic vascular resistance. *Semin Liver Dis* **19**, 4, pp. 411–426.

Winkler, W. (1995). *Matching and Record Linkage*, Business Survey Methods (J. Wiley), pp. 355–384.

Winkler, W. (2002). Record linkage and bayesian networks, in *Proceedings of the Section on Survey Research Methods, American Statistical Association*.

Witten, I. H. and Frank, E. (2005). *Data Mining: Practical Machine Learning Tools and Techniques* (Morgan Kaufmann Publishers, San Francisco, CA).

Wittig, U. and De Beuckelaer, A. (2001). Analysis and comparison of metabolic pathway databases, *Briefings in Bioinformatics* **2**, pp. 126–142.

Wolpert, D. H. (1992). Stacked generalization, *Neural Networks* **5**, pp. 241–259.

Wu, C. and Tai, X. (2009). Application of Gray Level Variation Statistic in Gastroscopic Image Retrieval, in *Proceedings of the IEEE/ACIS International Conference on Computer and Information Science (ICIS)*, pp. 342–346.

Xenarios, I., Salwinski, L., Duan, X. J., Higney, P., Kim, S. M. and Eisenberg, D. (2002a). DIP, the Database of Interacting Proteins: A Research Tool for Studying Cellular Networks of Protein Interactions, *Nucleic Acids Research* **30**, 1, pp. 303–305.

Xenarios, I., Salwnski, L., Duan, J., Higney, P., Kim, S. and Eisenberg, D. (2002b). Dip: The database of interacting proteins. a search tool for studying cellular networks of protein interactions, *Nucleic Acids Research* **30**, pp. 303–305.

Xiao, X. and Tao, Y. (2008). Dynamic anonymization: accurate statistical analysis with privacy preservation, in *Proc. of the ACM SIGMOD International Conference on Management of Data*, pp. 107–120.

Xu, Y., Wang, K., Fu, A. W.-C. and Yu, P. S. (2008). Anonymizing transaction databases for publication, in *Proc. of ACM SIGKDD Int. Conf. on Knowledge Discovery and Data Mining (KDD)*, pp. 767–775.

Yan, Q., Shan, L., Xin-Jun, M. and Zhi-Chang, Q. (2003). Romas: A role-based modeling method for multi agent systems, in *International Conference on Active Media Technology*.

Yan, X. and Han, J. (2002). gSpan: Graph-Based Substructure Pattern Mining. in *Proc. of IEEE Int. Conf. on Data Mining (ICDM)*, pp. 721–724.

Yan, X. and Han, J. (2003). CloseGraph: Mining Closed Frequent Graph Patterns. in *Proc. of ACM SIGKDD Int. Conf. on Knowledge Discovery and Data Mining (KDD)*, pp. 286–295.

Yang, Y., Webb, G. I., Korb, K. B. and Ting, K. M. (2007). Classifying under computational resource constraints: anytime classification using probabilistic estimators, *Machine Learning* **69**, 1.

Yao, C., Wang, X. S. and Jajodia, S. (2005). Checking for k-anonymity violation by views, in *Proc. of Int. Conf. on Very Large Databases (VLDB)*, pp. 910–921.

Yaziji, H., Goldstein, L. C., Barry, T. S., Werling, R. *et al.* (2004). HER-2 testing in breast cancer using parallel tissue-based methods, *Journal of the American Medical Assoc. (JAMA)* **291(16)**, pp. 1972–1977.

Youden, W. J. (1950). Index for rating diagnostic tests. *Cancer* **3**, 1, pp. 32–35.

Zadeh, L. A. (1965). Fuzzy sets, *Information and Control* **8(3)**, pp. 338–353.

Zaki, M. J., Parthasarathy, S., Ogihara, M. and Li, W. (1997). New algorithms for fast discovery of association rules. in *Proc. of ACM SIGKDD Int. Conf. on Knowledge Discovery and Data Mining (KDD)*, pp. 283–296.

Zamboulis, L., Poulovassilis, A. and Wang, J. (2008). Ontology-assisted data transformation and integration, in *Proc. 4th Intl. VLDB Workshop on Ontology-based Techniques for DataBases in Information Systems and Knowledge Systems (ODBIS)* (Auckland, New Zealand), pp. 29–36.

Zaniolo, C., Ceri, S., Snodgrass, R. T., Zicari, R. and Faloutsos, C. (1997). *Advanced Database Systems* (Morgan Kaufmann).

Zhang, H. and Padmanabhan, B. (2004). Using randomization to determine a false discovery rate for rule discovery, in *Proceedings of the Fourteenth Workshop On Information Technologies And Systems:2004*, pp. 140–145.

Zhang, N. and Zhao, W. (2005). Distributed privacy preserving information sharing, in *Proc. of Int. Conf. on Very Large Databases (VLDB)*, pp. 889–900.

Zhang, W. (1999). Mining fuzzy quantitative association rules, in *Proceedings of the 11th Int. Conf. on Tools with A.I.: 1999; Chicago, Illinois, USA*, pp. 99–102.

Zhou, X. S., Zillner, S., Moeller, M., Sintek, M., Zhan, Y., Krishnan, A. and Gupta, A. (2008). Semantics and cbir: A medical imaging perspective, in

ACM Int. Conf. on Image and Video Retrieval (CIVR), pp. 571–580.

Zien, A., Kueffner, R., Zimmer, R. and Lengauer, T. (2000). Analysis of gene expression data with pathway scores, in *Proceedings of the International Conference on Intelligent Systems for Molecular Biology*.